P9-BZL-703

Thrombolytic Therapy for Acute Stroke

Current Clinical Neurology

Daniel Tarsy, MD, Series Editor

Thrombolytic Therapy for Acute Stroke, Second Edition, edited by ***Patrick D. Lyden,*** *2005*

Psychiatry for Neurologists, edited by ***Dilip V. Jeste and Joseph H. Friedman,*** *2005*

Status Epilepticus: *A Clinical Perspective,* edited by ***Frank W. Drislane,*** *2005*

Parkinson's Disease and Nonmotor Dysfunction, edited by ***Ronald F. Pfeiffer and Ivan Bodis-Wollner,*** *2005*

Movement Disorder Emergencies: *Diagnosis and Treatment*, edited by ***Steven J. Frucht and Stanley Fahn,*** *2005*

Inflammatory Disorders of the Nervous System: *Pathogenesis, Immunology, and Clinical Management*, edited by ***Alireza Minagar and J. Steven Alexander,*** *2005*

Neurological and Psychiatric Disorders: *From Bench to Bedside*, edited by ***Frank I. Tarazi and John A. Schetz,*** *2005*

Multiple Sclerosis: Etiology, Diagnosis, and New Treatment Strategies, edited by ***Michael J. Olek,*** *2005*

Seizures in Critical Care: *A Guide to Diagnosis and Therapeutics,* edited by ***Panayiotis N. Varelas,*** *2005*

Vascular Dementia: *Cerebrovascular Mechanisms and Clinical Management,* edited by ***Robert H. Paul, Ronald Cohen, Brian R. Ott, Stephen Salloway,*** *2005*

Atypical Parkinsonian Disorders: *Clinical and Research Aspects*, edited by ***Irene Litvan,*** *2005*

Handbook of Neurocritical Care, edited by ***Anish Bhardwaj, Marek A. Mirski, and John A. Ulatowski,*** *2004*

Handbook of Stroke Prevention in Clinical Practice, edited by ***Karen L. Furie and Peter J. Kelly,*** *2004*

Clinical Handbook of Insomnia, edited by ***Hrayr P. Attarian,*** *2004*

Critical Care Neurology and Neurosurgery, edited by ***Jose I. Suarez,*** *2004*

Alzheimer's Disease: *A Physician's Guide to Practical Management,* edited by ***Ralph W. Richter and Brigitte Zoeller Richter,*** *2004*

The Visual Field: A Perimetric Atlas, edited by *Jason J. S. Barton and Michael Benatar, 2003*

Surgical Treatment of Parkinson's Disease and Other Movement Disorders, edited by *Daniel Tarsy, Jerrold L. Vitek, and Andres M. Lozano, 2003*

Myasthenia Gravis and Related Disorders, edited by *Henry J. Kaminski, 2003*

Seizures: *Medical Causes and Management,* edited by *Norman Delanty, 2002*

Clinical Evaluation and Management of Spasticity, edited by *David A. Gelber and Douglas R. Jeffery, 2002*

Early Diagnosis of Alzheimer's Disease, edited by *Leonard F. M. Scinto and Kirk R. Daffner, 2000*

Sexual and Reproductive Neurorehabilitation, edited by *Mindy Aisen, 1997*

Thrombolytic Therapy for Acute Stroke

Second Edition

Edited by

Patrick D. Lyden, MD

USCD Stroke Center, University of California, San Diego and Veteran's Affairs Medical Center San Diego, CA

HUMANA PRESS TOTOWA, NEW JERSEY

999 Riverview Drive, Suite 208
Totowa, New Jersey 07512

humanapress.com

This publication is printed on acid-free paper. ∞
ANSI Z39.48-1984 (American Standards Institute) Permanence of Paper for Printed Library Materials.

Cover design by Patricia F. Cleary

Production Editor: Robin B. Weisberg

For additional copies, pricing for bulk purchases, and/or information about other Humana titles, contact Humana at the above address or at any of the following numbers: Tel.: 973-256-1699; Fax: 973-256-8314; E-mail: orders@humanapr.com, or visit our Website: http://humanapress.com

Printed in the United States of America. 10 9 8 7 6 5 4 3 2 1

eISBN: 1-59259-933-8

Library of Congress Cataloging-in-Publication Data

Thrombolytic therapy for acute stroke / edited by Patrick D. Lyden.-- 2nd ed.
p. cm. -- (Current clinical neurology)
Includes bibliographical references and index.
ISBN 1-58829-398-X (alk. paper)
1. Cerebrovascular disease--Chemotherapy. 2. Thrombolytic therapy.
I. Lyden, Patrick D. II. Series.
RC388.5.T476 2005
616.8'10651--dc22

2005000628

Dedication

This book is again dedicated to our families, who daily cope with the vagaries, inconveniences, and turmoil surrounding our involvement in a Stroke Team. It is also dedicated to the patients who volunteered to participate in the placebo-controlled trials of thrombolytic stroke therapy: a more courageous and selfless group activity, on such a scale, may not be seen again in medical research.

Series Editor's Introduction

It often takes time for a new therapeutic modality to mature into an accepted treatment option. After initial approval, new drugs, devices, and procedures all go through this process until they become "vetted" by the scientific community as well as the medical community at large. Thrombolysis for treatment of stroke is no exception. *Thrombolytic Therapy for Acute Stroke, Second Edition* comes four years after the first edition and provides a very comprehensive, updated perspective on the use of intravenous rt-TPA in acute stroke. The authors provide longer term follow-up on the pivotal clinical trials that led to Food and Drug Administration approval, data concerning phase 4 trials in larger numbers of patients, and, most importantly, the community experience that has accumulated since its release. They add to this the latest promising information concerning intra-arterial thrombolysis, which is still under investigation and more speculative sections concerning possible new avenues of clinical research such as combining intravenous thrombolysis with neuroprotective therapies or intra-arterial thrombolysis. A wealth of factual information is supplemented by chapters containing sage opinion from Drs. Lyden and Caplan concerning the logistical, economic, and procedural issues that have been generated since the advent of this technology. Importantly, diagnosis does not take a back seat to therapeutics as illustrated by sections devoted to evaluation of the stroke patient, very useful illustrative cases and clinical comments, and chapters on the latest in imaging as applied to this field. Practical chapters concerning how to run a stroke code and hospital acute stroke protocols are especially helpful and are must reading for anyone contemplating this therapy for their institution.

As pointed out by Dr. Lyden, the implementation of thrombolytic therapy has been an uphill battle from the start. It is sobering to read about the disappointing results of early clinical trials, many of which startlingly were carried out without modern imaging. The pivotal NINDS trial for intravenous rt-TPA in stroke required unusual dedication and effort to succeed. Even after thrombolysis was demonstrated to be effective, concerns for its safety and skepticism regarding the logistics of speedy patient evaluation created some inertia and reluctance among clinicians. For example, neurologists on the front line were expected to provide more than "diagnose and adios" if this treatment was going to have an impact on stroke morbidity. In fact, however, this book makes it clear that the opposite has occurred. Neurologists and other health care providers, emergency room medical and nursing staffs, hospital administrators, health care officials on the local and national level and many others have been energized to create and nourish acute stroke teams throughout the country that have revolutionized the treatment of stroke. Presently, however, the proportion of acute stroke patients eligible to receive thrombolytic therapy who are actually treated remains very small. The wisdom and knowledge provided in this volume needs to be spread throughout the medical community and the public so as to maximize its benefit and fulfill its promise.

Daniel Tarsy, MD
Department of Neurology
Beth Israel Deaconess Medical Center
Harvard Medical School
Boston, MA

Preface

Thrombolytic Therapy for Acute Stroke, Second Edition remains intended for any physician seeking to learn to use thrombolytic therapy for acute stroke. As in the first edition, we present facts and data for the reader to consider; opinion is clearly segregated and labeled (*see* the debate chapters provided by Dr. Lou Caplan and myself.) We updated many chapters extensively, and added sections pertaining to new technology. Notably, some of the leading developers of stroke-magnetic resonance imaging contributed a key new chapter that hopefully will set the stage for improved patient selection. Yet, computed tomography will remain the most widely available imaging procedure for at least another decade, and Professor Rudiger von Kummer extensively revised this important chapter as well.

Patient selection remains the trick, and all chapters describing the background, use, and nuance of thrombolytic therapy were revised extensively. Everything one needs to know, and then some, is provided: rationale, preclinical trials, early trials, and pivotal trials. Practical how-to chapters will guide the reader in treating acute stroke patients, both with and without thrombolytic therapy. To enable the reader to practice the knowledge gained, we replaced all the case scenarios with new, detailed practice cases. Unique, I think, among stroke therapy books, this case section will allow the reader to put into play all of the facts and advice contained in the remainder of the book. Practicing these scenarios will enable practitioners to be as ready as possible for their first case.

The history of thrombolytic therapy for stroke makes for remarkable reading; as evidenced by the series of pilot experiments described in Chapter 6. The first uses of thrombolysis in humans were disasters, but no one knew going in that the risks were so high. Following those horrible results, nearly 20 years passed before the medical community again attempted thrombolytic therapy in stroke. That Greg del Zoppo, Justin Zivin, and especially John Marler were able to inspire the large, randomized trials of the early 1990s, based on critical animal experiments, is impressive.

As predicted in the preface to the first edition, to this day there remains no medical experiment of comparable size, complexity, or courage from patients and families as the NINDS rt-PA for Acute Stroke Trial. It is said, even now almost a decade after the landmark trial, that thrombolytic therapy can be used only in specialized centers full of "commandos" willing to take call and respond to Code Stroke calls on a moment's notice. As the case scenarios demonstrate, the commando model is certainly on the wane. Stroke patients now receive thrombolytic therapy in a variety of venues, and from a wide range of physicians, including emergency, internal, and family medicine practitioners. There is no doubt, however, that expertise and dedication to learning the protocol is required, as elegantly documented by the Cleveland Area survey, among other studies: a new chapter has been added that surveys the community implementation of thrombolytic stroke therapy.

The personal toll the original NINDS trial exacted from the authors—my friends and colleagues—is now nearly the stuff of legend in clinical neurology. In some ways, the legends both underplay and overstate the struggle we endured, but that is another story. The important point, to me, is that in many centers thrombolytic stroke therapy is now routine, as integrated in the daily functions of the medical center as Code Blue or cardiac transplantation. Getting us to this point required creativity, sacrifice, extreme effort, and in some cases heroism. The hard job is done now, and the task remains to diffuse the knowledge throughout the medical profession and in public: too few patients receive good stroke care, and during the time it took to read this preface, two more patients in the United States suffered disabling strokes. Thrombolytic therapy for stroke reduces disability; time is brain my friends, and the clock is ticking.

Patrick D. Lyden, MD

Acknowledgments

Editing a multiauthored book is a harrowing and gratifying experience, one that would be impossible without the able and noble efforts of others. I am grateful to the authors for diligently writing and revising their work. Without the expert and tireless assistance of Anthony DiLullo, I could never have begun this work. My special thanks go to the Fellows of the UCSD Stroke Center, for their dedicated hard work in implementing the principles of this book for many years during Code Strokes in San Diego, and to Dr. Justin Zivin, for years of mentoring. The nurses on staff at the UCSD Stroke Center, phenomenally dedicated to stroke research and patient care, include Nancy Kelly, Janet Werner, Teri McClean, and Jo Bell. I especially recognize my colleague in managing our multicentered trials, Karen Rapp, a nurse and clinical researcher of the highest caliber, motivation, and compassion and the co-director of the Stroke Center, Dr. Brett Meyer, a creative, indefatigable force of nature. My deepest gratitude goes to my colleague, partner, and companion, Dr. Christy Jackson, *sine qua non* at work and at home, and our children Hannah, Jessica, and Hillary, who have turned out to be quite able editorial assistants.

Contents

Contributors

ALEX ABOU-CHEBL, MD • Department of Neurology, Cleveland Clinic, Cleveland, OH
LAMA AL-KHOURY, MD • UCSD Stroke Center, San Diego, CA
JOSEPH BRODERICK, MD • Department of Neurology, University of Cincinnati, Cincinnati, OH
ASKIEL BRUNO, MD • Department of Neurology, Indiana University School of Medicine, Indianapolis, IN
LOUIS R. CAPLAN, MD • Neurology Department, Beth Israel Deaconess Medical Center, Boston, MA
YU D. CHENG, MD, PhD • Grossmont Medical Center, La Mesa, CA
GREGORY J. DEL ZOPPO, MD • Molecular and Experimental Medicine, The Scripps Research Institute, La Jolla, CA
SUSAN C. FAGAN, PharmD • Clinical Pharmacy Program, The Medical College of Georgia, Augusta, GA
MATTHEW L. FLAHERTY, MD• Department of Neurology, University of Cincinnati, Cincinnati, OH
ANTHONY J. FURLAN, MD • Head Section of Adult Neurology, Cleveland Clinic, Cerebrovascular Center, Cleveland, OH
JAMES C. GROTTA, MD • Department of Neurology, University of Texas-Houston Medical School, Houston, TX
E. CLARKE HALEY, MD • Department of Neurology, University of Virginia Health System, Charlottesville, VA
RANDALL HIGASHIDA, MD • UCSF-Radiology, University of California, San Francisco, CA
NAOHISA HOSOMI, MD • Molecular and Experimental Medicine, The Scripps Research Institute, La Jolla, CA
CHRISTY M. JACKSON, MD • UCSD Stroke Center, San Diego, CA
EDWARD C. JAUCH, MD, MS • Department of Emergency Medicine, University of Cincinnati Medical Center, Cincinnati, OH
IRENE KATZAN, MD • Department of Neurology, Cleveland Clinic, Cleveland, OH
CHELSEA S. KIDWELL, MD • Department of Neurology, Georgetown University, Washington, DC
RASHMI U. KOTHARI, MD • Borgess Research Institute, Michigan State University, Kalamazoo Center for Medical Studies, Kalamazoo, MI
THOMAS KWIATKOWSKI, PhD, MD • Department of Emergency Medicine, Long Island Jewish Medical Center, New Hyde Park, NY

LISE A. LABICHE, MD • Department of Neurology, University of Texas-Houston Medical School, Houston, TX
STEVEN R. LEVINE, MD • Stroke Program, Department of Neurology, The Mount Sinai School of Medicine and Medical Center, New York, NY
PATRICK D. LYDEN, MD • UCSD Stroke Center, University of California, San Diego, and Veteran's Affairs Medical Center, San Diego, CA
JOHN R. MARLER, MD • Neuroscience Center, National Institute of Neurological Disorders and Stroke, Rockville, MD
ANDREW N. RUSSMAN, MD • Department of Neurology, Cleveland Clinic, Cleveland , OH
PETER D. SCHELLINGER, MD • Department of Neurology, University Hospital at Heidelberg, Germany
RÜDIGER VON KUMMER, MD • Department of Neuroradiology, University of Technology Dresden, Germany
STEVEN WARACH, MD, PhD • National Institute of Neurological Disorders and Stroke, National Institutes of Health, Bethesda, MD

Color Plates

Color Plates follow p. 110.

Color Plate 1. *Fig. 4, Chapter 3:* γ-Aminobutyric acid-receptor activation leads to a hyperpolarizing influx of chloride that blocks voltage-gated calcium influx via the L-type voltage-sensitive calcium channel. (*See* complete caption on p. 50 and discussion on pp. 49–50.)

Fig. 5, Chapter 3: Following occlusion, granulocytes leave the circulation to enter ischemic brain. (*See* discussion on p. 53.)

Color Plate 2. *Fig. 9, Chapter 5:* The effect of caffeinol. (*See* complete caption on p. 92 and discussion on p. 91.)

Color Plate 3. *Fig. 2, Chapter 16:* (B) The time-to-peak map shows an area of delayed contrast and (D) the cerebral blood volume is diminshed within the right striatum and insular cortex. (*See* complete caption on p. 256 and discussion on pp. 253 and 256.)

Color Plate 4. *Fig. 7, Chapter 17:* Modified view of ischemic penumbra. (*See* complete caption on p. 291 and discussion on pp. 288–289.)

I

Background and Basic Investigations

1 Mechanisms of Thrombolysis

Gregory J. del Zoppo, MD
and Naohisa Hosomi, MD, PhD

Contents

INTRODUCTION

The pharmacological use of plasminogen activators is associated with symptomatic improvement in patients with coronary artery thrombosis, peripheral arterial occlusions, and thrombosis of the venous system. Based on prospective angiographic studies and planned programs *(1–5)*, thrombolysis is the only approved treatment of acute ischemic stroke *(6–8)* under limited circumstances. Currently, recombinant tissue plasminogen activator (rt-PA) is licensed in the United States and several other countries for the treatment of ischemic stroke within 3 h of onset *(6)*.

The development of agents that promote fibrinolysis by exogenous application stems from observations beginning in the 19th century *(9)* of the liquefaction of clotted blood and spontaneous dissolution of fibrin thrombi. Inquiry into the

From: *Current Clinical Neurology: Thrombolytic Therapy for Acute Stroke, Second Edition*
Edited by: P. D. Lyden © Humana Press Inc., Totowa, NJ

mechanisms of streptococcal fibrinolysis *(10)* paralleled a growing understanding of plasma proteolytic digestion of fibrin *(11)*. Streptokinase was first employed to dissolve closed space (intrapleural) fibrin clots *(12)*, but purified preparations were required for lysis of intravascular thrombi *(13)*. Development of plasminogen activators for therapeutic vascular thrombus lysis progressed in concert with insights into the mechanisms of thrombus formation and degradation.

The growth, dissolution, and migration of a thrombus depends on the relative contributions of platelet activation, coagulation system activation, and fibrinolysis. These processes are inextricably connected. Clinically, excess vascular fibrin or excess fibrin degradation may contribute to thrombosis or hemorrhage, respectively. Plasminogen activators are exploited clinically to dissolve significant (symptomatic) thrombi; however, all substances that promote plasmin formation may increase the risk of hemorrhage.

THROMBUS FORMATION

Thrombosis and thrombus growth involve the processes of endothelial injury, platelet adherence and aggregation, and thrombin generation. The relative contributions of these processes to the thrombus composition depend upon other factors including the degree of vascular injury, shear stress, and the presence of antithrombotic agents.

Thrombin is the central player in clot formation, acting as a link between platelet activation and coagulation. Thrombin cleaves fibrinogen, which contributes fibrin to the clot matrix. The growing fibrin matrix forms the scaffolding for the thrombus *(14)*. Inter-fibrin strand crosslinking is accomplished by factor XIII, a transglutaminase bound to fibrinogen, which is itself activated by thrombin and contributes to thrombus stabilization *(15)*. Thrombin mediates fibrin polymerization through the cleavage of the NH_2-terminal fragments of the Aα and Bβ chains of fibrinogen *(16,17)*. This leads to the generation of fibrin I and fibrin II monomers, and the release of fibrinopeptide A (FPA) and fibrinopeptide B (FPB), respectively.

Thrombin-mediated fibrin formation occurs simultaneously with platelet activation by several mechanisms. Thrombin is generated by extrinsic and intrinsic coagulation pathways that utilize platelet membrane receptors and phospholipid *(18)*. Additionally, platelets promote activation of the early stages of intrinsic coagulation using the factor XI receptor and high-molecular-weight kininogen (HMWK) *(19)*. Also, factors V and VIII interact with specific platelet membrane phospholipids (receptors) to facilitate the activation of factor X to Xa and the conversion of prothrombin to thrombin on the platelet surface *(20)*. Platelet-bound thrombin-modified factor V (factor Va) serves as a high-affinity platelet receptor for factor Xa *(21)*. Consequently, the rate of thrombin generation is significantly accelerated by a potent positive feedback mechanism, which leads to further fibrin network formation.

This process also leads to the conversion of plasminogen to plasmin and the activation of endogenous fibrinolysis. Thrombin provides one direct connection between thrombus formation and plasmin generation through localized generation of plasminogen activators from endothelial cells. Active thrombin has been shown, both in vitro and in vivo, to markedly stimulate tissue plasminogen activator (t-PA) release from endothelial stores *(22–24)*. In one experiment, infusion of factor Xa and phospholipid into nonhuman primates resulted in a pronounced increase in circulating t-PA activity *(25)*, suggesting that significant vascular stores of this plasminogen activator may be released by active components of coagulation. Other vascular and cellular stimuli may also augment plasminogen activator (PA) release, thereby pushing the balance toward thrombus lysis.

The relative platelet-fibrin composition of a specific thrombus is dependent on regional blood flow or shear stress. Thrombi are predominantly platelet rich at arterial flow rates, whereas activation of coagulation seems to predominate at lower shear rates, which are characteristic of venous flow. It has been suggested that the efficacy of pharmacological thrombus lysis is dependent on the relative fibrin content and the degree of fibrin crosslinking *(26,27)*. The latter may reflect thrombus age.

In situ thrombus development requires abrogation of the constitutive antithrombotic characteristics of the endothelial cell *(28)*. Alternatively, thrombus formation may occur following lodgment of a thrombus in a downstream vascular bed. In addition to both endothelial cell-derived antithrombotic characteristics and circulating anticoagulants (i.e., activated protein C, and protein S), thrombus growth is limited by the endogenous thrombus lytic system. The net effect of simultaneous *in situ* thrombus formation and fibrinolysis is to continually remodel the thrombus. This results from the preferential conversion of plasminogen to plasmin on the thrombus surface where fibrin binds t-PA in proximity to its substrate plasminogen, thereby accelerating local plasmin formation. In concert with local shear stress, these processes may lead to further embolization into downstream cerebral vasculature *(29)*. However, little is known about the endogenous generation and secretion of PAs within the cerebral vessels *(30)*. Exogenous application of pharmacologic doses of PAs accelerates conversion of thrombus-bound plasminogen to plasmin, and prevent thrombus formation as discussed below.

FIBRINOLYSIS

Plasmin formation is central to thrombus dissolution. The endogenous fibrinolytic system is comprised of plasminogen, PAs, and inhibitors of fibrinolysis. Fibrin (and fibrinogen) degradation requires plasmin generation. Plasminogen, its activators, and the inhibitors of the fibrinolytic components all contribute to the balance between hemorrhage and thrombosis (Tables 1 and 2).

Table 1
Plasminogen Activators

Plasminogen activators	M_R *(kDa)*	*Chains*	*Plasma concentration* $(mg\ dL^{-1})$	$t_{1/2}$	*Substrates*
Endogenous					
plasminogen	92	2	20	2.2 d	(Fibrin)
t-PA	68(59)	1→2	5×10^{-4}	5–8 min	Fibrin/plasminogen
scu-PA	54(46)	1→2	$2–20 \times 10^{-4}$	8 min	Fibrin/plasmin(ogen)
u-PA	54(46)	2	8×10^{-4}	9–12 min	Plasminogen
Exogenous					
streptokinase	47	1	0	41 and 30 min	Plasminogen/Fibrin(ogen)
APSAC	131	complex	0	70–90 min	Fibrin(ogen)
staphylokinase	16.5	0	Plasminogen		

Table 2
Plasminogen Activator Inhibitors

Inhibitor	M_R *(kDa)*	*Chains*	*Plasma concentration (mg dL^{-1})*	$t_{1/2}$	*Substrates*
Plasmin Inhibitors					
α_2-antiplasmin	65	1	7	3.3 min	Plasmin
α_2-macroglobulin (excess)	740	4	250	Plasmin	
Plasminogen Activator Inhibitors					
PAI-1	48–52	1	5×10^{-4}	7 min	t-PA, u-PA
PAI-2	47,70	1	$< \times 10^{-4}$	7 min	t-PA, u-PA
PAI-3	50	u-PA, t-PA			

Plasmin formation occurs in the plasma, where it can cleave circulating fibrinogen and fibrin, and on reactive surfaces such as thrombi or cells. The fibrin matrix—on the thrombus surface—offers one setting for plasminogen activation, and various cell types (i.e., polymorphonuclear [PMN] leukocytes, platelets, and endothelial cells), express receptors for plasminogen binding *(31)*. These cells express specific receptors that concentrate plasminogen and specific activators (e.g., urokinase plasminogen activator [u-PA]), which enhance local plasmin production. Similar receptors on tumor cells promote the dissolution of basement membranes and the metastatic process. Plasmin can also mediate the proteolytic cleavage of matrix ligands, which comprise basement membranes and vascular basal lamina.

Plasminogen

The naturally circulating PAs, single-chain t-PA, and single-chain urokinase plasminogen activator (scu-PA), catalyze plasmin formation from plasminogen *(32–35)*. Plasmin generated in the circulation degrades circulating fibrinogen and the fibrin lattice of thrombi into soluble products *(36)*.

Plasmin is derived from the zymogen, plasminogen, a single-chain 92 kDa glycosylated serine protease *(37,38)*. Plasminogen (Fig. 1) is present in two forms: glu-plasminogen, which has an NH_2-terminal glutamic acid and lys-plasminogen—lacking an 8 kDa peptide—which has an NH_2-terminal lysine. Plasmin cleavage of the NH_2-terminal fragment converts glu-plasminogen to lys-plasminogen *(39,40)*. Glu-plasminogen has a plasma clearance $t_{1/2}$ of approx 2.2 d, whereas lys-plasminogen has a $t_{1/2}$ of 0.8 d *(13)*. Both t-PA and u-PA catalyze the conversion of glu-plasminogen to lys-plasmin through either of two intermediates, glu-plasmin or lys-plasminogen *(41)*. Structurally, plasminogen contains five kringles, two of which (K_1 and K_5) mediate the binding of plasminogen to fibrin through characteristic lysine-binding sites *(37,42,43)*, and a protease domain (Fig. 1). The lysine-binding sites also mediate the binding of plasminogen to α_2-antiplasmin, thrombospondin, components of the vascular extracellular matrix (ECM), and histidine-rich glycoprotein *(38)*. α_2-Antiplasmin prevents binding of plasminogen to fibrin by this mechanism *(41)*. Partial degradation of the fibrin network enhances the binding of glu-plasminogen to fibrin, promoting further local fibrinolysis.

Plasminogen Activation

The activation of plasminogen is tied to thrombus formation by coagulation system activation (intrinsic activation) or augmented by the secretion of physiological PAs (extrinsic activation). It has been suggested that kallikrein, factor XIa, and factor XIIa in the presence of HMWK may directly activate plasminogen in the intrinsic activation method *(44,45)*. Several lines of evidence suggest that scu-PA may be an activator of plasminogen *(46–48)*. This pathway appears to be less important than the extrinsic pathway for physiological fibrinolysis

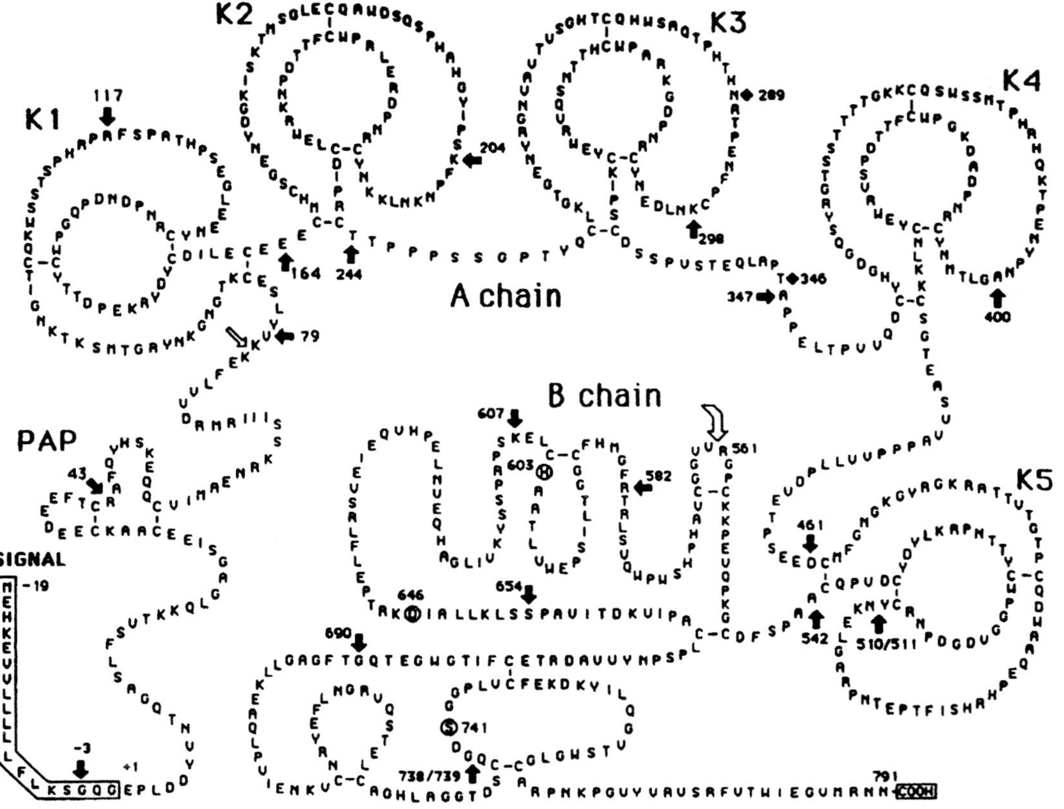

Fig. 1. The secondary structure of plasminogen. The molecule contains five kringle structures (K_1–K_5) in the A chain. Glycosylation sites are located at asn[289] and thr[346] (diamonds).

(13). The primary contributor to extrinsic activation appears to be t-PA, which is secreted from the endothelium and other cellular sources. Thrombin generated by either intrinsic or extrinsic coagulation stimulates t-PA secretion from endothelial stores *(22,49,50)*.

Several serine proteases can mediate the conversion of plasminogen to plasmin by cleaving the arg^{560}-val^{561} bond *(38,51,52)*. Serine proteases have common structural features including an NH_2-terminal "A" chain with substrate-binding affinity, a COOH-terminal "B" chain with the active site, and intra-chain disulfide bridges. Plasminogen-cleaving serine proteases include the coagulation proteins factor IX, factor X, prothrombin (factor II), protein C, chymotrypsin and trypsin, various elastases (of leukocyte origin), the plasminogen activators u-PA and t-PA, and plasmin itself *(38)*. t-PA activates plasminogen in accordance with models described by Collen and colleagues *(53,54)*. In the circulation, plasmin binds rapidly to the inhibitor α_2-antiplasmin and is thereby inactivated. Within the thrombus, plasminogen is protected from α_2-antiplasmin. Plasminogen activation by t-PA is markedly enhanced by the presence of fibrin through the ternary complex t-PA/fibrin/plasminogen *(54,55)*. Activation of thrombus-bound plasminogen also protects plasmin from the inhibitors α_2-antiplasmin and α_2-macroglobulin *(38)*. Here, the lysine-binding sites and catalytic site of plasmin are occupied by fibrin, thereby blocking its interaction with α_2-antiplasmin *(53,54)*. Furthermore, fibrin and fibrin-bound plasminogen render t-PA relatively inaccessible to inhibition by other circulating plasma inhibitors *(56)*. The net effect of these interactions is a preference for rt-PA to activate fibrin associated plasminogen, i.e., plasminogen bound into the thrombus matrix.

Thrombus Dissolution

Fibrinolysis occurs predominantly within the thrombus and at its surface *(57–60)*. Thrombus lysis is augmented by local blood flow. During thrombus consolidation, plasminogen bound to fibrin and to platelets allows local release of plasmin *(61)*. In the circulation, plasmin cleaves the fibrinogen Aα chain appendage, and generates fragment X (DED), Aα fragments, and Bβ 1–42. Further cleavage of fragment X leads to the generation of fragments DE, D, and E. In contrast, degradation of the fibrin network generates YY/DXD, YD/DY, and the unique DD/E (fragment X = DED and fragment Y = DE) *(36,57,62)*. Incorporation of some of these products into forming thrombus destabilizes the fibrin network. Crosslinkage of DD with fragment E is vulnerable to further cleavage allowing the generation of D-dimer fragments. The measurement of D-dimer levels may have clinical utility because D-dimers in plasma reflects the breakdown of fibrin-containing thrombi by plasmin. The absence of circulating D-dimer indicates the absence of massive thrombosis *(63)*. Ordinarily, in the setting of focal cerebral ischemia the thrombus load is small and the meaning of D-dimer elevations is uncertain. However, the alteration in circulating fibrinogen and the generation of breakdown products of fibrin(ogen) limits the protection from hemorrhage.

PLASMINOGEN ACTIVATORS

All fibrinolytic agents in current use are obligate PAs (Table 1). t-PA, scu-PA, and u-PA are considered endogenous PAs because they are involved in physiological fibrinolysis. t-PA and scu-PA have relative fibrin and thrombus specificity *(35,63)*. Recombinant t-PA, scu-PA, and u-PA as well as streptokinase (SK), acylated plasminogen streptokinase activator complex (APSAC), staphylokinase, PAs of vampire bat origin, and other novel agents have all been used clinically as exogenous PAs. Their conversion of plasminogen to plasmin in the circulation involves different mechanisms than those of the endogenous agents *(58–60)*.

Endogenous Plasminogen Activators

Tissue-Type Plasminogen Activator

t-PA is a 70 kDa single-chain glycosylated serine protease *(51,64)* (Fig. 2). It has four distinct domains, which include a finger (F-) domain, a growth factor (E-) domain, two kringle regions (K_1 and K_2), and a serine protease domain *(65)*. The finger domain residues 4–50 and the K_2 domain *(35,64,66)* are responsible for fibrin affinity. The growth-factor domain (residues 50–87) is homologous with epidermal growth factor (EGF), and the COOH-terminal serine protease domain contains the active site for plasminogen cleavage. The two kringle domains are homologous to the kringle regions of plasminogen.

The single-chain form is converted to the two-chain form by plasmin cleavage of the arg^{275}-isoleu^{276} bond. Both single-chain and two-chain species are enzymatically active and have relatively fibrin-selective properties. The catalytic efficiency of single-chain and two-chain t-PA for conversion of plasminogen to plasmin in vitro is stimulated to similar activity in the presence of fibrin *(64,67)*. Infusion studies in humans indicate that both single-chain and two-chain species have circulating plasma $t_{1/2}$s of 3–8 min *(35)*, although the biologic $t_{1/2}$s are longer on the thrombus surface. t-PA is considered to be fibrin-dependent because of its favorable binding constant for fibrin-bound plasminogen and its activation of plasminogen in association with fibrin *(35,65)*. Significant inactivation of circulating factors V and VIII does not occur with infused recombinant t-PA (rt-PA), and an anticoagulant state is generally not produced *(35)*. Sufficiently high doses, however, will produce clinically measurable fibrinogenolysis and plasminogen consumption.

t-PA may be secreted from cultured endothelial cells following stimulation by thrombin *(49,50,68)*, activated protein C (APC) *(69)*, histamine *(49)*, phorbol myristate esterase, and other mediators *(70–74)*, but the in vivo t-PA storage pool

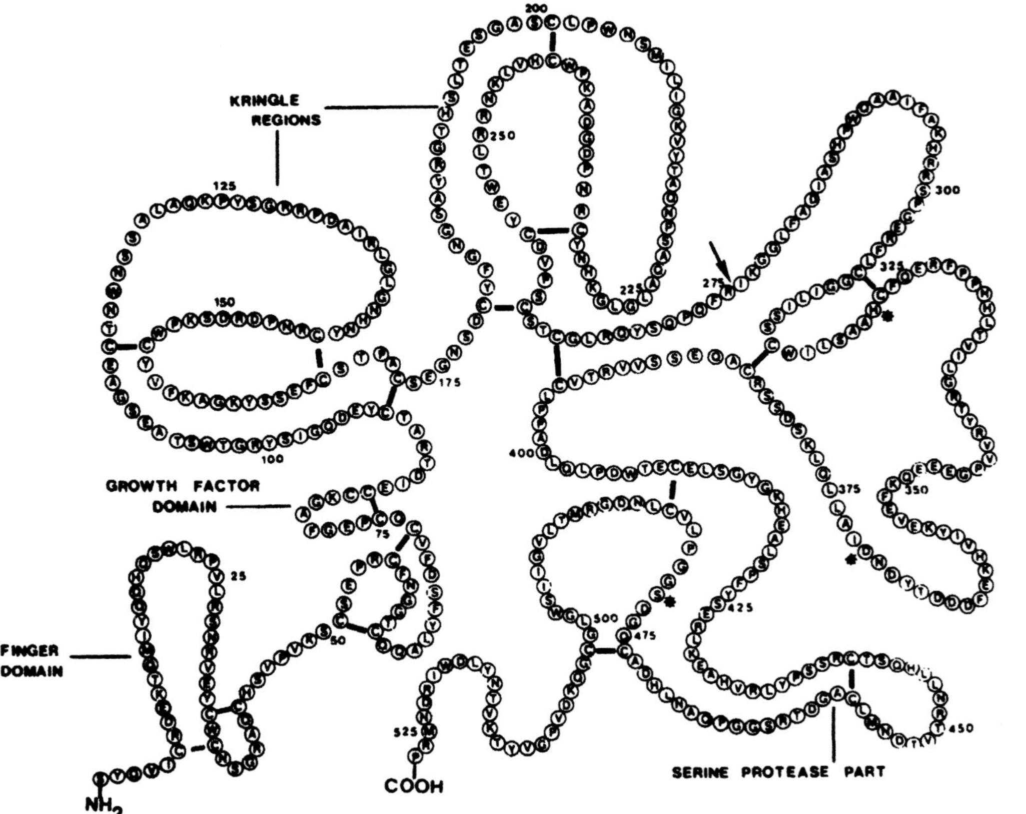

Fig. 2. The secondary structure of t-PA. The active site is formed by residues his^{322}, asp^{371}, and ser^{478} (asterisks). Conversion of single-chain t-PA to two-chain t-PA by plasmin occurs at the arg^{275}-isoleu^{276} bond (arrow). (Adapted and reproduced with permission of the publisher *[109]*, from the original source *[69]*).

location remains unclear. In patients, release or synthesis of t-PA may be enhanced by various stimuli, some of which probably release endothelial stores in vivo *(75–77)*. Physical exercise and certain vasoactive substances produce measurable increases in circulating t-PA levels. Desmopressin acetate (DDAVP) may produce a three- to fourfold increase in t-PA antigen levels within 60 min of parenteral infusion. Heparin and heparan sulfate have been associated with significant increases in t-PA activity, whereas synthetic anabolic steroids modestly potentiate fibrinolytic activity. t-PA is cleared by the liver *(78)*. t-PA and u-PA have been reported to be secreted by endothelial cells, neurons, astrocytes, and microglia in vivo or in vitro *(30,79–86)*. The reasons for this broad cell expression are uncertain.

UROKINASE PLASMINOGEN ACTIVATOR

Single-chain urokinase plasminogen activator (scu-PA or pro-UK) is a 54 kDa glycoprotein synthesized by endothelial and renal cells, as well as certain malignant cells (Fig. 3) *(31)*. This single-chain proenzyme of u-PA is unusual in possessing fibrin-selective plasmin-generating activity *(87,88)*. It has also been synthesized by recombinant techniques for use as an exogenous agent *(35,89)*.

The relationship of scu-PA to u-PA is complex; cleavage or removal of lys^{158} from scu-PA by plasmin produces high-molecular-weight (54 kDa) two-chain u-PA linked by the disulfide bridge at cys^{148} and cys^{279}. This consists of an A-chain (157 residues) and a glycosylated B-chain (253 residues). Further cleavages at lys^{135} and arg^{156} produce the low-molecular-weight (31 kDa) u-PA *(64)*. Both high- and low-molecular-weight u-PA species are enzymatically active.

High-molecular-weight (54 kDa) u-PA activates plasminogen to plasmin directly by first-order kinetics *(58,90)*. The two forms of u-PA exhibit measurable fibrinolytic and fibrinogenolytic activities in vitro and in vivo *(91,92)*, and have a plasma $t_{1/2}$ of 9–12 min. When infused as exogenous therapeutic agents, both u-PA species consume plasminogen and inactivate factors II (prothrombin), V, and VII. These latter changes constitute the systemic lytic state.

In hemostasis, t-PA and u-PA differ primarily in the domain organization of their noncatalytic regions, which regulate the function of these two PAs through co-factor binding that suggests they play quite different biological roles. Although both PAs can generate plasmin by cleavage of plasminogen, t-PA may be primarily involved in the maintenance of hemostasis through the dissolution of fibrin, whereas u-PA may be involved in generating pericellular proteolytic activity in relation to cells expressing u-PAR, needed for degradation of extracellular matrix. The roles of these two PAs in central nervous system (CNS) function are yet to be fully elucidated (*see* Plasminogen Activators in Cerebral Tissue).

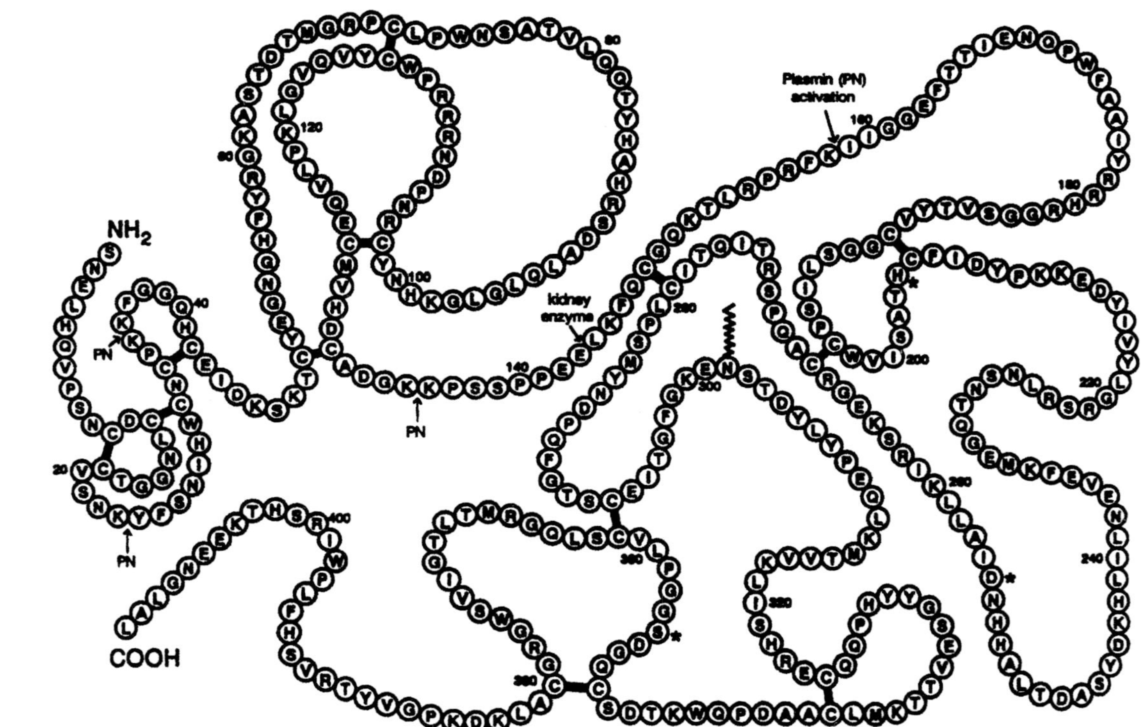

Fig. 3. The secondary structure of scu-PA (54kDa). The active site is formed by residues his^{204}, asp^{255}, and ser^{356} (asterisks). Activation by plasmin takes place at the 158–159 bind (arrow). The zig-zag line represents the glycosylation site. (With the kind permission of A. Sasahara.)

Exogenous Plasminogen Activators

STREPTOKINASE

Streptokinase (SK) is a 47 kDa single-chain polypeptide derived from group C β-hemolytic streptococci *(93)*. It combines stoichiometrically with plasminogen to form [streptokinase–plasminogen] complex, exposing an active site in the complexed plasminogen. The active [SK–plasminogen] complex converts circulating plasminogen directly to plasmin, and itself undergoes further intramolecular activation to form [SK–plasmin]. The [SK–plasminogen], [SK–plasmin], and plasmin species circulate together *(94)*. The [SK–plasmin] complex is not bound by the inhibitor α_2-antiplasmin, leaving this uninhibited form and free-circulating plasmin to degrade both fibrinogen and fibrin, and to inactivate prothrombin, and factors V and VIII *(61)*. The kinetics of elimination of SK are complex, with an initial $t_{1/2}$ of 4 min and a second $t_{1/2}$ of 30 min for the [SK–plasminogen] complex *(95)*. Because of the bacterial origin of SK, anti-streptococcal antibodies formed from antecedent infections neutralize infused SK. The anamnestic response is generally a maximum of 4–7 d following the initiation of the SK infusion. Neutralization of circulating antistreptococcal antibodies is necessary, and usually requires at least 3.5×10^5 U SK. However, because of the variable presence of anti-SK antibodies, the doses of SK required to achieve a steady-state plasminogen activation must be individualized. Depletion of plasminogen through conversion to plasmin and by, as yet poorly understood, clearance mechanisms for the [SK–plasminogen] complex can lead to hypoplasminogenemia. Generation of plasmin is then limited at low and high SK infusion dose-rates because of inadequate plasminogen conversion or depletion of plasminogen, respectively. In the latter case, an increase in SK infusion will not increase fibrinogenolysis.

ANISOYLATED PLASMINOGEN-STREPTOKINASE ACTIVATOR COMPLEX

Anisoylated plasminogen-streptokinase activator complex (APSAC [Anistreplase]) is an artificial activator constructed of plasminogen and SK bound noncovalently. It displays fibrin selectivity by virtue of the fibrin-attachment properties of the plasminogen kringle structures *(35)*. The activity of APSAC depends on the deacylation rate of the acyl-plasminogen component and the dissociation of SK from the complex. Hydrolytic activation of the acyl-protected active site of plasminogen allows plasmin formation by streptokinase within the complex in the presence of fibrin. The $t_{1/2}$ for deacylation of APSAC in plasma is approx 110 min, providing a $t_{1/2}$ for APSAC of 70 min *(96,97)*. From those observations and based on the terminal $t_{1/2}$ of SK, it is clear that APSAC has a longer circulation time than streptokinase. APSAC has not, despite its fibrin selectivity, found a place in the treatment of vascular thrombosis.

Staphylokinase

Staphylokinase (STK) is a 16.5 kDa polypeptide derived from certain strains of *Staphylococcus aureus (98–100)*. It combines stoichiometrically (1:1) with plasminogen to form an irreversible complex that activates free plasminogen. The binding of STK to plasmin has been worked out in detail *(100)*. The [STK–plasmin] complex has relative fibrin-specificity, based partly upon the observation that in the absence of fibrin the complex is inhibited by α_2-antiplasmin *(98,101)*. Recombinant STK has been prepared from the known gene nucleotide sequence, and has been tested in the setting of acute myocardial infarction (MI), but no there is no experience with STK in acute stroke.

Plasminogen Activators Derived From *Desmodus rotundus*

Recombinant PAs identical to those derived from the saliva of the vampire bat (*Desmodus rotundus*) have fibrin-dependent plasminogen-activating properties in vitro and in vivo. The α form of *Desmodus* salivary plasminogen activator (DSPA-α) and vampire bat salivary plasminogen activator (Bat-PA) are more fibrin-dependent than t-PA *(102,103)*. Fluid-phase plasmin is not produced *(104)*. Experimental studies suggest that rDSPA-α1 *(105)* and Bat-PA *(106)* may be superior to t-PA in terms of sustained recanalization without fibrinogenolysis. The plasma $t_{1/2}$ of DSPA is significantly longer than that of rt-PA *(102)*. With regard to fibrin selectivity, Bat-PA has a fastidious need for fibrin I and fibrin II polymer, which is unlike that of rt-PA *(103,107)*. Both novel PAs have not been vigorously tested for utility in CNS ischemia.

Novel Plasminogen Activators

Modifications of the deoxyribonucleic acid (DNA) sequences of u-PA and t-PA by point mutations and deletions have provided molecules with altered stability and specificity *(108,109)*. t-PA mutants lacking the K_1 and K_2 kringle domains (fibrin- and lysine-binding regions) exhibit fibrin specificity, normal specific activity, but reduced inhibition by PAI-1 *(66)*. Altered t-PAs containing deletions of F- (and/or E-) domain and single-site mutations with longer $t_{1/2}$, have been tested in various animal models of coronary artery thrombosis and pulmonary artery thrombosis *(110)*. Several mutant t-PAs with prolonged plasma $t_{1/2}$ are under study *(108,109)*.

Tenecteplase (TNK), an rt-PA mutant with delayed clearance and prolonged $t_{1/2}$, has been tested in small animal models *(111,112)*. TNK, in addition, has enhanced fibrin specificity and relative resistance to inhibition by PAI-1 compared to rt-PA *(112)*, which has been shown in modeling to produce superior recanalization. Development of this mutant t-PA has included application as bolus infusion in acute myocardial infusion where safety and coronary artery recanalization have been confirmed *(113–116)*. Application of TNK to clinical ischemic stroke is under study. However, it is unclear in this setting what advantages the delayed clearance will provide *(117)*. So far, there is no substantial evidence an increased risk of serious hemorrhage with extended PA circulation (given dose adjustments), but there is also no evidence of superior efficacy over rt-PA.

Other novel PA constructs have included single-site mutants and variants of rt-PA and recombinant scu-PA, t-PA/scu-PA and t-PA/u-PA chimerae *(118)*; u-PA/anti-fibrin monoclonal antibodies (MAbs) *(119)*, u-PA/anti-platelet MAbs *(120)* and bifunctional antibody conjugates *(121)*; and scu-PA deletion mutants *(122)*.

REGULATION OF ENDOGENOUS FIBRINOLYSIS

Endogenous fibrinolysis is modulated by several families of inhibitors of plasmin and of PAs. For streptokinase, APSAC, and staphylokinase, circulating neutralizing antibodies appear.

α_2-Antiplasmin is the primary inhibitor of fibrinolysis through direct plasmin inhibition. Excess plasmin is inactivated by covalent binding to α_2-macroglobulin. Thrombospondin interferes with fibrin-associated plasminogen activation by t-PA *(123)*. Inhibitors of the contact activation system and complement (C1 inhibitor) have an indirect effect on fibrinolysis. Histidine-rich glycoprotein (HRG) is a competitive inhibitor of plasminogen. Generally, however, these physiological modulators of plasmin activity are overwhelmed by pharmacological concentrations of PAs, leading to the thrombus lytic effect and fibrinogenolysis (e.g., with SK and u-PA).

Circulating plasmin generated in the plasma during fibrinolysis is bound by α_2-antiplasmin. Two forms of α_2-antiplasmin may be found in the plasma: (a) the native form that binds plasminogen, and (b) a second form that cannot bind plasminogen *(124)*. Ordinarily, α_2-antiplasmin is found in either plasminogen-bound or free circulating forms *(125)*. For fibrin-bound plasmin, as when t-PA activates fibrin-bound plasminogen, both the active site and the usual site of interaction with α_2-antiplasmin are already occupied. This confers some protection for fibrin-bound plasmin from the inhibitor.

Excess free plasmin is bound by α_2-macroglobulin. It is a relatively nonspecific inhibitor of fibrinolysis, inactivating plasmin, kallikrein, t-PA, u-PA, and APSAC *(126)*.

In addition to inhibitors of plasmin, specific PA inhibitors directly reduce the activity of t-PA, scu-PA, and u-PA (Table 2). Plasminogen activator inhibitor-1 (PAI-1) specifically inhibits both plasma t-PA and u-PA. PAI-1 is derived from both endothelial cell and platelet compartments *(127–129)*. Several lines of evidence indicate that K_2 of t-PA is responsible for the interaction between t-PA and PAI-1 and that this interaction is altered by the presence of fibrin *(130)*. PAI-1 is also an acute phase reactant *(131)*. Shut down of the fibrinolytic system following surgery is partially attributable to an increase in PAI-1 *(132)*, and deep venous thrombosis, septicemia, and type II diabetes mellitus are associated with elevated plasma PAI-1 levels. The potential risk of thrombosis then reflects the relative concentration of circulating PAI-1 and of t-PA.

PAI-2 is derived from placental tissue, granulocytes, monocytes/macrophages, and histiocytes *(133,134)*. The kinetics of PA inhibition by PAI-2 differs from that of PAI-1. PAI-2, which is found in a 70 kDa high-molecular-weight form and a 47 kDa low-molecular-weight form, has a lower K_i for u-PA and two-chain t-PA. This inhibitor probably plays little role in the physiological antagonism of t-PA, and is most important in the uteroplacental circulation *(135)*.

PAI-3 is a serine protease inhibitor of u-PA, t-PA, and APC found in plasma and urine *(136,137)*.

CONSEQUENCES OF THERAPEUTIC PLASMINOGEN ACTIVATION

Pharmacological concentrations (doses) of PAs can have significant effects on hemostasis. u-PA, SK, and occasionally t-PA produce systemic fibrinogen degradation, causing a fall in fibrinogen concentration. Rapid generation of plasmin in the circulation produces both a reduction in circulating plasminogen and α_2-antiplasmin. Inactivation of factors V and VIII may contribute to the systemic lytic state or anticoagulant state associated with the PAs u-PA and SK *(138)*. The systemic lytic state is marked by a decrease or depletion of circulating plasminogen, fibrinogen, and factors V and VIII with reciprocal generation of fragments of fibrin(ogen). The fragments interfere with fibrin multimerization and contribute to thrombus destabilization, whereas the circulating fragments, hypofibrinogenemia, and factor depletion produce a transient anticoagulant state that may limit thrombus extension as well as thrombus formation. For SK infusions, a severe hypoplasminogenemia may result, which makes dose adjustment particularly difficult. The clinical consequences of u-PA or SK infusion include a progressive decrease or depletion of measurable circulating plasminogen and fibrinogen, with prolongation of the activated partial thromboplastin time (aPTT) secondary to significant fibrinogen reduction and/or inactivation of factors V and VIII. The same phenomenon has been observed after rt-PA use in humans, rarely.

Certain PAs may also affect platelet function. Clinical studies of rt-PA in acute MI have demonstrated prolongation of standardized template bleeding times *(139)*. rt-PA infusion in experimental systems has been shown to produce prolonged hemorrhage or increased erythrocyte extravasation *(140,141)*. t-PA is known to cause disaggregation of human platelets, inhibitable by α_2-antiplasmin, through selective proteolysis of intraplatelet fibrin *(142)*. Lys- and glu-plasminogen can potentiate the disaggregation effect of rt-PA on platelets *(143)*. It is likely that the risk of intracerebral hemorrhage that attends PA infusion involves disruption of sustained platelet aggregation and dissolution of fibrin being formed at the site of vascular injury.

LIMITATION TO THE CLINICAL USE OF FIBRINOLYTIC AGENTS

The clinical setting in which PAs are used is an important and relevant variable in risk reduction. Intracerebral hemorrhage is a known feature of PA exposure. The use of fibrinolytic agents in pharmacological doses in clearly defined thrombotic disorders should conform to criteria established by a National Institutes of Health (NIH) Consensus Conference *(144)*, which attempts to limit the risk of hemorrhagic events. An abbreviated summary of strict contraindications to the use of fibrinolytic agents includes a history of previous intracranial hemorrhage, septic embolism, malignant hypertension or sustained diastolic or systolic blood pressure in excess of 180/110, conditions consistent with ongoing parenchymal hemorrhage (e.g., gastrointestinal source), pregnancy or parturition, history of recent trauma or surgery, and known hemorrhagic diatheses (for details, *see* Chapter 18). These contraindications apply for the use of rt-PA in select ischemic stroke patients less than 3 h from symptom onset *(6)*, as well as other approved indications for the use of pharmacological rt-PA, u-PA, or SK.

PLASMINOGEN ACTIVATORS IN CEREBRAL TISSUE

Although current clinical interests focus on the use of PAs as therapeutic agents for vascular reperfusion, cerebral tissue also expresses endogenous PAs. Various roles for specific PAs have been suggested. For instance, PA activity has been associated with development, vascular remodeling, cell migration, and tumor development and vascular invasion in the CNS. In normal cerebral tissue, t-PA antigen is associated with microvessels of a size similar to those of the vasa vasorum of the aorta *(30)*. Expression of PA activity has been reported in nonischemic tissues of mouse, spontaneously hypertensive rats, and primates *(145,146)*.

Resident nonvascular cells of the CNS have been reported to variously express t-PA, u-PA, or PAI-1. t-PA and u-PA have been reported to be secreted by endothelial cells, neurons, astrocytes, and microglia in vivo or in vitro *(79–86)*.

PAs may be involved in cell migration, development, vascular remodeling, and neuron viability in the CNS. u-PA mRNA is expressed in neurons and oligodendrocytes during process outgrowth in rodent brain *(147)*. t-PA is expressed by neurons in many brain regions, but extracellular proteolysis seems confined to specific discrete brain regions *(148)*. Recent studies suggesting that t-PA may co-mediate hippocampal neurodegeneration during excitotoxicity or following focal cerebral ischemia *(149)*, have opened a discussion that PAs may play roles in cellular viability outside the fibrinolytic system. However, conflicting evidence of increasing injury by t-PA has been balanced against credible reports of no effect or reductions in infarct volume in rodent focal cerebral ischemia models *(149,150)*. Recent experimental studies suggested that rt-PA can augment or cause neuron injury in the hippocampus of rodents *(151,152)*. Differences in arterial supply and structure of the target tissues between rodent models and human stroke patients raise the clinical relevancy of those findings *(153)*. However, at the high doses of rt-PA applied in the rodent models, in concert with studies of urokinase and t-PA knockout constructs, it appears that under limited conditions rt-PA could alter neuron behavior *(153)*.

REFERENCES

1. del Zoppo GJ, Ferbert A, Otis S, et al. Local intra-arterial fibrinolytic therapy in acute carotid territory stroke: A pilot study. *Stroke* 1988;19:307–313.
2. Mori E, Tabuchi M, Yoshida T, Yamadori A. Intracarotid urokinase with thromboembolic occlusion of the middle cerebral artery. *Stroke* 1988;19:802–812.
3. del Zoppo GJ, Poeck K, Pessin MS, Wolpert SM, Furlan AJ, Ferbert A. Recombinant tissue plasminogen activator in acute thrombotic and embolic stroke. *Ann Neurol* 1992;32:78–86.
4. Mori E, Yoneda Y, Tabuchi M, Yoshida T, Ohkawa S, Ohsumi Y. Intravenous recombinant tissue plasminogen activator in acute carotid artery territory stroke. *Neurology* 1992;42: 976–982.
5. Yamaguchi T, Hayakawa T, Kikuchi H. Intravenous tissue plasminogen activator ameliorates the outcome of hyperacute embolic stroke. Cerebrovasc Dis 1993;3:269–272.
6. The National Institutes of Neurological Disorders and Stroke rt-PA Stroke Study Group. Tissue plasminogen activator for acute ischemic stroke. *N Engl J Med* 1995;333:1581–1587.
7. Hacke W, Kaste M, Fieschi C, Toni D, Lesaffre E, von Kummer R, for the ECASS Study Group. Intravenous thrombolysis with recombinant tissue plasminogen activator for acute hemispheric stroke. The European Cooperative Acute Stroke Study (ECASS). *JAMA* 1995;274:1017–1025.
8. Hacke W, Kaste M, Fieschi C, von Kummer R, Davalos A, Meier D, for the Second European-Australasian acute Stroke Study Investigators. Randomised double-blind placebo-controlled trial of thrombolytic therapy with intravenous alteplase in acute ischaemic stroke (ECASS II). *Lancet* 1998;352:1245–1251.
9. Sherry S. The history and development of thrombolytic therapy. In: *Thrombolytic Therapy for Peripheral Vascular Disease*, Comerota AJ, ed. J. B. Lippincott Co: Philadelphia. 1995; pp. 67–86.
10. Kaplan MH. Nature and role of the lytic factor in hemolytic streptococcal fibrinolysis. *Proc Soc Exp Biol Med* 1944;57:40–43.
11. Christensen LR, MacLeod CM. A proteolytic enzyme of serum: Characterization, activation, and reaction with inhibitors. *J Gen Physiol* 1945;28:559–583.
12. Tillett WS, Sherry S. The effect in patients of streptokinase fibrinolysis (streptokinase) and streptococcal deoxyribonuclease on fibrinous, purulent and sanguineous pleural exudations. *J Clin Invest* 1949;28:173–190.
13. Johnson AJ, Tillett WS. Lysis in rabbits of intravascular blood clots by the streptococcal fibrinolytic system (streptokinase). *J Exp Med* 1952;95:449–464.
14. Hermans J, McDonagh J. Fibrin: Structure and interactions. *Semin Thromb Hemost* 1982;8:11–24.

15. Davie EW, Fujikawa K, Kisiel W. The coagulation cascade: Initiation, maintenance, and regulation. *Biochemistry* 1991;30:10,363–10,370.
16. Nossel HL. Relative proteolysis of fibrin B-beta chain by thrombin and plasmin as a determinant of thrombosis. *Nature* 1981;291:754–762.
17. Alkjaersig N, Fletcher AP. Catabolism and excretion of fibrinopeptide A. *Blood* 1982; 60:148–156.
18. Majerus PW, Miletich JP, Kane WP, Hoffmann SL, Stanford N, Jackson CM. The formation of thrombin on platelet surface. In: *The Regulation of Coagulation*, Mann KG, Taylor FB, eds. Elsevier/North Holland: New York. 1980; pp. 215–215.
19. Kaplan AP. Initiation of the intrinsic coagulation and fibrinolytic pathways of man: The role of surfaces, Hageman factor, prekallikrein, high molecular weight kininogen, and factor XI. *Prog Hemost Thromb* 1978;4:127–175.
20. Nesheim ME, Hibbard LS, Tracy PB, Bloom JW, Myrmel KH, Mann KA: Participation of factor Va in prothrombinase. In: *The Regulation of Coagulation*, Mann KG, Tayler FB, eds. Elsevier/North Holland: New York. 1980; pp. 145–159.
21. Miletich JP, Jackson CM, Majerus PW. Properties of the factor Xa binding site on human platelets. *J Biol Chem* 1978;253:6908–6916.
22. Levin EG, Marzec U, Anderson J, Harker LA. Thrombin stimulates tissue plasminogen activator release from cultured human endothelial cells. *J Clin Invest* 1984;74:1988–1995.
23. Van Hinsbergh VWM. Regulation of the synthesis and secretion of plasminogen activators by endothelial cells. *Haemostasis* 1988;18:307–327.
24. Liesi P, Kirkwood T, Vaheri A. Fibronectin is expressed by astrocytes cultured from embryonic and early postnatal rat brain. *Exp Cell Res* 1986;163:175–185.
25. Giles AR, Nosheim ME, Herring SW, Hoogendoorn H, Stump DC, Heldebrant CM. The fibrinolytic potential of the normal primate following the generation of thrombin in vivo. *Thromb Haemost* 1990;63:476–481.
26. Schwartz ML, Pizzo SV, Hill RL, McKee PA. Human factor XIII from plasma and platelets. Molecular weight, subunit structures, proteolytic activation and cross-linking of fibrinogen and fibrin. *J Biol Chem* 1973;248:1395–1407.
27. Gaffney PJ, Whittaker AN. Fibrin cross-links and lysis rates. Thromb Res 1979;14:85–94.
28. Nawroth PP, Stern DM. Endothelial cells as active participants in procoagulant reactions. In: *Vascular Endothelium in Hemostasis and Thrombosis*, Gimbrone MA, ed. Churchill-Livingstone: Edinburgh. 1986; pp. 14–39.
29. Collen D, de Maeyer L. Molecular biology of human plasminogen. I. Physiocochemical properties and microheterogeneity. *Thromb Diath Haemorhag* 1975;34:396–402.
30. Levin EG, del Zoppo GJ. Localization of tissue plasminogen activator in the endothelium of a limited number of vessels. *Am J Pathol* 1994;144:855–861.
31. Plow EF, Felez J, Miles LA. Cellular regulation of fibrinolysis. *Thromb Haemost* 1991;66:132–136.
32. Bachmann F, Kruithof IEKO. Tissue plasminogen activator: Chemical and physiological aspects. *Semin Thromb Hemost* 1984;10:6–17.
33. Aoki N, Harpel PC. Inhibitors of the fibrinolytic enzyme system. *Semin Thromb Hemost* 1984;10:24–41.
34. Collen D, Lijnen HR. New approaches to thrombolytic therapy. *Arteriosclerosis* 1984;4: 579–585.
35. Verstraete M, Collen D. Thrombolytic therapy in the eighties. *Blood* 1986;67:1529–1541.
36. Gaffrey PJ, Lane DA, Kakkar VV, Brahser M. Characterization of a soluble D-dimer-E complex in cross-linked fibrin digests. *Thromb Res* 1975;7:89–99.
37. Forsgren M, Raden B, Israelsson M, Larsson K, Heden LO. Molecular cloning and characterization of a full-length cDNA clone for human plasminogen. *FEBS Lett* 1987;213: 254–260.

38. Bachmann F. Molecular aspects of plasminogen, plasminogen activators and plasmin. In: *Haemostasis and Thrombosis*, Bloom AL, Forbes CD, Thomas DP, Tuddneham EGD, eds. Churchill Livingstone: Edinburgh. 1994; pp. 575–613.
39. Wallen P, Wiman B. Characterization of human plasminogen. II. Separation and partial characterization of different molecular forms of human plasminogen. *Biochim Biophys Acta* 1973;257:122–134.
40. Holvoet P, Lijnen HR, Collen D. A monoclonal antibody specific for lys-plasminogen. Application to the study of the activation pathways of plasminogen in vivo. *J Biol Chem* 1985;260:12,106–12,111.
41. Thorsen S, Mullertz S, Svenson E, Kok P. Sequence of formation of molecular forms of plasminogen and plasminogen-inhibitor complexes in plasma activated by urokinase or tissue-type plasminogen activator. *Biochem J* 1984;223:179–187.
42. Peterson LC, Serenson E. Effect of plasminogen and tissue-type plasminogen activator on fibrin gel structure. *Fibrinolysis* 1990;5:51–59.
43. Tran-Thong C, Kruithof EKO, Atkinson J, Bachmann F. High-affinity binding sites for human glu-plasminogen unveiled by limited plasmic degradation of human fibrin. *Eur J Biochem* 1986;160:559–604.
44. Miles LA, Greengard JS, Griffin JH. A comparison of the abilities of plasma kallikrein, Beta-Factor XIIa, Factor XIa and urokinase to activate plasminogen. *Thromb Res* 1983;29:407–417.
45. Kluft C, Dooijewaard G, Emeis JJ. Role of the contact system in fibrinolysis. *Semin Thromb Hemost* 1987;13:50–68.
46. Wun TC, Ossowski L, Reich E. A proenzyme of human urokinase. *J Biol Chem* 1982;257: 7262–7276.
47. Wun TC, Schleuning E, Reich E. Isolation and characterization of urokinase from human plasma. *J Biol Chem* 1982;257:3276–3287.
48. Ichinose A, Fujikawa K, Suyama T. The activation of pro-urokinase by plasma kallikrein and its inactivation by thrombin. *J Biol Chem* 1986;261:3486–3489.
49. Hanss M, Collen D. Secretion of tissue-type plasminogen activator and plasminogen activator inhibitor by cultured human endothelial cells: Modulation by thrombin endotoxin and histamine. *J Lab Clin Med* 1987;109:97–104.
50. Levin EG, Stern DM, Nawrath PP, et al. Specificity of the thrombin-induced release of tissue plasminogen activator from cultured human endothelial cells. *Thromb Haemost* 1986;56: 115–119.
51. Robbins KC, Summaria L, Hsieh B, Shah RJ. The peptide chains of human plasmin. *J Biochem* 1967;242:2333–2342.
52. Robbins KC. The plasminogen-plasmin system. In: *Thrombolytic Therapy for Peripheral Vascular Disease* , Comerota AJ, ed. J. B. Lippincott: Philadelphia. 1995; pp. 41–65.
53. Wiman B, Collen D. Molecular mechanism of physiological fibrinolysis. *Nature* 1979;272: 549–550.
54. Collen D. On the regulation and control of fibrinolysis. *Thromb Haemost* 1980;43:77–89.
55. Hoylaerts M, Rijken DC, Lijnen HR, Collen D. Kinetics of the activation of plasminogen by human tissue plasminogen activator. Role of fibrin. *J Biol Chem* 1982;257:2912–2919.
56. Wun T-C, Capugno A. Initiation and regulation of fibrinolysis in human plasma at the plasminogen activator level. *Blood* 1987;69:1354–1362.
57. Bloom AL, Thomas DP. *Haemostasis and Thrombosis*. Edinburgh, Churchill-Livingstone, 1987.
58. Kakkar VV, Scully MF. Thrombolytic therapy. *Br Med Bull* 1978;34:191–199.
59. Sharma GVRK, Cella G, Parish AF, Sasahara AA. Drug therapy: Thrombolytic therapy. *N Engl J Med* 1982;306:1268–1276.

60. Verstraete M. Biochemical and clinical aspects of thrombolysis. *Semin Hematol* 1978; 15:35–54.
61. Castellino FJ. Biochemistry of human plasminogen. *Semin Thromb Hemost* 1984;10:18–23.
62. Yasaka M, Yamaguchi T, Miyashita T, Tsuchiya T. Regression of intracardiac thrombus after embolic stroke. *Stroke* 1990;21:1540–1544.
63. Bounameaux H, de Moerloose P, Perrier A, Reber G. Plasma measurement of D-dimer as diagnostic aid in suspected venous thromboembolism: An overview. *Thromb Haemost* 1994;71:1–6.
64. Rijken DC. Structure/function relationships of t-PA. In: *Tissue Type Plasminogen Activator (t-PA): Physiological and Clinical Aspects Vol. 1*, Kluft C, ed. CRC Press: Boca Raton. 1988; pp. 101–122.
65. Pennica D, Holmes WE, Kohr WJ, Harkins RN, Vehar GA, Ward CA. Cloning and expression of human tissue-type plasminogen activator cDNA in *E coli*. *Nature* 1983;301:214–221.
66. Ehrlich HJ, Bang NW, Little SP, et al. Biological properties of a kringleless tissue plasminogen activator (t-PA) mutant. *Fibrinolysis* 1987;1:75–81.
67. Ranby M, Bergsdorf N, Norrman B, Svenson E, Wallen P. *Tissue plasminogen activator kinetics. In: Progress in Fibrinolysis Vol. VI*, Davison JF, Bachmann F, Bouvier CA, Kruithof EKO, eds. Churchill-Livingstone: New York. 1982; pp. 182–182.
68. Gelehrter TD, Sznycer-Laszuk R. Thrombin induction of plasminogen activator-inhibitor in cultured human endothelial cells. *J Clin Invest* 1986;77:165–169.
69. Sakata Y, Curriden S, Lawrence D, et al. Activated protein C stimulates the fibrinolytic activity of cultured endothelial cells and decreases antiactivator activity. *Proc Natl Acad Sci USA* 1985;82:1121–1125.
70. Moscatelli D. Urokinase-type and tissue-type plasminogen activators have different distributions in cultured bovine capillary endothelial cells. *J Cell Biochem* 1986;30:19–29.
71. Bulens F, Nelles L, Van den Panhuyzen N, Collen D. Stimulation by retinoids of tissue-type plasminogen activator secretion in cultured human endothelial cells: Relations of structure to effect. *J Cardiovasc Pharmacol* 1992;19:508–514.
72. Thompson EA, Nelles L, Collen D. Effect of retinoic acid on the synthesis of tissue-type plasminogen activator and plasminogen activator inhibitor-I in human endothelial cells. *Eur J Biochem* 1991;201:627–632.
73. Saksela O, Moscatelli D, Rifkin DB. The opposing effects of basic fibroblast growth factor and transforming growth factor beta on the regulation of plasminogen activator activity in capillary endothelial cells and decreases antiactivator activity. *J Cell Biol* 1987;105: 957–963.
74. Levin EG, Marotti KR, Santell L. Protein kinase C and the stimulation of tissue plasminogen activator release from human endothelial cells. Dependence on the elevation of messenger RNA. *J Biol Chem* 1989;264:16,030–16,036.
75. Smith D, Gilbert M, Owen WG. Tissue plasminogen activator release in vivo in response to vasoactive agents. *Blood* 1985;66:835–839.
76. Brommer EJP. Clinical relevance of t-PA levels of fibrinolytic assays. In: *Tissue-Type Plasminogen Activator (t-PA): Physiological and Clinical Aspects Part 2*, Kluft C, ed. CRC Press: Boca Raton. 1988; pp. 89–89.
77. Agnelli G. The pharmacological basis of thrombmolytic therapy. In: *Thrombolysis Yearbook 1995*, Agnelli G, ed. Excerpta Medica: Amsterdam. 1995; pp. 31–61.
78. Verstraete M, Bounameaux H, de Cock F, Van de Loerf F, Collen D. Pharmacokinetics and systemic fibrinogenolytic effects of recombinant human tissue-type plasminogen activator (rt-PA) in humans. *J Pharmacol Exp Ther* 1986;235:506–512.
79. Krystosek A, Seeds NW. Normal and malignant cells, including neurons, deposit plasminogen activator on growth substrata. *Exp Cell Res* 1986;166:31–46.

80. Pittman RN. Release of plasminogen activator and a calcium-dependent metalloprotease from cultured sympathetic and sensory neurons. *Dev Biol* 1985;110:91–101.
81. Vincent VA, Lowik CW, Verheijen JH, de Bart AC, Tilders FJ, Van Dam AM. Role of astrocyte-derived tissue-type plasminogen activator in the regulation of endotoxin-stimulated nitric oxide production by microglial cells. *GLIA* 1998;22:130–137.
82. Toshniwal PK, Firestone SL, Barlow GH, Tiku ML. Characterization of astrocyte plasminogen activator. *J Neurol Sci* 1987;80:277–287.
83. Tsirka SE, Rogove AD, Bugge TH, Degen JL, Strickland S. An extracellular proteolytic cascade promotes neuronal degeneration in the mouse hippocampus. *J Neurosci* 1997;17: 543–552.
84. Masos T, Miskin R. Localization of urokinase-type plasminogen activator mRNA in the adult mouse brain. *Brain Res Mol Brain Res* 1996;35:139–148.
85. Tranque P, Naftolin F, Robbins R. Differential regulation of astrocyte plasminogen activators by insulin-like growth factor-I and epidermal growth factor. *Endocrinology* 1994;134: 2606–2613.
86. Nakajima K, Tsuzaki N, Shimojo M, Hamanoue M, Kohsaka S. Microglia isolated from rat brain secrete a urokinase-type plasminogen activator. *Brain Res* 1992;577:285–292.
87. Lijnen HR, Zamarron C, Blaber M, Winkler ME, Collen D. Activation of plasminogen by pro-urokinase. I. Mechanism. *J Biol Chem* 1986;261:1253–1258.
88. Peterson LC, Lund LR, Nielsen LS, Dano K, Shriver L. One-chain urokinase-type plasminogen activator from human sarcoma cells is a proenzyme with little or no intrinsic activity. *J Biol Chem* 1988;263:11,189–11,195.
89. Gunzler WA, Steffens GJ, Otting F, Buse G, Flohe L. Structural relationship between human high and low molecular mass urokinase. Hoppe Seylers Z *Physiol Chem* 1982;563:133–141.
90. White FW, Barlow GH, Mozen MM. The isolation and characterization of plasminogen activators (urokinase) from human urine. *Biochemistry* 1966;5:2160–2169.
91. Fletcher AP, Alkjaersig N, Sherry S, Genton E, Hirsh J, Bachmann F. The development of urokinase as a thrombolytic agent. Maintenance of a sustained thrombolytic state in man by its intravenous infusion. *J Lab Clin Med* 1965;65:713–731.
92. Stump DC, Mann KH. Mechanisms of thrombus formation and lysis. *Ann Emerg Med* 1988;17:1138–1147.
93. Davies MC, Englert ME, De Rezo EC. Interaction of streptokinase and human plasminogen observed in the ultracentrifuge under a variety of experimental conditions. *J Biol Chem* 1964;239(8):2651–2656.
94. Reddy KN, Marcus B. Mechanisms of activation of human plasminogen by streptokinase. *J Biol Chem* 1972;246:1683–1691.
95. Fletcher AP, Alkjaersig N, Sherry S. The clearance of heterologous proteins from the circulation of normal and immunized man. *J Clin Invest* 1958;37(9):1306–1315.
96. Standing R, Fears R, Ferres H. The protective effect of acylation on the stability of APSAC (Eminase) in human plasma. *Fibrinolysis* 1988;2:157.
97. Ferres H. Preclinical pharmacological evaluation of Eminase (APSAC). *Drugs* 1987; 33(Suppl 3):33–50.
98. Lignen HR, de Cock F, Matsuo O, Collen D. Comparative fibrinolytic and fibrinogenolytic properties of staphylokinase and streptokinase in plasma of different species in vitro. *Fibrinolysis* 1992;6:33–37.
99. Collen D. Staphlyokinase: a potent, uniquely fibrin-selective thrombolytic agent. *Nature Medicine* 1998;4(3):279–282.
100. Jespers L, Vanwetswinkel S, Lijnen HR, Van Herzeele N, Van Hoef B, Demarsin E, et al. Structural and functional basis of plasminogen activation by staphylokinase. *Thromb Haemost* 1999;81(4):479–484.

101. Lijnen HR, Van Hoef B, Matsuo O, Collen D. On the molecular, interactions between plasminogen- staphylokinase, α2-antiplasmin and fibrin. *Biochim Biophys Acta* 1992;1118: 144–148.
102. Witt W, Maass B, Baldus B, Hildebrand M, Donner P, Schleuning WD. Coronary thrombosis with Desmodus salivary plasminogen activator in dogs. Fast and persistent recanalization by intravenous bolus administration. *Circulation* 1994;90:421–426.
103. Bergum PW, Gardell SJ. Vampire bat salivary plasminogen activator exhibits a strict and fastidious requirement for polymeric fibrin as its cofactor, unlike human tissue-type plasminogen activator. A kinetic analysis. *J Biol Chem* 1992;267:17,726–17,731.
104. Hare TR, Gardell SJ. Vampire bat salivary plasminogen activator promotes robust lysis of plasma clots in a plasma milieu without causing fluid phase plasminogen activation. *Thromb Haemost* 1992;68:165–169.
105. Witt W, Baldus B, Bringmann P, Cashion L, Donner P, Schleuning WD. Thrombolytic properties of Desmodus rotundus (vampire bat) salivary plasminogen activator in experimental pulmonary embolism in rats. *Blood* 1992;79:1213–1217.
106. Mellot MJ, Stabilito II, Holahan MA, et al. Vampire bat salivary plasminogen activator promotes rapid and sustained reperfusion without concomitant systemic plasminogen activation in a canine model of arterial thrombosis. *Arterioscler Thromb* 1992;12:212–221.
107. Gardell SJ, Ramjit DR, Stabilito II, Fujita T, Lynch JJ, Cuca GC, et al. Effective thrombolysis without marked plasminemia after bolus intravenous administration of vampire bat salivary plasminogen activator in rabbits. *Circulation* 1991;84:244–253.
108. Lijnen HR, Collen D. Development of new fibrinolytic agents. In: *Haemostasis and Thrombosis*, Bloom AL, Forbes CD, Thomas DP, Tuddenham EGD, eds. Churchill-Livingstone: Edinburgh. 1994; pp. 625–637.
109. Van de Werf F. New thrombolytic strategies. *Aust N Z J Med* 1993;23:763–765.
110. Barnathan ES, Kuo A, Van der Keyl H, McCrae KR, Larsen GR, Cines DB. Tissue-type plasminogen activator binding to human endothelial cells. *J Biol Chem* 1988;263: 7792–7799.
111. Smalling RW. Pharmacological and clinical impact of the unique molecular structure of a new plasminogen activator. *Eur Heart J* 1997;18(F):F11–F16.
112. Benedict CR, Refino CJ, Keyt BA, et al. New variant of human tissue plasminogen activator (TPA) with enhanced efficacy and lower incidence of bleeding compared with recombinant human TPA. *Circulation* 1995;92(10):3032–3040.
113. Cannon CP, McCabe CH, Gibson CM, Ghali M, Sequeira RF, McKendall GR, et al. TNK-tissue plasminogen activator in acute myocardial infarction. Results of the Thrombolysis in Myocardial Infarction (TIMI) 10A dose-ranging trial. *Circulation* 1997;95(2):351–356.
114. Cannon CP, Gibson CM, McCabe CH, Adgey AA, Schweiger MJ, Sequeira RF, et al. TNK-tissue plasminogen activator compared with front-loaded alteplase in acute myocardial infarction: results of the TIMI 10B trial. Thrombolysis in Myocardial Infarction (TIMI) 10B Investigators. *Circulation* 1998;98(25):2805–2814.
115. Van de Werf F, Cannon CP, Luyten A, Houbracken K, McCabe CH, Berioli S, et al. Safety assessment of single-bolus administration of TNK tissue-plasminogen activator in acute myocardial infarction: the ASSENT-1 trial. The ASSENT-1 Investigators. *Am Heart J* 1999;137(5):786–791.
116. Gibson CM, Cannon CP, Murphy SA, et al. Weight-adjusted dosing of TNK-tissue plasminogen activator and its relation to angiographic outcomes in the thrombolysis in myocardial infarction 10B trial. TIMI 10B Investigators. *Am J Cardiol* 1999;84(9):976–980.
117. Modi NB, Eppler S, Breed J, Cannon CP, Braunwald E, Love TW. Pharmacokinetics of a slower clearing tissue plasminogen activator variant, TNK-tPA, in patients with acute myocardial infarction. *Thromb Haemost* 1998;79(1):134–139.

118. Pierard L, Jacobs P, Gheysen D, Hoylaerts M, Andre B, Topisirovic L, et al. Mutant and chimeric recombinant plasminogen activators. *J Biol Chem* 1987;262:11,771–11,778.
119. Runge MS, Bode C, Matsueda GR, Haber E. Antibody-enhanced thrombolysis: Targeting of tissue plasminogen activator in vivo. *Proc Natl Acad Sci USA* 1987;84:7659–7662.
120. Bode C, Meinhardt G, Runge MS, et al. Platelet-targeted fibrinolysis enhances clot lysis and inhibits platelet aggregation. *Circulation* 1991;84:805–813.
121. Jones RD, Donaldson IM, Parkin PJ. Impairment and recovery of ipsilateral sensory-motor function following unilateral cerebral infarction. *Brain* 1989;112:113–132.
122. Kasper W, Meinertz T, Hohnloser S, Engler H, Hasler C, Rossler W, et al. Coronary thrombolysis in man with prourokinase: Improved efficacy with low dose urokinase. *Klin Wochenschr* 1988;66:109–114.
123. Bachmann F. Fibrinolysis. In: *Thrombosis and Haemostasis*, Verstraete M, Vermylen J, Lijnen HR, Arnout J, eds. Leuven, ISTH/University of Leuven Press: 1987; pp. 227–265.
124. Kluft C, Los N. Demonstration of two forms of α_2-antiplasmin in plasma by modified crossed immunoelectrophoresis. *Thromb Res* 1981;21:65–71.
125. Winman B, Nilsson T, Cedergren B. Studies on a form of α_2-antiplasmin in plasma which does not interact with the lysine-binding sites in plasminogen. *Thromb Res* 1982; 28: 193–200.
126. Aoki N, Harpel P. Inhibitors of the fibrinolytic enzyme system. *Semin Hemostat Thromb* 1984;10:24–39.
127. Philips M, Juul AG, Thorsen S. Human endothelial cells produce a plasminogen activator inhibitor and a tissue-type plasminogen activator-inhibitor complex. *Biochim Biophys Acta* 1984;802:99–110.
128. Loskutoff DJ, van Mourik JA, Erickson LA, Lawrence DA. Detection of an unusually stable fibrinolytic inhibitor produced by bovine endothelial cells. *Proc Natl Acad Sci USA* 1983;80:2956–2960.
129. Thorsen S, Philips M, Selmer J, Lecander I, Astedt B. Kinetics of inhibition of tissue-type and urokinase-type plasminogen activator by plasminogen-activator inhibitor type 1 and type 2. *Eur J Biochem* 1988;175:33–39.
130. Wilhelm OG, Jaskunas SR, Vlahos CJ, Bang NU. Functional properties of the recombinant kringle-2 domain of tissue plasminogen activator produced in Escherichia coli. *J Biol Chem* 1990;265:14,606–14,611.
131. Juhan-Vague I, Moerman B, de Cock F, Aillaud MF, Collen D. Plasma levels of a specific inhibitor of tissue-type plasminogen activator (and urokinase) in normal and pathological conditions. *Thromb Res* 1984;33:523–530.
132. Kluft C, Verheihen J-H, Jie AFH, et al. The postoperative fibrinolytic shutdown: A rapidly reverting acute-phase pattern for the fast-acting inhibitor of tissue-type plasminogen activator after trauma. *Scand J Clin Lab Invest* 1985;45:605–610.
133. Schleuning W-D, Medcalf RL, Hession C, RothenbŸhler R, Shaw A, Kruithof EKO. Plasminogen activator inhibitor 2: Regulation of gene transcription during phorbol ester-mediated differentiation of U-937 human histiocytic lymphoma cells. *Mol Cell Biol* 1987;7:4564–4567.
134. Kruithof EKO, Tran-Thang C, Gudinchet A, et al. Fibrinolysis in pregnancy: A study of plasminogen activator inhibitors. *Blood* 1987;69:460–466.
135. Bonnar J, Daly L, Sheppard BL. Changes in the fibrinolytic system during pregnancy. *Semin Thromb Hemost* 1990;16:221–229.
136. Stump D, Thienpoint M, Collen D. Purification and characterization of a novel inhibitor of urokinase from human urine: Quantitation and preliminary characterization in plasma. *J Biol Chem* 1986;261:12,759–12,766.

137. Heeb MJ, Espana F, Geiger M, Collen D, Stump D, Griffin JH. Immunological identity of heparin-dependent plasma and urinary protein C inhibitor and plasminogen activator inhibitor-3. *J Biol Chem* 1987;262:15,813–15,816.
138. Marder VJ, Sherry S. Thrombolytic therapy. Current status. *N Engl J Med* 1988;388: 1512–1520.
139. Gimple LW, Gold HK, Leinbach RC, et al. Correlation between template bleeding times and spontaneous bleeding during treatment of acute myocardial infarction with recombinant tissue plasminogen activator. *Circulation* 1989;80:581–588.
140. Agnelli G, Buchanan MR, Fernandez F, et al. A comparison of the thrombolytic and hemorrhagic effects of tissue-type plasminogen activator and streptokinase in rabbits. *Circulation* 1985;72:178–182.
141. Marder VJ, Shortell CK, Fitzpatrick PG, Kim C, Oxley D. An animal model of fibrinolytic bleeding based on the rebleed phenomenon: Application to a study of vulnerability of hemostatic plugs of different age. *Thromb Res* 1992;67(1):31–40.
142. Loscalzo J, Vaughan DB. Tissue plasminogen activator promotes platelet disaggregation in plasma. *J Clin Invest* 1987;79:1749–1755.
143. Chen LY, Muhta JL. Lys- and glu-plasminogen potentiate the inhibitory effect of recombinant tissue plasminogen activator on human platelet aggregation. *Thromb Res* 1994;74:555–563.
144. NIH Consensus Conference. Thrombolytic therapy in treatment. *Br Med J* 1980;280: 1585–1587.
145. Danglet G, Vinson D, Chapeville F. Qualitative and quantitative distribution of plasminogen activators in organs from healthy adult mice. *FEBS Lett* 1986;194:96–100.
146. Matsuo O, Okada K, Fukao H, Suzuki A, Ueshima S. Cerebral plasminogen activator activity in spontaneously hypertensive stroke-prone rats. *Stroke* 1992;23:995–999.
147. Dent MA, Sumi Y, Morris RJ, Seeley PJ. Urokinase-type plasminogen activator expression by neurons and oligodendrocytes during process outgrowth in developing rat brain. *Eur J Neurosci* 1993;5:633–647.
148. Sappino A-P, Madani R, Huarte J, et al. Extracellular proteolysis in the adult murine brain. *J Clin Invest* 1993;92:679–685.
149. Wang YF, Tsirka SE, Strickland S, Stieg PE, Soriano SG, Lipton SA. Tissue plasminogen activator (t-PA) increases neuronal damage after focal cerebral ischemia in wild-type and t-PA-deficient mice. *Nature Medicine* 1998;4:228–231.
150. del Zoppo GJ. t-PA: A neuron buster, too? (editorial). *Nature Medicine* 1998;4:148–150.
151. Tsirka SE, Rogove AD, Strickland S. Neuronal cell death and tPA. *Nature* 1996; 384:123–124.
152. Tsirka SE, Gualandris A, Amaral DG, Strickland S. Excitotoxin-induced neuronal degeneration and seizure are mediated by tissue plasminogen activator. *Nature* 1995;377:340–344.
153. del Zoppo GJ. tPA: A neuron buster, too?. *Nature Medicine* 1998;4:148–149 .

2 Pathology of Cervico-Cranial Artery Occlusion

Louis R. Caplan, MD

CONTENTS

INTRODUCTION

Brain ischemia is caused by a heterogeneous array of different vascular disorders. The general categories of vascular disorders most often used are embolism, "thrombosis" (referring to a local *in situ* process that narrows and often occludes an artery or vein), and systemic hypoperfusion. Systemic disorders that lead to brain ischemia include cardiac disorders (cardiac arrest, arrythmias, low cardiac output), conditions that cause hypovolemia and lack of adequate oxygen-carrying blood (blood loss, severe anemia, shock, carbon monoxide poisoning, hypotension), and acute pulmonary conditions (i.e., pulmonary embolism). Because patients with systemic disorders are not candidates for thrombolysis and there are usually no associated intracranial vascular occlusions, this large category is not discussed here. This chapter, therefore, focuses entirely on embolic and thrombotic disorders.

BRAIN EMBOLISM

Embolism has been variously defined and categorized. Although some use this category to include only cardiac-origin embolism, the author urges a more general approach. An embolus refers to a particle that originates in one place and moves to another site; a traveling particle rather than one that stays at the place

From: *Current Clinical Neurology:Thrombolytic Therapy for Acute Stroke, Second Edition*
Edited by: P. D. Lyden © Humana Press Inc., Totowa, NJ

it originated (thrombus). Embolism is the process of particle migration within the vascular bed.

There are three main descriptors of embolism: (a) the *donor site* that is the source of the embolus, (b) the *material* that makes up the embolus, and (c) the *recipient site* where the embolus rests or remains. All are important determinants when considering treatment *(1–3)*.

Donor Sources

The donor sites for embolic material are the heart, aorta, and extracranial and intracranial arteries. Emboli originating from the heart are usually called cardiogenic, whereas emboli originating within the aorta or proximal arteries are called intra-arterial or artery-to-artery emboli but are sometimes referred to as local emboli.

Some emboli arise in the venous system and simply pass through the heart to reach the brain and other systemic arteries. These emboli traverse communications between the right heart-pulmonary system and the left heart-systemic circulation. The most common such communications are intra-atrial septal defects and patent foramen ovales. Occasionally incriminated are ventricular septal defects and pulmonary arteriovenous malformations. These emboli are often referred to as *paradoxical emboli*. Studies have shown that paradoxical embolism is much more common than previously thought.

A variety of different cardiac disorders can provide the source for embolism. The most common categories are listed in Table 1. In all published series, arrhythmias—especially atrial fibrillation and coronary artery disease-related conditions—are the most common sources, followed in frequency by valve disorders. Table 2 enumerates the most frequent cardiac sources in the Stroke Data Bank *(1,4,5)* and designates the Stroke Data Bank's categorization of high- and medium-risk heart conditions with respect to their importance in serving as sources of emboli. Table 3 lists the most frequent potential cardiac sources of embolism in the Lausanne Stroke Registry *(1,6,7)*.

The aorta is now also recognized as a very important source of emboli to the brain, especially during and after cardiac surgery *(8–10)*. Clamping an atheromatous aortic arch often leads to release of particles into the brain and systemic arteries. Atherosclerosis is often severe in the aorta and the plaques are often located in the ascending aorta and the arch proximal to the origins of the carotid and brachiocephalic arteries *(11)*. Particles released can consist of cholesterol crystals, calcified plaque debris, white clots, and red thrombi. Protuberant mobile large plaques are most often associated with brain embolism.

Arterial sources of embolism are also quite varied. Emboli arise from a variety of different disorders and from a variety of different sites. Although atherosclerosis is by far the most common condition that leads to intra-arterial embolism, other vascular diseases also can serve as donor sources. Trauma and dissections

Table 1
Most Frequent Cardiac Disorders Associated With Brain Embolism

Arrythmias
Atrial fibrillation
Sick-sinus syndrome (brady-tachy syndrome)
Valve diseases
Rheumatic mitral and aortic valve disease
Calcific aortic and mitral valve disease
Prosthetic valves
Bacterial endocarditis
Nonbacterial thrombotic endocarditis (marantic endocarditis)
(most common causes: lupus erythematosis, cancer, antiphospholipid antibody syndrome)
myxomatous valve degeneration (mitral valve prolapse)
mitral annulus calcification
? valve strands
Myocardial disorders
Myocardial infarction
Hypokinetic regions
Myocardial aneurysms
Myocarditis
Myocardopathies
Septal lesions
Patent foramen ovale
Atrial septal defects
Ventricular septal defects
Atrial septal aneurysms
Cardiac chamber lesions
Cardiac tumors (myxomas, rhabdomyomas, fibroelastomas)
Ball thrombi
"Spontaneous echo contrast"

of arteries leads to local thrombus formation and embolism. Occasionally inflammatory diseases of the brachiocephalic branches of the aortic arch, such as temporal arteritis and Takayasu's disease, are sources of intra-arterial embolism. Thrombi sometimes form within arterial aneurysms, saccular, dissecting, and fusiform dolicocephalic aneurysms, and can then break off and embolize to distal branch arteries. Fibromuscular dysplasia (FMD) is an important but relatively uncommon vascular disease that affects the pharyngeal and occasionally the intracranial portions of the carotid and vertebral arteries; stenosis resulting from FMD can occasionally serve as a source of distal intra-arterial embolism.

Table 2
Patients in the Stroke Data Bank With Selected Cardiac Characteristics in High and Medium Cardiac-Risk Groups

Cardiac-risk categories	*High-risk (n = 250)*	*Medium-risk (n = 166)*
High-risk categories		
Valve surgery	15	
A-fib, A-flutter, sick sinus with valve disease	28	
A-fib, A-flutter, sick sinus but no valve disease	162	
Ventricular aneurysm*	5	
Mural thrombus*	12	
Cardiomyopathy or left ventricle hypokinesis*	7	
Akinetic region*	52	
Medium-risk categories		
Myocardial infarct within 6 mo	25	18
Valve disease without A-fib, A-flutter, sick sinus	31	19
Congestive heart failure	92	95
Decreased left ventricle function*	0	3
Hypokinetic segment*	0	12
Mitral valve prolapse (by history or echocardiogram	5	13
Mitral annulus calcification*	14	46

* Determined by echocardiography. Some patients had more than one characteristic. (Modified from ref. *5* with permission.)

Table 3
Potential Cardiac Sources of Embolism in the Lausanne Stroke Registry

Cardiac abnormalities	*n patients (%)*
Isolated myocardial abnormalities	84 (27.5%)
Focal left ventricle akinesia without thrombus	61 (20%)
Focal left ventricle akinesia with thrombus	7 (2.3%)
Global ventricular hypokinesia	7 (2.3%)
Patent foramen ovale	6 (2%)
Left atrial myxoma	2 (0.7%)
Left ventricle thrombus	1 (0.3%)
Isolated valve abnormalities	71 (23.3%)
Mitral valve prolapse	51 (16.7%)
Mitral stenosis or insufficiency	10 (3.3%)
Prosthetic mitral or aortic valve	10 (3.3%)
Isolated arrythmia	127 (41.6%)
Atrial fibrillation	118 (38.7%)
Sick-sinus syndrome	9 (2.9%)

(continued)

Table 3 (*Continued*)
Potential Cardiac Sources of Embolism in the Lausanne Stroke Registry

Cardiac abnormalities	*n patients (%)*
Arrythmias plus myocardial abnormalities	12 (3.9%)
Atrial fibrillation plus focal left ventricular akinesia without thrombus	6 (2%)
Atrial fibrillationplus focal left ventricular akinesia with thrombus	1 (0.3%)
Atrial fibrillation plus global hypokinesia	3 (1%)
Atrial fibrillation plus left ventricular thrombus	2 (0.7%)
Arrythmias plus valve abnormalities	11 (3.6%)
Atrial fibrillation plus mitral valve prolapse	6 (2%)
plus mitral stenosis	2 (0.7%)
plus prosthetic valve	3 (1%)

Modified from ref. *7* with permission.

Table 4
Embolic Materials

Cardiac origin	*Arterial origin*
Red erythrocyte-fibrin clots	Red erythrocyte-fibrin clots
White platelet-fibrin clots	White platelet-fibrin clots
Calcific particles	Calcific particles
Bacteria	Cholesterol chrystals
Fibrous strands	Parts of plaques
Myxomatous tumors	
Prosthetic valve parts	

Thrombi can, on occasion, form within large arteries in the absence of important arterial disease in patients with cancer and other causes of hypercoagulability *(12)*.These luminal thrombi then embolize to intracranial arteries causing strokes.

These conditions are discussed further in the section, Disorders—"*In Situ* Arterial Thrombosis."

Embolic Material

The actual "stuff" that embolizes is of great importance *(1–3)*. As far as is known, thrombolytic drugs lyse so-called "red" erythrocyte-rich thrombi. The mechanism relates to breaking or relaxing the fibrin bridges and bonds that hold the thrombus together. Fresh, soft, red thromboemboli are more easily lysed than old, organized, fibrotic thromboemboli. There are a variety of different particles that can embolize from cardiac and arterial sources. These are listed in Table 4.

Recipient Sites and Resultant Infarct Patterns

About 80% of emboli that arise from the heart go into the anterior (carotid artery) circulation, equally divided between the left and right sides. The remaining 20% of emboli go into the posterior (vertebrobasilar) circulation, a rate roughly equal to the proportion of the blood supply that goes into the vertebrobasilar arteries. The recipient artery destination depends on the size and nature of the particles. Calcific particles from heart valves or mitral annular calcifications are less mobile and adapt less well to the shape of their recipient artery resting places than red (erythrocyte-fibrin) and white (platelet-fibrin) thrombi. The circulating blood stream seems to be able to somehow bypass obstructing cholesterol crystal emboli, especially in the retinal arteries.Within the anterior and posterior circulations there are predilection sites for the destination of embolic particles. Large emboli entering a common carotid artery may become lodged in the common or internal carotid artery, especially if atheromatous plaques have already narrowed the lumens of these vessels. If the emboli were able to pass through the carotid arteries in the neck, the next common lodging place is the intracranial bifurcation of the internal carotid arteries (ICAs) into the anterior cerebral (ACA) and middle cerebral arteries (MCAs). Bifurcations are common resting places for emboli. Emboli that pass through the carotid intracranial bifurcations most often go into the MCAs and their branches. Gacs et al. showed that balloon emboli placed in the circulation nearly always followed the same pathway and ended up in the MCAs and their branches *(13)*. Embolism in experimental animals produced by the introduction of silicone cylinders or spheres, elastic cylinders, and autologous blood clots, also showed a very high incidence of MCA territory localization *(14)*. Emboli often pass into the superior and inferior divisions of the MCA and the cortical branches of these divisions. The superior division supplies the cortex and white matter above the sylvian fissure including the frontal and superior parietal lobes. The inferior division supplies the area below the sylvian fissure including the temporal and inferior parietal lobes. The ACA supplies the paramedian frontal lobe. Emboli seldom go into the penetrating artery (lenticulostriate arteries) branches of the MCAs or the penetrators from the ACAs because these vessels originate at about a 90° angle from the parent arteries.Embolism into the MCAs causes a variety of different patterns of infarction *(1,15)*. Blockage of the mainstem MCA before the lenticulostriate branches can cause a large infarct that encompasses the entire MCA territory including the deep basal ganglia and internal capsule as well as the cerebral cortex and subcortical white matter of both the suprasylvian and infrasylvian MCA territories. In some patients, an embolus has blocked the intracranial ICA causing infarction of the ACA territory as well as the entire MCA territory. In young patients, when the mainstem MCA is blocked, the rapid development of collateral circulation over the convexity of the brain often leads to sparing of the superficial territory of the MCA. The lenticulostriate branches are blocked by the clot in the mainstem MCA and collateral circulation to the deep MCA territory is poor. The resultant infarct is limited to the basal ganglia and surrounding cerebral white matter and is usually referred to as a striatocapsular infarct. Passage of an embolus into the superior division of the MCA leads to a cortical/subcortical infarct in the region of the suprasylvian convexity and embolism to the inferior division leads to an infarct limited to the temporal and inferior parietal lobes below the sylvian fissure. When an embolus rests first in the mainstem MCA and then travels to one of the divisional branches, infarction involves the deep territory and cortex above or below the sylvian fissure. Small emboli block cortical branches and cause small cortical/subcortical infarcts involving one or several gyri. Occasionally emboli block the ACA or its distal branches. This causes an infarct in the paramedian area of one frontal lobe.

Emboli that enter the posterior circulation can block the vertebral arteries in the neck or intracranially. Emboli that pass through the intracranial vertebral arteries (ICVAs) will usually be able to pass through the proximal and middle portions of the basilar artery which are wider than the ICVAs. The basilar artery becomes narrower as it courses craniad. Emboli often block the distal basilar artery bifurcation—"top of the basilar"—or one of its branches *(16–18)*. The main branches of the basilar artery bifurcation are penetrating arteries to the medial portions of the thalami and midbrain, the superior cerebellar artery that supplies the upper surface of the cerebellum, and the posterior cerebral arteries (PCAs), which supply the lateral portions of the thalami and the temporal and occipital lobe territories of the PCAs. The most frequent brain areas infarcted are the posterior inferior portion of the cerebellum in the territory of the posterior inferior cerebellar artery (PICA) branch of the ICVA; the superior surface of the cerebellum in the territory of the superior cerebellar artery; the thalamic and hemispheral territories of the PCAs. The clinical and imaging findings in patients with these lesions are described in detail elsewhere *(16)*. Table 5 notes the most frequent locations of brain infarction in the Lausanne Stroke Registry in patients with potential cardiac sources of embolism *(7)*.

When emboli arise from arteries, the emboli can of course, only go into more distal portions of that artery. Emboli that originate in the ICA usually go into the MCA and its branches but occasionally must go into the anterior cerebral, and anterior choroidal arteries and their branches. Occasional emboli go into penetrating artery branches. Within the posterior circulation, emboli that originate from the vertebral arteries in the neck go to the ipsilateral intracranial vertebral artery and its PICA branch and more distally into the basilar artery and any of the branches on either side of the basilar artery and the SCAs and PCAs.

Ultrasound studies show that microembolic particles often pass through the intracranial arteries without causing symptoms or brain infarcts. The adequacy

Table 5
Location and Distribution of Infarcts in the Lausanne Stroke Registry in Patients With Potential Cardiac Sources of Embolism

Anterior circulation	213 (70%)
Global MCA	33 (11%)
Superior division MCA	60 (20%)
Inferior division MCA	54 (18%)
Deep subcortical	56 (18%)
Anterior cerebral artery (ACA)	9 (3%)
ACA and MCA together	1 (0.3%)
Posterior circulation	69 (23%)
Brainstem	18 (6%)
Thalamus (deep PCA)	12 (4%)
Superficial PCA	21 (7%)
Superficial and deep PCA	3 (1%)
Cerebellum	10 (3%)

MCA, middle cerebral artery; PCA, posterior cerebral artery.

of flow through proximal arteries undoubtedly effects the fate of artery-to-artery emboli. When there are proximal vascular occlusive lesions that diminish flow, particles may not be cleared (washed out) as adequately as when the circulation is normal *(19)*. These particles are often distributed within the distal fields causing so-called border-zone ischemia between intracranial arterial territories.

IN SITU ARTERIAL DISORDERS —THROMBOSIS

Atherosclerosis of Large Arteries

Atherosclerosis is by far the most common condition leading to stenosis and occlusion of large extracranial and intracranial arteries. The initial arterial lesion is a fatty streak that develops in the intima and then enlarges into a raised atherosclerotic plaque. Athrosclerotic plaques have been more thoroughly studied within the coronary arteries but the process is similar in the carotid arteries *(20–23)*. Plaques contain a mixture of lipid, smooth muscle, fibrous and collagen tissues, macrophages, and other inflammatory cells. Plaques can enlarge quickly when hemorrhages occur within the plaques *(23)*. When a critical plaque size and reduction in the lumen are reached, the atherosclerotic process accelerates. Reduced luminal area and the bulk of the protruding plaque alter the physical and mechanical properties of blood flow and create regions of local turbulence and stasis. Platelets adhere to the irregular surfaces of plaques. Secretion of chemical mediators within platelets and within the underlying vascular endothelium causes aggregation and further adherence of platelets to the endothelium. A "white clot" composed of platelets and fibrin develops and, at first, is rather loosely adherent to the vascular wall. Plaques often interrupt the endothelium, ulcerate, and rupture. Breaches in the endothelium allow cracks and fissures to form allowing contact of the constituents of the plaque with the luminal contents. The coagulation cascade is activated by this contact and a "red thrombus" composed of erythrocytes and fibrin forms within the lumen. Platelet secretion can also activate the serine proteases that form the body's coagulation system and promote red clot formation. When thrombi first form they are poorly organized and only loosely adherent. They often then propagate and embolize. Within a period of 1 to 2 wk, thrombi organize and become more adherent. Fragments are less likely to break off and embolize from organized thrombi. There are important sex and racial differences in the distribution of atherosclerotic occlusive lesions *(24–28)*. In white men, the predominant cerebrovascular occlusive lesions are in the carotid and vertebral arteries in the neck *(15,21,29–31)*. African-Americans, individuals of Asian origin, and women are more likely to have occlusive lesions in the large intracranial arteries of the circle of Willis and their main branches, and less likely to have severe occlusive vascular lesions in the neck. Caucasian men who have carotid artery disease in the neck also have a high frequency of coexisting coronary artery and occlusive lower limb artery disease, as well as hypertension, hypercholesterolemia, and a history of smoking. After menopause, the frequency of extracranial occlusive disease increases in women.

Within the anterior circulation, the most frequent and important occlusive lesion in Caucasian men is within the ICA in the neck. Atherosclerotic lesions usually begin within the common carotid artery (CCA) along the posterior wall of that vessel opposite the flow-divider between the ICA and the external carotid artery (ECA) *(19,20,25)*. Atherosclerotic plaques grow in diameter and often spread rostrally within the CCA, and the proximal ICA, and ECAs. The next most common atherosclerotic lesions in white men are found within the intracranial ICA in the proximal intracranial portion of the artery, the carotid siphon, and within the proximal portions of the MCAs. These lesions all produce symptoms by causing hypoperfusion of supplied brain territories or by clot-fragment embolism.

Women, African-Americans, and Asians often develop occlusive lesions within the MCAs and their branches *(25–28,32)*. ICA siphon and neck lesions are found less often. African-Americans, Asians, and women who develop occlusive neck lesions usually smoke and have important co-existing atherosclerotic risk factors such as hypertension and hypercholesterolemia. Asian patients who have stenosing neck atherosclerotic lesions often have accompanying intracranial disease *(28,32)*.

Within the posterior circulation among Caucasian men, occlusive lesions are found most often at the origins of the vertebral arteries in the neck and within the adjacent subclavian artery. The next most common site is within the ICVAs and the basilar artery. Caucasian men with occlusive extracranial vertebral artery (ECVA) disease also have a high frequency of co-existing carotid artery disease *(16,30,31)* as well as hypertension and hypercholesterolemia. Intracranial posterior circulation lesions are also common in Caucasian men and women, African-Americans, and Asians. The predominant lesions are within ICVAs. Atherosclerotic lesions within the ICVAs are often bilateral. Atherosclerotic lesions involving the posterior cerebral arteries are more common in women, African-Americans, and Asians *(16)*.

Arterial Dissections

Arterial dissection is probably the second most common disease that leads to thrombi forming within arteries. Dissections are often related to mechanical injury. When there is an obvious direct injury the dissections are usually called traumatic, but even so-called "spontaneous" dissections usually involve some mechanical perturbation of the arterial wall. Stretching or tearing within the arterial media causes formation of an intramural hematoma. Blood within the media dissects longitudinally along the vessel wall and expansion of the arterial wall subsequently compromises the lumen. The expanding intramural hematoma can tear through the intima and inject fresh, congealed, hematoma-containing, thrombus-like material into the arterial lumen. This material is, at first, not adherent to the endothelium and often embolizes. The intimal tear and the underlying medial hematoma cause some irritation of the endothelium, which in turn causes activation of platelets and the coagulation cascade, promoting the formation of a luminal thrombus *in situ*. Compromise of the lumen by the expanding intramural lesion alters blood flow, which also promotes thrombus formation. Thus, thrombus can form *in situ* within the dissected artery or reach the lumen by introduction of the intramural contents. In either case, the acute lumenal thrombus is poorly organized and nonadherent and readily embolizes distally *(15,16)*.

Arterial dissections most often involve the pharyngeal portions of the extracranial carotid and vertebral arteries *(15,16,33–36)*. The pharyngeal portions of the neck arteries are relatively mobile whereas the origins of the arteries and their penetrations into the cranial cavity are relatively anchored and much less mobile. Tearing most often occurs in portions of arteries that are flexible and stretch with motion. Within the ECVAs, the most common site of dissection is the most distal portion of the artery, which emerges from the intervertebral foramina and courses around the atlas to penetrate the dura mater and enter the foramen magnum *(16,34,35)*. Dissections also occur in the mobile part of the proximal portion of the ECVAs above the origin of the arteries from the subclavian arteries but before the arteries enter the vertebral column at the intervertebral foramen of the sixth or fifth cervical vertebrae.

Intracranial dissections are much less common than extracranial dissections. In the anterior circulation, dissections most often affect the intracranial ICA and extend into the middle and anterior cerebral arteries *(37)*. Within the posterior circulation, the most common site is the intracranial vertebral artery *(16,35,38)*. Dissections within the ICVAs often spread into the basilar artery. Occasionally the basilar artery is the primary site of dissection *(16,35)*.

OTHER LARGE-ARTERY DISEASES

Other vascular conditions cause large-artery occlusions at a much lower frequency than atherosclerosis and arterial dissections. FMD is a heterogeneous condition characterized mostly by abnormalities in the smooth muscle and connective tissue within the arterial media *(15,16)*. The lesions can occur in the pharyngeal carotid artery and in the vertebral arteries within the vertebral column. Occasionally, the lesions involve the intracranial large arteries. Thrombi can develop in regions of narrowing of arteries related to FMD. Various types of arteritis can, on rare occasions, cause arterial occlusions. The most important such disorder is arteritis related to the Herpes zoster-varicella virus *(39)*. The virus can spread from the trigeminal ganglion to the middle cerebral artery and cause endothelial lesions that promote thrombus formation. Although other forms of arteritis are frequently mentioned as part of obligatory differential diagnoses, they are extremely rare causes of brain infarction and are not often complicated by thrombosis of sizable intracranial arteries. Migraine can be accompanied by arterial vasoconstriction. Narrowing of intracranial arteries, especially the PCA, and perturbation of the endothelium can promote thrombus formation *(16,40)*.

Hypercoagulable States (41,42)

Occasionally, occlusion of extracranial arteries is caused by hypercoagulability. There may also be an underlying endothelial lesion (e.g., a plaque within the carotid or vertebral arteries). Polycythemia, thrombocytosis, hereditary and acquired deficiencies of coagulation factors (antithrombin III, protein C, and protein S), cancer, increased serum levels of fibrinogen, and deficiencies of fibrinolytic factors can all cause or contribute to hypercoagulability. Cancer—especially mucinous adenocarcinomas and inflammatory diseases such as Crohn's and ulcerative colitis—can also lead to increased coagulability. Acute and chronic infections induce an increase in acute phase reactants that increase coagulability.

In hypercoagulable patients, thrombi can form anywhere. Thrombi can form in regions of endothelial abnormalities. Often, there are multiple small intracranial thrombi.

Penetrating Artery Disease

The arteries that penetrate into the deeper regions of the brain are susceptible to somewhat different disease processes than the superficial branches of the same intracranial arteries. These vessels supply the basal ganglia, caudate nuclei, thalami, pons, portions of the midbrain and medulla, as well as regions of the internal capsules, corona radiata, and centrum semi-ovale. The small, penetrating artery branches arise mostly at nearly right angles from the anterior, middle, and posterior cerebral arteries and the basilar artery. The predominant conditions that affect these penetrating arteries are lipohyalinosis *(43–45)* and intracranial atheromatous branch disease *(46–48)*.

Lipohyalinotic arteries have walls thickened by the deposition of hyaline material and lipids. This process can lead to arterial narrowing with subsequent brain infarction in tissue supplied by the compromised penetrating artery *(43–45)*. Because few patients die immediately after lacunar infarction, the precipitating pathology has not been defined. Choking off of the lumen by progressive medial wall hypertrophy is possible as is a superimposed occlusive white or red thrombus. Atheromas can also develop within the parent arteries and block or extend into the orifices of the penetrating branches *(46–48)*. Microatheromas can also form within the proximal portion of the branches. Pathological studies are scant and it is not well known how often microthrombi form in these penetrating arteries. Microdissections have been discovered at necropsy within the proximal portions of relatively large penetrating arteries *(47)*.

REFERENCES

1. Caplan LR. *Brain Embolism in Practical Clinical Neurocardiology,* Caplan LR, Chimowitz M, Hurst JW, eds. Marcel Dekker: Marcel Dekker, 2000.
2. Caplan LR. Brain embolism, revisited. *Neurology* 1993;43:1281–1287.
3. Caplan LR. Of birds, and nests and brain emboli. *Rev Neurol* (Paris)1991;147:265–273.
4. Foulkes MA, Wolf PA, Price TR, Mohr JP, Hier DB. The stroke data bank: design, methods, and baseline characteristics. *Stroke* 1988;19:547–554.
5. Kittner SJ, Sharkness CM, Price TR, et al. Infarcts with a cardiac source of embolism in the NINCDS Stroke Data Bank: historical features. *Neurology* 1990;40:281–284.
6. Bogousslavsky J, van Melle G, Regli F. The Lausanne stroke registry: analysis of 1000 consecutive patients with first stroke. *Stroke* 1988;19:1083–1092.
7. Bogousslavsky J, Cachin C, Regli F, et al. Cardiac sources of embolism and cerebral infarction. Clinical consequences and vascular concomitants. *Neurology* 1991;41:855–859.
8. Amarenco P, Duyckaerts C, Tzourio C, et al. The prevalence of ulcerated plaques in the aortic arch in patients with stroke. *N Engl J Med* 1992;326:221–225.
9. Amarenco P, Cohen A, Baudrimont M, Bousser M-G. Transesophageal echocardiographic detection of aortic arch disease in patients with cerebral infarction. *Stroke* 1992;23: 1005–1009.

10. The French Study of Aortic Plaques in Stroke Group. Atherosclerotic disease of the aortic arch as a risk factor for recurrent ischemic stroke. *N Engl J Med* 1996;334:1216–1221.
11. Tobler HG, Edwards JE. Frequency and location of atherosclerotic plaques in the ascending aorta. *J Thor Cardiovasc Surg* 1988;96:304–306.
12. Caplan LR, Stein R, Patel D, et al. Intraluminal clot of the carotid artery detected radiographically. *Neurology* 1984;34:1175–1181.
13. Gacs G, Merer FT, Bodosi M. Balloon catheter as a model of cerebral emboli in humans. *Stroke* 1982;13:39–42.
14. Helgason C. Cardioembolic stroke topography and pathogenesis. *Cerebrovasc Brain Metab Rev* 1992;4:28–58.
15. Caplan LR. *Stroke: A Clinical Approach, 3rd ed.* Butterworth-Henemann: Boston, 2000.
16. Caplan LR. *Posterior Circulation Disease: Clinical Findings, Diagnosis, and Management.* Blackwell Science: Boston, 1996.
17. Caplan LR. Top of the basilar syndrome: selected clinical aspects. *Neurology* 1980;30:72–79.
18. Caplan LR, Tettenborn B. Vertebrobasilar occlusive disease: review of selected aspects. 2. Posterior circulation embolism. *Cerebrovasc Dis* 1992;2:320–326.
19. Caplan LR, Hennerici M. Impaired clearance of emboli "washout" is an important link between hypoperfusion, embolism, and ischemic stroke. *Arch Neurol* 1998;55:1475–1482.
20. Hennerici M, Sitzer G, Weger H-D. *Carotid Artery Plaques.* Basel:Karger, 1987.
21. Fisher CM, Ojemann RG. A clinico-pathologic study of carotid endarterectomy plaques. *Rev Neurol(Paris)* 1986;142:573–589.
22. Heistad DD. Unstable coronary-artery plaques. *N Engl J Med* 2003;349:2285–2287.
23. Kolodgie FD, Gold HK, Burke AP, et al. Intraplaque hemorrhage and progression of coronary atheroma. *N Engl J Med* 2003;349(24),2316–2325.
24. Gillum RF, Gorelick PB, Cooper ES. *Stroke in Blacks: A Guide to Management and Prevention.* Karger: Basel, Switzerland, 1999.
25. Caplan JR, Gorelick PB, Hier DB. Race, sex, and occlusive cerebrovascular disease: a review. *Stroke* 1986;17:648–655.
26. Gorelick PB, Caplan LR, Hier DB, et al. Racial differences in the distribution of anterior circulation occlusive disease. *Neurology* 1984;34:54–59.
27. Gorelick PB, Caplan LR, Hier DB, et al. Racial differences in the distribution of posterior circulation occlusive disease. *Stroke* 1985;16:785–790.
28. Feldmann E, Daneault N, Kwan E, et al. Chinese-White differences in the distribution of occlusive cerebrovascular disease. *Neurology* 1990;40:1541–1545.
29. Fisher CM, Gore I, Okabe N, White PD. Atherosclerosis of the carotid and vertebral arteries-extracranial and intracranial. *J Neuropathol Exp Neurol* 1965;24:455–476.
30. Hutchinson EC, Yates PO. Carotico-vertebral stenosis. *Lancet* 1957;1:2–8.
31. Hutchinson EC, Yates PO. The cervical portion of the vertebral artery. a clinicopathological study. *Brain* 1956;79:319–331.
32. Lee SJ, Cho S-J, Moon H-S, et al. Combined extracranial and intracranial atherosclerosis in Korean patients. *Arch Neurol* 2003;60:1561–1564.
33. Fisher CM, Ojemann R, Roberson G. Spontaneous dissection of cervicocerebral arteries. *Can J Neuro Sci* 1978;5:9–19.
34. Caplan LR, Zarins C, Hemmatti M. Spontaneous dissection of the extracranial vertebral artery. *Stroke* 1985;16:1030–1038.
35. Caplan LR, Tettenborn B. Vertebrobasilar occlusive disease: review of selected aspects. 1. Spontaneous dissection of extracranial and intracranial posterior circulation arteries. *Cerebrovasc Dis* 1992;2:256–265.
36. Selim M, Caplan LR. Carotid artery dissection in the neck. *Curr Treat Options Cardiovasc Med.* 2004;, 249–253.
37. Chaves C, Estol C, Esnaola MM, et al. Spontaneous intracranial internal carotid artery dissection. *Arch Neurol* 2002;59:977–981.

38. Caplan LR, Baquis G, Pessin MS, et al. Dissection of the intracranial vertebral artery. *Neurology* 1988;38:868–877.
39. Hilt DC, Buchholz D, Krumholz A, et al. Herpes zoster opthalmicus and delayed contralateral hemiparesis caused by cerebral angiitis: diagnosis and management approaches. *Ann Neurol* 1983;14:543–553.
40. Caplan LR, Migraine and vertebrobasilar ischemia. *Neurology* 1991;41:55–61.
41. Markus HS, Hambley H. Neurology and the blood: haematological abnormalities in ischaemic stroke. *J Neurol Neurosurg Psychiatry* 1998;64:150–159.
42. Feinberg WM. Coagulation in Brain Ischemia: Basic Concepts and Clinical rRelevance, Caplan LR, ed. Springer-Verlag: London, 1995, pp 85–96.
43. Fisher CM, The arterial lesions underlying lacunes, *Acta Neuropathol* 1969;12:1–15.
44. Fisher CM, Cerebral miliary aneurysms in hypertension. *Am J Pathol* 1972;66:313–324.
45. Rosenblum WJ, Miliary aneurysms and "fibrinoid" degeneration of cerebral blood vessels, *Hum Pathol* 1977;8:133–139.
46. Fisher CM, Caplan LR, Basilar artery branch occlusion: a cause of pontine infarction, *Neurology* 1971;21:900–905.
47. Fisher CM, Bilateral occlusion of basilar artery branches, *J Neurol Neurosurg Psychiatry* 1977;40:1182–1189.
48. Caplan LR, Intracranial branch atheromatous disease: a neglected, understudied, and underused concept, *Neurology* 1989;39:1246–1250.

3 The Ischemic Penumbra and Neuronal Salvage

Patrick Lyden, MD

CONTENTS

INTRODUCTION

The majority of focal cerebral ischemic events result from arterial occlusion caused by embolism or *in situ* thrombosis. This interruption in blood flow, if severe and prolonged, leads to cerebral infarction. Brain infarction results from a disruption in blood flow, which causes a reduction in oxygen and glucose supplied to the tissue. Glucose and oxygen deprivation causes a metabolic shift toward the production of lactic acidic. Coincident with this impairment of the Na^+/Ca^{++} exchange pump, excessive glutamate release causes an unregulated amount of calcium to enter the cells. Intracellular calcium increases trigger a variety of processes that result in the breakdown of membranes and nucleic acids. In addition, the release of free radicals, the breakdown of the blood–brain barrier and development of the inflammatory response all work together to promote further cellular injury.

For centuries, the brain was believed to tolerate no more than a few minutes of ischemia; brain cell death was considered irreversible. A series of investigations conducted in the 1980s proved that only a portion of the brain tissue is irreparably damaged so quickly after focal ischemia. The surrounding region

From: *Current Clinical Neurology: Thrombolytic Therapy for Acute Stroke, Second Edition*
Edited by: P. D. Lyden © Humana Press Inc., Totowa, NJ

may remain viable for several hours. This concept has been referred to as the "ischemic penumbra" *(1–6)*. Restoration of blood flow to this area within a certain period of time may salvage the "viable" cells and diminish the degree of neurological deficits. One way to re-establish blood flow is by dissolution of the thrombus. This concept led to thoughts about thrombolysis as a possible treatment for stroke. The clinician contemplating the use of thrombolysis is acknowledging *de facto* the existence of a penumbra that cannot be measured or documented. Using somewhat circular logic, the successful thrombolytic trials support the notion that some portion of ischemic brain remains salvageable for hours after symptom onset. Limited direct evidence suggests that salvageable brain cells may reside in penumbral zones. It is critical to understand the genesis of the penumbra concept prior to cerebral thrombolysis.

THE ISCHEMIC PENUMBRA

After vascular occlusion, there is a heterogeneous depression of cerebral blood flow (CBF) in the territory of the occluded artery. The *penumbra* is identified as the brain region receiving regional CBF (rCBF) between two critical values *(2,5)*. The first, higher critical value is associated with neuronal paralysis; brain areas receiving rCBF less than 18–20 mL/100 g/min do not function. The second, lower critical value is associated with cell death; brain areas receiving less than 8–10 mL/100 mg/min do not survive, and this area becomes the *core* of the infarction *(2)*. Neurons in the penumbra are sometimes identified as "idling" to suggest that they are salvageable, although the mechanism of such a phenomenon is unknown. The time course of cell death in the core is rapid whereas cells in the penumbra may survive up to several hours *(7)*.

Soon after the original description of the penumbra, it was recognized that cells do not survive forever, idling in the penumbra *(8,9)*. Thus, it became clear that the penumbra involved two different parameters: blood flow and time. In baboons, for example, cells in a zone of blood that is receiving 20 cc/100 g/min will survive for a few hours, but cell receiving 12 cc/100 g/min may only survive for 2 h. This idea suggests that over time the "core" of the infarct enlarges, eventually subsuming the penumbra, giving rise to the clinical dictum that "time is brain." In other words, an increasing fraction of brain loses blood flow below the critical threshold for neuronal survival.

In rats, temporary occlusion of the middle cerebral artery (MCA) longer than 30 min results in varying degrees of infarction *(10)*. Reperfusion after 30 min of occlusion will result in some diminution of the infarct, compared to permanent occlusion, up to 120 min. After 2 h, however, reperfusion does not alter infarction volume. Around the infarction, there is a variable amount of neuronal loss *(11)*. Degenerating neurons can be detected within about 3 mm of the infarction border for up to 3 wk after stroke. After that, no further cell loss can be seen using routine stains. In cats, a similar phenomenon has been documented *(12)*. There was a close correlation between rCBF and neuron density around the infarction: the farther away from the edge of the cyst, the greater the blood flow and density of neurons. In humans, it is difficult to document a similar loss of neurons within a few millimeters of areas of complete infarction, or cyst formation *(11)*. These data are consistent with the interpretation that over the long term, there is no survival of penumbral tissue. If reperfusion begins early, however, penumbral tissue may survive; otherwise, the marginal tissue is eventually included in the cyst formed by the core of the infarct.

Baron and colleagues have obtained elegant data using positron emission tomography (PET) scanning to explore the penumbra concept. They showed that over time after stroke an area of excessive oxygen extraction, perhaps reflecting the core, does in fact enlarge *(13)*. Unfortunate for those designing therapy however, was that the temporal evolution of the penumbra was highly variable. In some patients a penumbra could be identified as late as 16 h after stroke onset, but in others there was no penumbra by 5 h. In another, similar study, possibly viable tissue could be identified in the penumbra for up to 48 h in some patients *(14)*. Mosely and colleagues at Stanford conducted similar sorts of experiments using magnetic resonance imaging (MRI) of water diffusion, a possible marker of the core, and blood perfusion, a possible marker of the penumbra. In such studies, some patients do indeed exhibit patterns to indicate a core that is smaller than the penumbra. In untreated patients, the ultimate size of the infarction is comparable to the size of the "penumbra," suggesting that the core did enlarge to subsume the penumbra. In some patients who underwent recanalization, the ultimate infarct was smaller, only the size of the core, suggesting that thrombolysis in fact prevented enlargement of the core. The MRI conceptualization of the penumbra was also documented in rats by Fisher and colleagues *(15)*. After 1 h occlusion, a core diffusion-weighted image abnormality was surrounded by a larger follow-flow area. After 2 h of occlusion, the core and penumbra were identical and outcome was much poorer.

Until very recently, the concept of the penumbra simply included two zones, one surrounding the other, as shown in Fig. 1. There are a number of problems with the simple penumbra concept. Despite the interesting data obtained by some groups, the vast majority of patients with focal ischemia do not exhibit such consistent patterns. Many more patients who respond to thrombolysis with a gratifying recovery do *not* show a pattern on PET or MRI consistent with a presumed core and a larger penumbra. It is increasingly clear that the penumbra concept should be expanded to include more complicated flow patterns. For example, Fig. 2 illustrates a possible scenario in which a central core is surrounded by patches of penumbral flow, some of which include additional zones of very low, or core, flow. It is quite likely that variable areas of brain receive

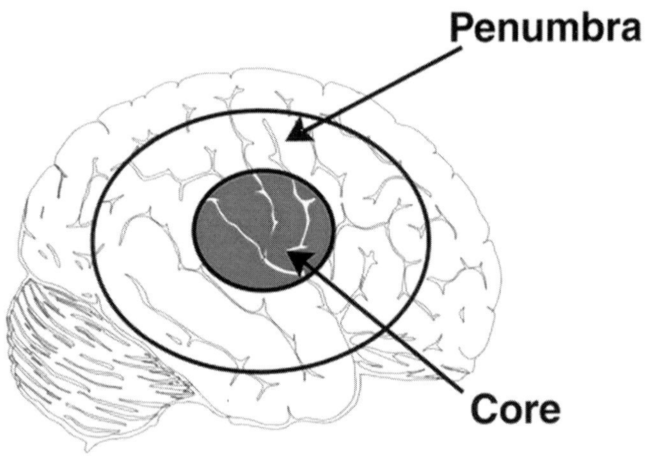

Fig. 1. Traditional concept that the infarct core is surrounded by an enveloping penumbra.

penumbral levels of flow and that the distribution of these areas in the brain is determined by variable degrees of collateralization from other blood vessels. Such collaterals generally connect in the pia between end-branches of the larger arteries. There is some limited pathological data to support this concept of "islands" of penumbral flow near to areas of complete infarction *(16)*.

No matter what the spatial pattern of blood flow changes, it is clear that cells in penumbral regions do not survive indefinitely. The exact duration of survival is unknown, and likely it is different under differing circumstances. Cells in zones receiving from 10 to 20 cc/100 g/min likely survive for hours, but the number of hours is not known. Many factors may reduce the time such marginally perfused cells might survive. For example, it is known that hyperthermia of 1 or 2°C will accelerate cell death *(17)*. Elevations of serum glucose also accelerate cell death *(18)*. Such marginal levels of blood flow do not support neuronal survival indefinitely, but could be sufficient to deliver neuroprotectants into the ischemic zone. Therefore, pending recanalization and restoration of blood flow, a number of therapies could be directed at idling neurons in the penumbra. Such neuroprotectants might salvage brain by preserving neurons until blood flow is restored. The possible mechanisms of neuroprotection include interrupting ischemic excitotoxicity, blocking apoptosis, and blocking the inflammatory response that follows ischemia

EXCITOTOXICITY AND NEUROINHIBITORY THERAPY

The elucidation of the excitotoxic cell death mechanism advanced stroke neurology considerably. An understanding of the biochemical events outlined below spawned a plethora of therapeutic trials. As of 2005, no agent had yet

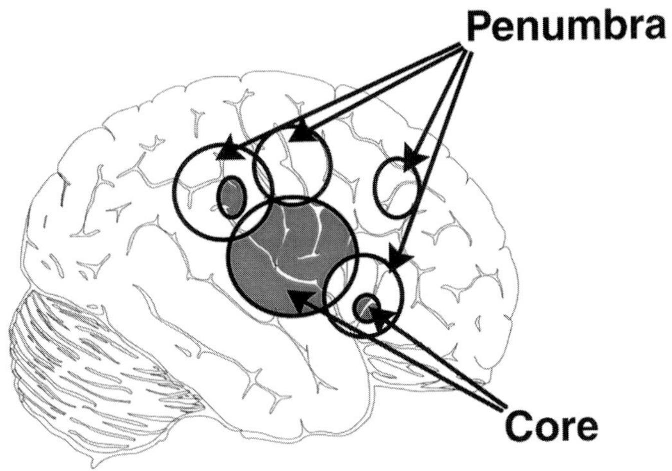

Fig. 2. Alternative concept that regions corresponding to core and penumbra may be heterogenous.

proven successful in humans, despite considerable excitement from laboratory studies. The first treatment for amyotrophic lateral sclerosis, riluzole, is thought to protect spinal neurons by blocking excitotoxicity. Future successful neuroprotection depends on further delineation of the steps in the ischemic cascade, and identifying candidate points for intervention.

The Ischemic Cascade and the Role of Intracellular Calcium

The sudden deprivation of oxygen and glucose sets into motion a set of events called the ischemic cascade. The use of the term cascade implies that ischemia proceeds in an orderly manner from the beginning of the cascade to the end. Alternatively, it is becoming clear that the several steps in the cascade occur simultaneously, rather than sequentially and in addition there appear to be multiple feed-forward, feed-back, and amplification steps (for example, *see* refs. *19–21*). A simple sketch of some of these phenomena is presented as Fig. 3.

Glutamate exposure is associated with cell death and degeneration in cell culture *(22–24)* (reviewed in ref. *25*) and glutamate receptor antagonists protect cultured cells from exposure to glutamate, hypoglycemia and hypoxia *(26,27)*. At least three glutamate receptor subtypes are identified based on ligand binding studies: *N*-methyl-D-aspartate (NMDA), α-amino-3-hydroxy-5-methyl-4-isoxazoleproionate (AMPA)-kainate, and metabotropic *(28)*. Of these subtypes, the NMDA receptor appears to be critical in mediating the effects of ischemia, although interest in AMPA/kainate receptors continues, especially in studies of global ischemia *(27,29)* and the role of the metabotropic receptor subtype remains unclear *(30)*.

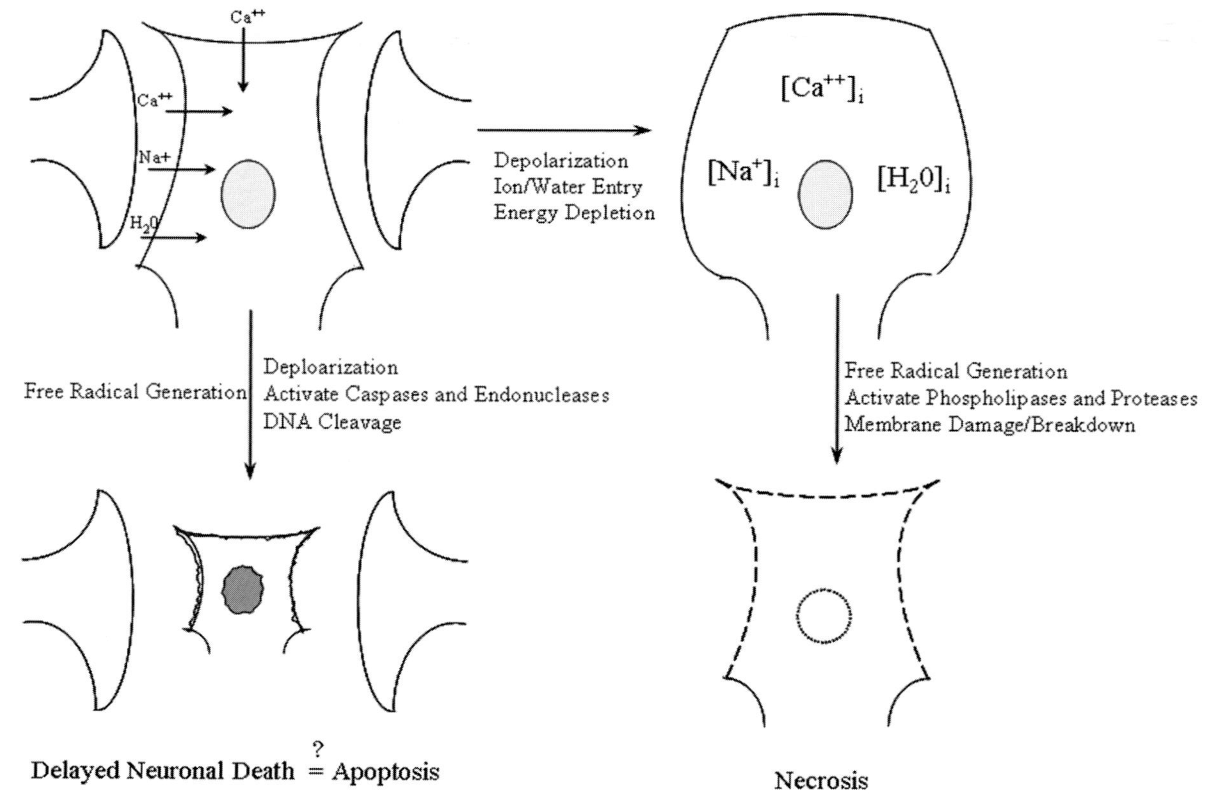

Fig. 3. Depolarization and ion flux may lead to cell death by apoptosis or necrosis pathways.

Depolarization of the post-synaptic cell occurs in response to application of glutamate, and appears to be a necessary step in the sequence of events leading to cell death *(23,24)*. During excitation of the post-synaptic membrane, there is an influx of sodium, chloride, calcium, and water into the cell *(27,31,32)*. Inflow of ions and water leads to edema, and, if severe or prolonged, such edema may lead to cell lysis and death *(32)*. Glutamate does not cause edema or lysis of mature neurons in culture unless sodium and/or chloride are present in the culture medium *(32)*. Inflow of calcium may lead to delayed neuronal death through unknown mechanisms after comparatively brief exposure to ischemia or excitotoxins *(31,33)*. There is some evidence, albeit preliminary and often contradictory, that this delayed cell death may be mediated through apoptotic mechanisms *(34,35)*. This effect persists in culture if sodium is not present in the medium but is blocked by MG^{++} or by removing calcium from the medium *(24,32)*.

During ischemia, intracellular calcium concentrations increase through mechanisms other than the ligand-gated channels previously described. Some calcium channels are voltage-gated, and depolarization to a membrane voltage that opens some of these channels may be a critical determinant of calcium influx *(24,31)*. However, because calcium appears to enter the cell through the NMDA receptor itself, ligand-gated influx appears to continue even in voltage-clamped cells *(24,36)*. Nevertheless, it seems reasonable to suspect that prevention of glutamate-stimulated depolarization should prevent some of the early cellular edema caused by sodium, chloride, and water movement, and some of the calcium flow that leads to delayed toxicity. In support of this expectation, it was observed that hyperpolarization reduced or blocked calcium inflow into neurons *(37)* and reduced the probability of discharge *(38)*. Other routes of influx include the release of calcium from intracytoplasmic stores *(39)* (mediated in part via metabotropic receptors linked to protein kinase C) and loss of adenosine triphosphate (ATP)-dependent calcium extrusion mechanisms *(40)*. Also, with membrane damage there is influx of calcium down an electrochemical gradient *(41)*.

There is now a growing consensus that the increase in intracellular calcium sets into motion a variety of events that lead to cell death, most especially the activation of cytosolic phospolipases, and proteases *(19,42)*. Proteases may play a central role in activating programmed cell death (PCD) and phospholipases may be critically involved in both further excitotoxin release and the generation of reactive oxygen species. A vicious cycle is created that causes spread of the core zone of infarction as a direct result of early glutamate-mediated increases in intracellular calcium *(19)*.

Several direct glutamate antagonists (MK-801, CGS-19755, and dextrophan) and indirect agents that bind at the NMDA glycine site (ACEA1021, felbamate, GV150526a) appear to protect brain during focal ischemia *(43–51)*. The direct agents resemble dissociative anesthetics such as ketamine and phencyclidine and humans experience significant side effects during treatment with NMDA

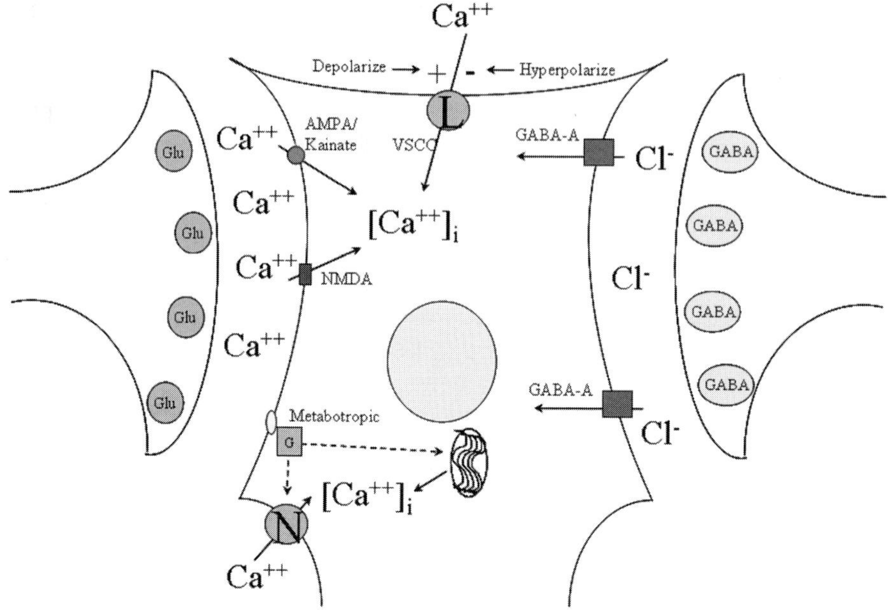

Fig. 4. γ-Aminobutyric acid-receptor activation leads to a hyperpolarizing influx of chloride that blocks voltage-gated calcium influx via the L-type voltage-sensitive calcium channel (VSCC). There may also be inhibition of the N-type calcium channel. *See* color insert following p.110.

antagonists that ended development efforts for some agents. Therefore, others have chosen to pursue an alternative strategy for brain protection during cerebral ischemia and use agents that block the effect of excitotoxins without causing such severe side effects. We chose γ-aminobutyric acid (GABA) agonists for this purpose. The events discussed here are sketched in Fig. 4.

In mammalian brain, GABA is considered the principal inhibitory neurotransmitter *(52)*. Inhibitory neurotransmitters increase chloride conductance, lower the resting membrane potential of the neuron and reduce the probability that glutamate stimulation leads to action potential *(38,52,53)*. GABA mediates its effects through two receptor subtypes, A and B. The GABA-A receptor is a ligand-gated chloride channel found throughout the brain that mediates a fast inhibitory response *(54,55)*. The GABA-B receptor appears to participate in presynaptic release of several neurotransmitters and post-synaptically to mediate the late inhibitory post-synaptic potential *(56)*. When GABA or a suitable analog occupies the post-synaptic GABA-A receptor, the resting membrane potential may not increase and voltage-gated calcium channels are prevented from opening *(37,38,57)*. Also, GABA-A agonists reduce the cerebral metabolic rate for glucose at doses that do not cause sedation or impair respiration or cardiac function *(58,59)*. GABA-A receptors are found on cerebral blood vessels and cause dilation of cerebral, but not extracranial, vessels. This effect is blocked by competitive antagonists of the GABA receptor *(60)*. GABA-B agonists reduce the pre-synaptic release of glutamate and should be neuroprotective via a pre-synaptic mechanism. Despite this rationale, and the preliminary work presented here, there may be conditions under which GABA is neurotoxic *(61,62)* A new strategy for utilizing GABAergic mechanisms emerged with the development of GABA modulators. Some steroid molecules have nongenomic actions on cells that appear to be mediated via binding sites on membrane-bound ionophores *(63,64)* (for review, *see* refs. *65* and *66*). Of particular relevance are the 5-reduced, 3α-hydroxylated pregnane steroids that appear to be potent modulators of chloride flux through the GABA-A ion channel *(67)*. On the other hand, other neurosteroids, such as pregnenolone sulfate, may have GABA-antagonist actions, and some have agonist or antagonist properties at the NMDA receptor. Pregnanolone and allopregnanolone are potent sedatives and anticonvulsants *(68)*. We are unaware of any studies of neurosteroids in ischemia.

Apoptosis and Necrosis

Despite the obvious difference in blood flow between the core and the penumbra, the mechanisms of cell death in the two regions are not fully known. *Necrosis* is obviously one mechanism for cell death in both the penumbra and the core. During necrosis, the cell initially swells, then shrinks and can be observed as a small, pyknotic form on sections *(69)*. Finally, microglia and macrophages remove the debris of the dead cell. If necrosis includes the adjacent glia and structural matrix, a cyst is formed and the process is termed *pannecrosis*. Recently, *apoptosis*, or PCD, has been observed in ischemic brain *(70)*. In this type of cell death, ischemia is thought to activate "suicide" proteins that are latent in all cells. These proteins are normally expressed during embryogenesis and enable the organism to remove cells that will not be needed during further development. The morphometry of apoptosis is quite different from necrosis, and special techniques are available to study the two forms of cell death *(71)*. The role of apoptotic cell death in the core and in the penumbra is not known. Figure 3 illustrates the factors involved in these two forms of cell death. How cells end up "choosing" one form of death over the other is not known.

The cellular and molecular events leading to cell death have been described in cell culture systems. Relating these findings to living subjects, and to ischemia in particular, is problematic. A thorough review of recent in vitro findings is available and not repeated here *(71–73)*. A few pertinent findings are described.

Injuries such as hypoglycemia, anoxia, and excitotoxin exposure kill cells via necrosis. Necrotic cell death is clearly associated with elevations of intracellular calcium, which has been demonstrated in culture, brain slices, and intact brain. The histopathological sequence of cellular changes leading to necrosis has been documented *(69,74)*. After focal or global ischemia swollen, eosinophilic neurons appear within 2–8 h. Pyknotic, shrunken neurons appear within 24–36 h. Phagocytosis of neurons, astrocytes, and surrounding matrix occurs over days. Once the necrotic cell death pathway begins, it probably cannot be interrupted easily. In areas of severe ischemia (core) a cyst is formed after phagocytosis and removal of all brain elements. In the surrounding brain (penumbra) some cells are removed and astrocytes may proliferate, leaving a zone of "incomplete" infarction that is depleted of neurons but not cystic. The behavioral consequences of this incomplete infarction are unknown.

Another mechanism of cell death has been proposed *(71)*. PCD via a series of events that may represent apoptosis can also be simulated in neuronal cell culture. The initial events are shrinkage of the nucleus and cytoplasm, chromatin condensation followed by nuclear fragmentation, and the separation of cell membrane protuberances (blebs). A hallmark is the cleavage of deoxyribonucleic acid (DNA) by endonucleases into segments of nonrandom length, which results in "laddering" on DNA isolation gels. Ultimately, the cell separates into small, pyknotic bodies that are phagocytosed by cells resident in the tissue. There is little or no inflammatory infiltrate associated with apoptosis *(71)*. During some phases, it is difficult to distinguish apoptotic from necrotic cells using morphological criteria *(71)*. There is a suggestion that the morphological changes may not occur simultaneously with endonuclease cleavage of DNA *(75)*. Following focal cerebral injury, including MCA occlusion, apoptotic-like changes can be documented in brain *(70,76–79)*. Specifically, focal ischemia is associated with DNA nicking as documented with labels specific for free DNA strands, nonrandom DNA fragmentation as documented by the "laddering" phenomenon on DNA extraction gels, and ultrastructural findings consistent with apoptosis. It is not clear if apoptotic-like cell death occurs in the core, the penumbra or both. It is also not clear whether this pathway can be interrupted. Of most concern, it is not clear whether apoptotic-like cell death occurs separately from necrotic death, or whether the two phenomena represent different manifestations of one underlying cell death process *(80)*. It is very clear that necrotic and apoptotic appearing cells can be found in the same regions of brain at the same time *(76)*.

There is some evidence supporting the existence of apoptosis as a separate event in the central nervous system. Deprivation of growth factors (adrenalectamized rats) results in apoptotic-like death of some populations of hippocampal neurons *(81)*. Administration of cycloheximide, an inhibitor of protein synthesis required for apoptotic cell death, blocks the death of spinal cord cells after trauma and hippocampal cells after 2VO forebrain ischemia *(82,83)*. In the spinal cord study this histopathologic finding was correlated with amelioration of the behavioral sequelae of the trauma, paraparesis *(82)*. These findings suggest that blocking steps related to apoptotic cell death might ameliorate the functional sequelae of ischemia. Candidate treatments have yet to emerge or enter clinical trials.

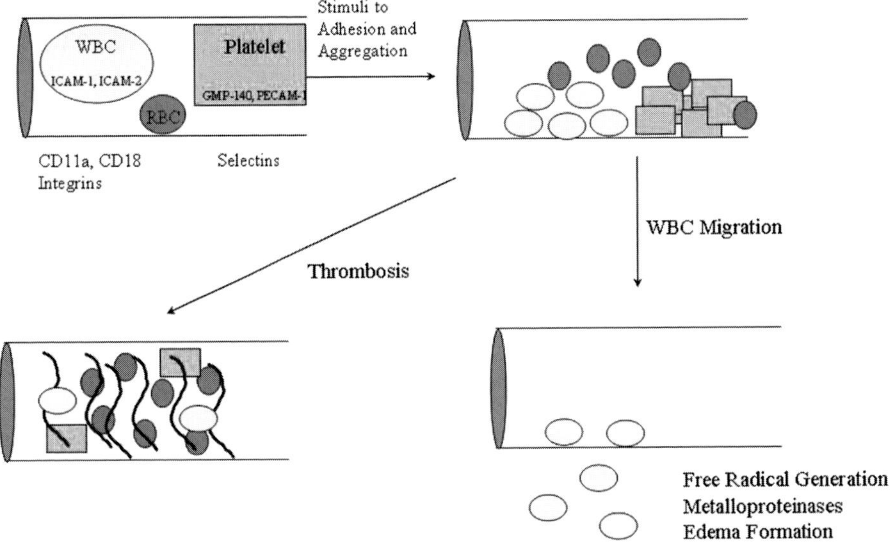

Fig. 5. Following occlusion, granulocytes leave the circulation to enter ischemic brain. *See* color insert following p.110.

THE ROLE OF GRANULOCYTES

Restoration of arterial blood flow after several hours of occlusion may not result in complete tissue reperfusion, the so-called "no-reflow phenomenon" *(84,85)*. The mechanism is not certain, but may involve endothelial swelling, occlusion of microvessels with platelet-fibrin aggregates, red cell microthrombi, or perivascular swelling. The no-reflow effect does not occur if white blood cells are removed from the circulation *(85)*. Granulocytes may adhere to ischemic endothelium, blocking capillaries and stimulating platelet aggregation and formation of micro-thrombi, as illustrated in Fig. 5. The receptor complex on the granulocyte that mediates adherence is composed of the integrins CD18/CD11 (for review, *see* ref. *86*). This complex binds to the intercellular adhesion molecule (ICAM) on the endothelial cell.

In addition to mediating the no-reflow phenomenon, granulocytes may have direct toxic effects in the brain. After adhesion, granulocytes migrate into the brain (diapedesis), and can be observed in the peri-ischemic zone within hours of permanent or transient arterial occlusion *(87)*. Once in the brain, granulocytes release phagocytic chemotactic factors as well as cytokines that may promote cellular destruction. Granulocytes also release enzymes that lead to the formation of free radicals, which leads to an increase in hypochlorous acid and chloramines *(88)*. These compounds then activate granulocytic serine proteases and metalloproteinases, which together begin to destroy surrounding tissue. These events proceed independently of the energy status of the brain cells and may be augmented by early reperfusion, the reperfusion injury syndrome. Granulocytes have been detected in the penumbra in multiple animal models *(89,90)*. There is very little evidence of reperfusion injury in humans after cerebral thrombolysis, however. A monoclonal antibody directed against the ICAM receptor effectively blocks granulocyte adherence to endothelial cells, prevents the no-reflow phenomenon, and trans-migration into brain *(89,90)*. In animal models anti-ICAM reduces neurological injury after focal ischemia *(90–92)*. The anti-ICAM-1 antibody (dose of 1 mg/kg given intravenously 2 h after ischemia onset, plus 0.5 mg/kg 24 h after ischemia onset) has been tested previously in the suture occlusion model in rats *(90)* where it was effective in reducing infarction volume by 41%. In this study, all animals were subjected to the same 120-min occlusion duration; infarction volume in vehicle treated subjects was 171±38 mm^3 or 17% of cerebrum *(90)*. This was associated with a significant reduction in the numbers of granulocytes found in the cortex ipsilateral to the occlusion.

COMBINATORIAL NEUROPROTECTION

As outlined previously, there are a variety of interacting events proceeding simultaneously during ischemia and it now seems unlikely that a single agent will prove sufficient to salvage most of the ischemic brain in most patients. On the other hand, multiple agents targeted at different receptors or events in the ischemic cascade may cooperatively improve outcome. Attempts have been made to design a combination of neuroprotective agents, with some success, but it is difficult to predict the doses of the two agents to use. Furthermore, the combination may manifest benefit as increased potency compared to the single agents or it may lengthen the treatment delay time window, or both. A study of nimodipine (0.25 μg/min × 24-h iv infusion) plus MK-801 (5 mg/kg iv), or both together, showed that the calcium channel blocker added to efficacy in the rat four-vessel occlusion model *(93)*. In an MCA occlusion model, the combination (MK-801 2 mg/kg and nimodipine 5 μg/kg/min × 3 min and 1 μg/kg/min for 230 min) resulted in lower levels of intracellular calcium and less histological damage, compared to MK-801 treatment alone *(94)*. In neither study were higher doses of the single agents used so no truly synergistic effect could be demonstrated. Zivin et al. found that adding MK-801 to tissue plasminogen activator (t-PA) resulted in a significant increase in ED_{50} for the combination *(95)*. In this study, 1.0 mg/kg MK-801 was given 5 min and t-PA was given 60 min after ischemia. The ED_{50} for the combination was significantly greater than that for t-PA alone. However, the combination was not effective if t-PA was delayed to 90 min. The combination of a free radical scavenger plus MK-801 plus insulin plus diazepam appeared to be more effective that the single drug, but no effort was made to simulate the benefit of the combination by increasing the doses of the single agents *(96)*. Bowes et al. attempted to delay the use of thrombolysis by combining t-PA and anti-ICAM-1 in a rabbit cerebral embolism model *(91)*. When both treatments were given 30 min after ischemia onset, each was effective, as was the combination. After a treatment delay of 90 min t-PA and the combination were effective, but the ED_{50}s were the same (no synergistic benefit). After a delay of 180 min, t-PA was not effective when used alone, nor when combined with anti-ICAM given either 5 or 175 min after ischemia. In this study, no evidence of treatment interaction could be found, either by examining the potencies of single vs combined treatments, or by examining the maximum effective treatment delay. In a follow-up study, the same group studied longer time intervals *(97)*. In this study, t-PA given 2 h after embolization was not effective but the combination of anti-ICAM 15 min after and t-PA 2 h after embolization was quite effective. Again, the dose of t-PA alone was not increased to see whether a maximal dose of the single agent was equipotent to the combination. However, this is highly unlikely because the dose of t-PA used, 3 mg/kg, is known to thrombolyse the majority of the injected emboli. Therefore, this study suggests that the use of the two agents conferred a benefit that could not be obtained from higher doses of either agent alone (i.e., synergism).

HEMORRHAGIC INFARCTION AND INTRACEREBRAL HEMMORHAGE

Ischemic etiologies account for the majority of stroke cases *(98)*. On the other hand, cerebral hemorrhage accounts for about 12% of all stroke cases, yields a much higher mortality and morbidity than ischemia, may be responsible for a disproportionate share of the neurological disability attributed to stroke, and responds to no known effective therapy. Experience with hyperacute treatment of ischemic stroke suggests that of all "911" strokes (emergency transport to hospital within 60 min of stroke onset) a higher fraction may be hemorrhagic *(99)*. Thus, of the population that presents early to hospital, a large proportion suffer from an etiology for which there is no known treatment and few clinical trials.

Cerebral hemorrhage can be identified as one of two forms that probably occupy opposite ends of one pathophysiological continuum *(100)*. Hematoma is a large, homogenous, solid collection of blood that occupies space, displaces, and destroys surrounding brain tissue. Hemorrhagic infarction, also called transformation, is the leakage of blood cells into adjacent, ischemic brain tissue without displacing or necessarily destroying brain cells.

Spontaneous hematoma probably results from a ruptured blood vessels rather than from brain ischemia primarily. There is much speculation about the factors that lead to vessel wall rupture, and chronic hypertensive vasculopathy is often noted in such patients *(101)*. Other illnesses that affect the vessel wall are also associated with hematoma, such as diabetes, polyarteritis nodosa, and amyloid angiopathy. There is some evidence that matrix metalloproteinases play a role in the genesis of hematoma, and this observation lead to the development of the intracerebral collagenase model of hematoma. The factors that cause the bleeding to start and then stop, and the time course of hemorrhage development are not known. After the hematoma has occurred, however, there are extensive areas of ischemia around the expanding mass.

There is no treatment for hematoma. Removal of the hematoma by aspiration seems to improve neurologic outcome in animals, if the clot is removed soon enough after stroke onset *(102)*. All of the effects of the mass begin to resolve after its removal—intracranial pressure declines toward normal, blood flow increases toward normal, and edema begins to resorb. In humans, however, aspiration or prompt removal of the mass has not been shown to be effective. This is very likely a result of the logistical difficulty of transporting patients from the field, through radiology, and into the operating room rapidly *(103,104)*. Therefore, there is a very great need to develop a strategy that protects brain long enough for the patient to undergo removal of the hematoma. Since the subcortical hematoma causes cortical ischemia *(105)* it seems reasonable to suggest that anti-ischemia therapy directed at protecting the cortex may be successful, even though the hematoma itself is subcortical.

Thrombolytic therapy for acute ischemic stroke produces an increase in the native rate of hemorrhagic transformation. Asymptomatic hemorrhage was noted in about 20% of patients in a recent trial of t-PA for acute stroke and in nearly 40% of patients receiving streptokinase for acute stroke in the Australian and European multicenter stroke trials *(106,107)*. Hematoma with symptomatic deterioration occurred in 6% of the National Institutes of Neurological Disorders and Stroke (NINDS) trial *(108)*. The factors that may promote transformation are poorly understood, although suspects include hypertension, anticoagulation, and timing of reperfusion after stroke onset.

Neuroprotectants could be useful during thrombolysis in a number of ways. As mentioned previously, neuroprotectants might preserve neurons in the penumbra longer, pending recanalization. That is, neuroprotection might delay the time at which areas of penumbra become irretrievably damaged. Also, neuroprotectants might limit the incidence of hemorrhagic transformation after ischemia. That is, neuroprotection might prevent hemorrhages that occur because a portion of the ischemic brain dies prior to recanalization. To date there have been no completed studies of thrombolytic plus neuroprotectant combinations, although such studies are underway. For the time being, then, such combinations remain experimental.

REFERENCES

1. Astrup J, Siesjo BK, Symon L. Thresholds in cerebral ischemia: The ischemic penumbra. *Stroke* 1981;12:723–725.
2. Astrup J, Symon L, Branston NM, Lassen NA. Cortical evoked potential and extracellular K+ and H+ at critical levels of brain ischemia. *Stroke* 1977;8:51–57.
3. Garcia JH, Liu K-F, Ye Z-R, Gutierrez JA. Incomplete infarct and delayed neuronal death after transient middle cerebral artery occlusion in rats. *Stroke* 1997;28:2303–2310.
4. Heiss W-D. Experimental evidence of ischemic thresholds and functional recovery. *Stroke* 1992;23:1668–1672.
5. Heiss W-D. Progress in cerebrovascular disease: flow thresholds of functional and morphological damage of brain tissue. *Stroke* 1983;14:329–331.
6. Hossmann K-A. Viability thresholds and the penumbra of focal ischemia. *Ann Neurol* 1994;36:557–565.
7. Kaplan B, Brint S, Tanabe J, Jacewicz M, Wang X-J, Pulsinelli W. Temporal thresholds for neocortical infarction in rats subjected to reversible focal cerebral ischemia. *Stroke* 1991;22:1032–1039.
8. Jones TH, Morawetz RB, Crowell RM, et al. Thresholds of focal cerebral ischemia in awake monkeys. *J Neurosurg* 1981;54:773–782.
9. Heiss WD, Rosner G. Functional recovery of cortical neurons as related to degree and duration of ischemia. *Ann Neurol* 1983;14:294–301.
10. Memezawa H, Smith M-L, Siesjo BK. Penumbral tissues salvaged by reperfusion following middle cerebral artery occlusion in rats. *Stroke* 1992;23:559.
11. Nedergaard M. Neuronal injury in the infarct border: a neuropathologicsl study in the rat. *Acta Neuropathol*1987;73:267–274.
12. Mies G, Auer LM, Ebhardt G, Traupe H, Heiss W-D. Flow and neuronal density in tissue surrounding chronic infarction. *Stroke* 1983;14:22–27.
13. Baron JC. Mapping the Ischaemic Penumbra with PET: implications for acute stroke treatment. *Cerebrovasc Dis* 1999;9:193–201.
14. Heiss W-D, Huber M, Fink GR, et al. Progressive derangement of periinfarct viable tissue in ischemic stroke. *J Cereb Blood Flow Metab* 1992;12:193–203.
15. Minematsu K, Li L, Sotak CH, Davis MA, Fisher M. Reversible focal ischemic injury demonstrated by diffusion-weighted magnetic resonance imaging in rats. *Stroke* 1992; 23:1311.
16. Clark WM, Madden KP, Rothlein R, Zivin JA. Reduction of central nervous system ischemic injury in rabbits using leukocyte adhesion antibody treatment. *Stroke* 1991;22:877–883.
17. Busto R, Dietrich W, Mordecai G. Small differences in intraischemic brain temperature critically determines the extent of neuronal injury. *J Cereb Blood Flow Metab* 1987;7: 729–738.
18. Bruno A, Biller J, Adams HP, Clarke WR, Woolson RF, Williams LS, Hansen MD, TOAST Investigators. Acute blood glucose level and outcome from ischemic stroke. *Neurology* 999;52:280–284.
19. Strijbos PJLM, Leach MJ, Garthwaite J. Vicious cycle involving Na^+ channels, glutamate release, and NMDA receptors mediates delayed neurodegeneration through nitric oxide formation. *J Neurosci* 1996;16:5004–5013.
20. Pellegrini-Giampietro DE, Cherici G, Alesiani M, Carla V, Moroni F. Excitatory amino acid release and free radical formation may cooperate in the genesis of ischemia-induced neuronal damage. *J Neurosci* 1990;10:1035–1041.
21. Lu YM, Yin HZ, Chiang J, Weiss JH. Ca^{2+}-permeable AMPA/kainate and NMDA channels: High rate of Ca^{2+} influx underlies potent induction of injury. *J Neurosci* 1996;16:5457–5465.

22. Choi DW, Maulucci-Gedde M, Kriegstein AR. Glutamate neurotoxicity in cortical cell culture. *J.Neurosci.* 1987;7:357–368.
23. Rothman SM. Synaptic activity mediates death of hypoxic neurons. *Science* 1983;220: 536–537.
24. Rothman SM, Thurston JH, Hauhart RE. Delayed neurotoxicity of excitatory amino acids in vitro. *Neuroscience* 1987;22:471–480.
25. Rothman SM, Olney JW. Glutamate and the pathophysiology of hypoxic-ischemic brain damage. *Ann Neurol* 1986;19:105–111.
26. Weiss J, Goldberg MP, Choi DW. Ketamine protects cultured neocortical neurons from hypoxic injury. *Brain Res* 1986;380:186–190.
27. Hartley DM, Kurth MC, Bjerkness L, Weiss JH, Choi DW. Glutamate receptor-induced $^{45}Ca^{2+}$ accumulation in cortical cell culture correlates with subsequent neuronal degeneration. *J Neurosci* 1993;13:1993–2000.
28. Nakanishi S. Molecular diversity of glutamate receptors and implications for brain function. Science 1992;258:597–603.
29. Carriedo SG, Yin HZ, Weiss JH. Motor neurons are selectively vulnerable to AMPA/kainate receptor-mediated injury in vitro. *J Neurosci* 1996;16:4069–4079.
30. Choi S, Lovinger DM. Metabotropic glutamate receptor modulation of voltage-gated Ca^{2+} channels involves multiple receptor subtypes in cortical neurons. *J Neurosci* 1996;16:36–45.
31. Choi DW. Glutamate neurotoxicity in cortical cell culture is calcium-dependent. *Neurosci Lett* 1985;58:293–297.
32. Choi DW. Ionic dependence of glutamate neurotoxicity. *J Neurosci* 1987;7:369–379.
33. Goldberg MP, Choi DW. Combined oxygen and glucose deprivation in cortical cell culture: Calcium-dependent and calcium-independent mechanisms of neuronal injury. *J Neurosci* 1993;13:3510–3524.
34. Bhat RV, DiRocco R, Marcy VR, et al. Increased expression of IL-1β converting enzyme in hippocampus after ischemia: Selective localization in microglia. *J Neurosci* 1996;16: 4146–4154.
35. Schulz JB, Weller M, Klockgether T. Potassium deprivation-induced apoptosis of cerebellar granule neurons: A sequential requirement for new mRNA and protein synthesis, ICE-like protease activity, and reactive oxygen species. *J Neurosci* 1996;16:4696–4706.
36. MacDermott AB, Mayer ML, Westbrook GL, Smith SJ, Barker JL. NMDA-receptor activation increases cytoplasmic calcium concentration in cultured spinal cord neurones. *Nature* (Lond) 1986;321:519–522.
37. Riveros N, Orrego F. *N*-Methylaspartate-activated calcium channels in rat brain cortex slices. Effect of calcium channel blockers and of inhibitory and depressant substances. *Neuroscience* 1986;17:541–546.
38. Hirayama T, Ono H, Fukuda H. Effects of excitatory and inhibitory amino acid agonists and antagonists on ventral horn cells in slices of spinal cord isolated from adult rats. *Neuropharmacology* 1990;29:1117–1122.
39. Frandsen A, Schousboe A. Mobilization of dantrolene-sensitive intracellular calcium pools is involved in the cytotoxicity induced by quisqualate and *N*-methyl-D-aspartate but not by 2-amino-3-(3-hydroxy-5-methylisoxazol-4-yl)propionate and kainate in cultured cerebral cortical neurons. *Proc Natl Acad Sci USA* 1992;89:2590–2594.
40. Katchman AN, Hershkowitz N. Early anoxia-induced vesicular glutamate release results from mobilization of calcium from intracellular stores. *J Neurophysiol* 1993;70:1–7.
41. Bickler PE, Hansen BM. Causes of calcium accumulation in rat cortical brain slices during hypoxia and ischemia: Role of ion channels and membrane damage. *Brain Res* 1994;664: 269–276.

42. O'Regan MH, Smith-Barbour M, Perkins LM, Phillis JW. A possible role for phospholipases in the release of neurotransmitter amino acids from ischemic rat cerebral cortex. *Neurosci Lett* 1995;185:191–194.
43. Ozyurt E, Graham D, Woodruff G, McCullogh J. Protective effect of the glutamate antagonist MK-801 in focal cerebral ischemia in the cat. *J Cereb Blood Flow Metab* 1988;8: 138–143.
44. Yum SW, Faden AI. Comparison of the neuroprotective effects of the *N*-methyl-D- aspartate antagonist MK-801 and the opiate-receptor antagonist nalmefene in experimental spinal cord ischemia. *Arch Neurol* 1990;47:277–281.
45. Park CK, Nehls DG, Graham DI, Teasdale GM, McCulloch J. The glutamate antagonist MK-801 reduces focal ischemic brain damage in the rat. *Ann Neurol* 1988;24:543–551.
46. Boast CS, Gerhardt B, Pastor G, Lehmann J, Etienne PE, Liebman JM. The *N*-methyl-D-aspartate antagonist CGS19755 and CPP reduce ischemic brain damage in gerbils. *Brain Res* 1988;442:345–348.
47. George CP, Goldberg MP, Choi DW, Steinberg GK. Dextromethorphan reduces neocortical ischemic neuronal damage in vivo. *Brain Res* 1988;440:375–379.
48. Prince DA, Feeser HR. Dextromethorphan protects against cerebral infarction in a rat model of hypoxia-ischemia. *Neurosci Lett* 1988;85:291–296.
49. Steinberg GK, Saleh J, Kunis D. Delayed treatment with dextromethorphan and dextrophan reduces cerebral damage after transient focal ischemia. *Neurosci Lett* 1988;89:193–197.
50. Newell DW, Barth A, Malouf AT. Glycine site NMDA receptor antagonists provide protection against ischemia-induced neuronal damage in hippocampal slice cultures. *Brain Res* 1995;675:38–44.
51. Tsuchida E, Bullock R. The effect of the glycine site-specific *N*-Methyl-D-Aspartate antagonist ACEA1021 on ischemic brain damage caused by acute subdural hematoma in the rat. *J Neurotrauma* 1995;12:279–288.
52. Roberts E. γ-Aminobutyric acid and nervous system function—a perspective. *Biochem Pharmacol* 1974;23:2637–2649.
53. Bachelard HS. Biochemistry of centrally active amino acids. In: Mandel P, DeFeudis FV, eds. *Advances in Biochemical Psychopharmacology*. New York: Raven Press, 1981: 475–498.
54. Albin RL, Sakurai SY, Makowiec RL, Higgins DS, Young AB, Penney JB. Excitatory amino acid, $GABA_A$, and $GABA_B$ binding sites in human striate cortex. *Cerebral Cortex*. 1991;1:499–509.
55. Jansen KLR, Faull RLM, Dragunow M, Leslie RA. Distribution of excitatory and inhibitory amino acid, sigma, monoamine, catecholamine, acetylcholine, opioid, neurotensin, substance P, adenosine and neuropeptide Y receptors in human motor and somatosensory cortex. *Brain Res* 1991;566:225–238.
56. Karlsson G, Olpe H-R. Late inhibitory postsynaptic potentials in rat prefrontal cortex may be mediated by GABA-B receptors. *Experientia* 1989;45:157–148.
57. Scharfman HE, Sarvey JM. Responses to γ-aminobutric acid applied cell bodies and dendrites of rat visual cortical neurons. *Brain Res* 1985;358:385–389.
58. Kelly PAT, McCulloch J. Effects of the putative GABAergic agonists, muscimol and THIP, upon local cerebral glucose utilisation. *J Neurochem* 1982;39:613–624.
59. Kelly PAT, McCulloch J. The effects of the GABAergic agonist muscimol upon the relationship between local cerebral blood flow and glucose utilization. *Brain Res* 1983;258:338–342.
60. Edvinsson L, Krause DN. Pharmacological characterization of GABA receptors mediating vasodilation of cerebral arteries in vitro. *Brain Res* 1979;173:89–97.
61. Erdo SL, Michler A, Wolff JR. GABA accelerates excitotoxic cell death in cortical cultures: Protection by blockers of GABA-gated chloride channels. *Brain Res* 1991;542:254–258.

62. van den Pol AN, Obrietan K, Chen G. Excitatory actions of GABA after neuronal trauma. *J Neurosci* 1996;16:4283–4292.
63. Akhondzadeh S, Stone TW. Potentiation by neurosteroids of muscimol/adenosine interactions in rat hippocampus. *Brain Res* 1995;677:311–318.
64. Frye CA. The neurosteroid 3α,5α-THP has antiseizure and possible neuroprotective effects in an animal model of epilepsy. *Brain Res* 1995;696:113–120.
65. Gee KW, McCauley LD, Lan NC. A putative receptor for neurosteroids on the $GABA_A$ receptor complex: The pharmacological properties and therapeutic potential of epalons. *Crit Revs Neurobiology* 1995;9:207–227.
66. Lambert JJ, Belelli D, Hill-Venning C, Peters JA. Neurosteroids and $GABA_A$ receptor function. *Trends Pharmacol Sci* 1995;16:295–303.
67. Devaud LL, Purdy RH, Morrow AL. The Neurosteroid, 3α-hydroxy-5α-pregnan-20-one, protects against bicuculline-induced seizures during ethanol withdrawal in rats. *Alcohol Clin Exp Resp* 1995;19:350–355.
68. Hauser CAE, Wetzel CHR, Rupprecht R, Holsboer F. Allopregnanoline acts as an inhibitory modulator on α_1-and α_6-containing $GABA_A$ receptors. *Biochem Biophys Res Commun* 1996;219:531–536.
69. Brown AW, Brierley JB. The nature, distribution, and earliest stages of anoxic-ischemic nerve cell damage in the rat brain as defined by the optical microscope. *Br J Exp Pathol* 1968;49:87–106.
70. Linnik MD, Zobrist RH, Hatfield MD. Evidence supporting a role for programmed cell death in focal cerebral ischemia in rats. *Stroke* 1993;24:2002–2009.
71. Wyllie AH, Kerr JFR, Currie AR. Cell Death: The Significance of Apoptosis. *Int Rev Cytol* 1980;68:251–305.
72. Oppenheim RW. Cell death during development of the nervous system. *Annu Rev Neurosci* 1991;14:453–501.
73. Clarke PGH. Developmental cell death: morphological diversity and multiple mechanisms. *Anat Embryol* 1990;181:195–213.
74. Pulsinelli WA, Brierley JB, Plum F. Temporal profile of neuronal damage in a model of transient forebrain ischemia. *Ann Neurol* 1982;11:491–498.
75. Cohen GM, Sun X-M, Snowden RT, Dinsdale D, Skilleter DN. Key morphological features of apoptosis may occur in the absence of internucleosomal DNA fragmentation. *Biochem J* 1992;286:331–334.
76. Charriaut-Marlangue C, Margaill I, Represa A, Popovici T, Plotkine M, Ben-Ari Y. Apoptosis and necrosis after reversible focal ischemia: an *in situ* DNA fragmentation analysis. *J Cereb Blood Flow Metab* 1996;16:186–194.
77. Tominaga T, Kure S, Narisawa K, Yoshimoto T. Endonuclease activation following focal ischemic injury in the rat brain. *Brain Res* 1993;608:21–26.
78. Li Y, Sharov VG, Jiang N, Zaloga C, Sabbah HN, Chopp M. Ultrastructural and light microscopic evidence of apoptosis after middle cerebral artery occlusion in the rat. *Am J Pathol* 1995;146:1045–1051.
79. MacManus JP, Hill IE, Huang Z-G, Rasquinha I, Xue D, Buchan AM. DNA damage consistent with apoptosis in transient focal ischaemic neocortex. *NeuroReport* 1994;5:493–496.
80. van Lookeren Campagne M, Gill R. Ultrastructural morphological changes are not characteristic of apoptotic cell death following focal cerebral ischaemia in the rat. *Neurosci Lett* 1996;213:111–114.
81. Zhongting H, Kazunari Y, Hitoshi O, Haiping L, Mitsuhiro K. The in vivo time course for elimination of adrenalectomy-induced apoptotic profiles from the granule cell layer of the rat hippocampus. *J Neurosci* 1997;17:3981–3989.
82. Liu XZ, Xu XM, Hu R, et al. Neuronal and glial apoptosis after traumatic spinal cord injury. *J Neurosci* 1997;17:5395–5406.

83. Goto K, Ishige A, Sekigushi Ket al. Effects of cycloheximide on delayed neuronal death in rat hippocampus. *Brain Research* 1990;534:299–302.
84. Ames AI, Wright LW, Kowada M, Thurston JM, Majno G. Cerebral ischemia. II. The no-reflow phenomenon. *Am J Pathol* 1968;52:437–447.
85. Schmid-Schönbein GW. Capillary plugging by granulocytes and the no-reflow phenomenon in the microcirculation. *Proc Fed Amer Soc Exp Biol* 1987;46:2397–2401.
86. Harlan JM, Vedder NB, Winn RK, Rice CL. Mechanisms and consequences of leukocyte-endothelial interaction. *West J Med* 1991;155:365–369.
87. Hallenbeck JM, Dutka AJ, Tanishima T, et al. Polymorphonuclear leukocyte accumulation in brain regions with low blood flow during the early postischemic period. *Stroke* 1986;17:246–253.
88. Menger MD, Lehr H-A, Messmer K. Role of oxygen radicals in the microcirculatory manifestations of postischemic injury. *Klin Wochenschr* 1991;69:1050–1055.
89. del Zoppo G, Schmid-Schönbein GW, Mori E, Copeland BR, Chang C-M. Polymorphonuclear leukocytes occlude capillaries following middle cerebral artery occlusion and reperfusion in baboons. *Stroke* 1991;22:1276–1283.
90. Zhang RL, Chopp M, Li Y, et al. Anti-ICAM-1 antibody reduces ischemic cell damage after transient middle cerebral artery occlusion in the rat. *Neurology* 1994;44:1747–1751.
91. Bowes MP, Zivin JA, Rothlein R. Monoclonal antibody to the ICAM-1 adhesion site reduces neurological damage in a rabbit cerebral embolism stroke model. *Exp Neurol* 1993; 119:215–219.
92. Clark WM, Madden KP, Rothlein R, Zivin JA. Reduction of central nervous system ischemic injury by monoclonal antibody to intercellular adhesion molecule. *J Neurosurg* 1991; 75:623–627.
93. Rod MR, Auer RN. Combination therapy with nimodipine and dizocilpine in a rat model of transient forebrain ischemia. *Stroke* 1992;23:725–732.
94. Uematsu D, Araki N, Greenberg JH, Sladky J, Reivich M. Combined therapy with MK-801 and nimodipine for protection of ischemic brain damage. *Neurology* 1991;41:88–94.
95. Zivin JA, Mazzarella V. Tissue plasminogen activator plus glutamate antagonist improves outcome after embolic stroke. *Arch Neurol* 1991;48:1235–1238.
96. Auer RN. Combination therapy with U74006F (tirilazad mesylate), MK-801, insulin and diazepam in transient forebrain ischaemia. *Neurol Res* 1995;17:132–136.
97. Bowes MP, Rothlein R, Fagan SC, Zivin JA. Monoclonal antibodies preventing leukocyte activation reduce experimental neurologic injury and enhance efficacy of thrombolytic therapy. *Neurology* 1995;45:815–819.
98. American Heart Association. *Heart and Stroke Facts and Figures*. Dallas: American Heart Association, 1992.
99. Lyden PD, Rapp K, Babcock T, Rothrock J. Ultra-rapid identification, triage, and enrollment of stroke patients into clinical trials. *J Stroke Cerebrovasc Dis* 1994;4:106–113.
100. Lyden PD, Zivin JA. Hemorrhagic transformation after cerebral ischemia: Mechanisms and incidence. *Cerebrovasc Brain Met Rev* 1993;5:1–16.
101. Kaufman HH. *Intracerebral Hematomas*. New York: Raven Press, 1992:1–240.
102. Kanno T, Sano H, Shinomiyo Y, Katada K, Nagata J, Hoshino M, Mitsuyama F. Role of surgery in hypertensive intracerebral hematoma. *J Neurosurg* 1985;61:1091–1099.
103. Broderick J, Brott T, Tomsick T, Tew J, Duldner J, Huster G. Management of intracerebral hemorrhage in a large metropolitan population. *Neurosurgery* 1994;34:882–887.
104. Lisk DR, Pasteur W, Rhoades H, Putnam RD, Grotta JC. Early presentation of hemispheric intracerebral hemorrhage: prediction of outcome and guidelines for treatment allocation. *Neurology* 1994;44:133–139.
105. Yang G-Y, Betz AL, Chenevert TL, Brunberg JA, Hoff JT. Experimental intracerebral hemorrhage: relationship between brain edema. blood flow, and blood–brain barrier permeability in rats. *J Neurosurg* 1994;81:93–102.

106. Brott TG, Haley EC, Jr, Levy DEet al. Urgent therapy for stroke: Part 1. Pilot study of tissue plasminogen activator administered within 90 minutes. *Stroke* 1992;23:632–640.
107. Hommel M, Boissel JP, Cornu C, et al. Termination of streptokinase in severe acute ischaemic stroke. *Lancet* 1995;345:57–57.
108. NINDS rt-PA Stroke Study Group. Tissue plasminogen activator for acute ischemic stroke. *N Engl J Med* 1995;333:1581–1587.

II Scientific Rationale and Clinical Trials

4 Preclinical Testing of Thrombolytic Therapy for Acute Ischemic Stroke

Steven R. Levine, MD

Contents

INTRODUCTION

Prior to definitive human trials, considerable effort was expended in the laboratory perfecting thrombolytic therapy. The essential literature that provided the experimental impetus for proceeding to human trials is summarized in this chapter. From this experience, two important lessons emerged. First, thorough exploration of drug risks and benefits should be performed in relevant animal models prior to human trials. Second, animal models can predict human results accurately, but only if the correct models are chosen, and the results handled rigorously. For example, the experimental data clearly predicted the efficacy, and the side effects, of thrombolytic therapy with tissue plasminogen activator (t-PA). Furthermore, the excessive risk associated with streptokinase (SK) was predicted by the animal models. These data serve to illuminate an approach to studying putative stroke therapies in the future.

From: *Current Clinical Neurology: Thrombolytic Therapy for Acute Stroke, Second Edition*
Edited by: P. D. Lyden © Humana Press Inc., Totowa, NJ

EARLY EXPERIMENTAL STUDIES OF THROMBOLYSIS FOR STROKE USING PLASMIN, UROKINASE, OR STREPTOKINASE

The experimental and basic early studies of thrombolytics for ischemic stroke are summarized in Table 1 *(1–9)*. Meyer et al. *(10)* created pumice emboli with subsequent platelet and thrombi adherence to the regions of damaged endothelium in cats and monkeys. Intravenous (iv) or intra-arterial injection of either bovine or human plasmin resulted in lysis of the thrombi in every experiment. Intra-arterial infusion caused more rapid clot dissolution and the SK-activated human plasmin was believed to be minimally more effective than the bovine-fibrinolysin. Clot lysis began 4 to 18 min after intra-arterial infusion and 8 to 30 min after dosing. Hemorrhagic infarction did not appear to be increased by fibrinolytic therapy. However, 2 to 4 h post-fibrinolysis infusion the thrombus usually started to reform and propagate. This did not occur if heparin was given 30 min to 1 h prior to fibrinolytics. Distal emboli resulting from the parent clot dissolution was documented in five experiments. These smaller emboli were then also dissolved.

Del Zoppo et al. *(1)* demonstrated that after 3 h of reversible eccentric balloon (inflatable silastic placed transorbitally) compression of the baboon middle cerebral artery (MCA) proximal to the lenticulostriate arteries (n = 5), intra-carotid urokinase (12 × 106 international units [IU] over 1 h started 30 min after balloon deflation), improved neurological function and reduced infarct size without evidence of macroscopic intracerebral hemorrhage (ICH) compared with untreated animals (n = 6).

DeLey et al. *(11)* showed that very early treatment with intra-carotid SK (500,000 IU) in conjunction with flunarizine prevented the lowering of the cerebral metabolic rate of oxygen as determined by positron emission tomography scanning in a dog MCA occlusion (autologous blot clot) model.

PRECLINICAL TRIALS OF TISSUE PLASMINOGEN ACTIVATOR

Table 2 shows the basic studies of t-PA for ischemic stroke. Intense effort went into establishing the efficacy of thrombolytics, especially tissue t-PA, for experimental cerebral ischemia *(12–14)*. If t-PA is administered immediately after experimental embolic occlusion, significant reduction in neurological damage occurs *(12)*. t-PA may reduce neurological damage in rabbit embolic stroke models as late as 45 min after the cerebral embolic occlusion *(15)*. t-PA-related ICH did not occur when therapy was started 4 h after the onset of vascular occlusion. However, there was no benefit when treatment was delayed for 1 h *(15)*. In both a small- and a large-clot rabbit embolic stroke model, there was no evidence that t-PA changed the histological appearance of lesions compared with

Table 1
Experimental and Basic Studies of Thrombolytics for Ischemic Stroke

Author (reference)	*Year*	*UK/SK/plasmin animal model*	*Main results (compared with controls when applicable)*
Whisnant *(2)*	1960	Clot in internal carotid artery	No increased risk of hemorrhagic infarction compared with controls
Centero *(3)*	1985	Rabbit autologous clot	Variable and no statistical differences with controls, no gross ICH
Del Zoppo *(1)*	1986	Baboon MCA balloon	Improved neurological function, reduced infarct size, no macroscopic ICH
Hirschberg *(4–6)*	1987	Dog MCA occlusion	Thrombolysis, no ICH, five petechial hemorrhages
Slivka *(7)*	1987	Rabbit CCA/MCA occlusion	Two gross ICH; petechial hemorrhage same as controls
Deley *(8)*	1988	Dog MCA clot	Thrombolysis without improved tissue perfusion or infarct reduction if treatment 30 min after 3-h-old clot injected.
			Normalization of cerebral blood flow and salvaged tissue if treatment within 5 min of insult
Clark *(9)*	1989	Rabbit autologous clot	>50% hemorrhage

Abbr: ICH, intracranial hemorrhage; MCA, middle cerebral artery; CCA, common carotid artery.

Table 2
Experimental and Basic Studies of Thrombolytics for Ischemic Stroke: t-PA

Author (reference)	*Year*	*Animal model*	*Treatment onset*	*Main results (compared with controls when applicable)*
Zivin *(12)*	1985	Rabbit autologous clot	<2 min up to 45 min, 1 h	Neurological improvement, no large ICH, no protection
Del Zoppo *(14)*	1986	Baboon reversible MCA occlusion	3 h	Improved neurological function
Penar *(55)*	1987	Rat autologous clot	–	No effect on vessel patency, no ICH, less "low-flow" regions, untreated groups, change in fibrinogen
no				
Kissel *(56)*	1987	Rabbit autologous clot	–	Improved CBF at 90 min but not at 30 min
Watson *(57)*	1987	Rat with laser-induced thrombosis	–	Segmental recanalization, decreased lesion volume in 6 of 9, no ICH
Papadopolous *(58)*	1987	Rat with human clot	2 h	Increased CBF, within 30 min, improved EEG, thrombolysis achieved, no ICH
Slivka *(7)*	1987	Rabbit CCA/MCA occlusion	24 h	ICH
Chehrazi *(59)*	1988	Rabbit autologous clot	30 min, 2 h, 4 h	Reduced infarct size in zomin treatment on-set group, no ICH
Philips *(60,61)*	1988	Rabbit autologous clot	15 min	Rapid reperfusion, no macroscopic ICH, no difference in infarct extent
Clark *(9)*	1989	Rabbit autologous clot	≤60 min, 6 h	14% hemorrhages (37% in controls) 30 hemorrhage (21 in controls)
Lyden *(17)*	1989	Rabbit embolism	10 min	100% lysis at 5 mg/kg, no increased ICH
Bednar *(62)*	1990	Rabbit embolism	< 60 min	Restored CBF, reduced final infarct size
Benes *(20)*	1990	Rabbit embolism	30 min	Reduced infarct incidence, no ICH
Terashi *(63)*	1990	Hypertensive rats	t-PA preischemia	Higher brain ATP and lower lactate t-PAI-1 than vehicle treated rats, no hemorrhagic lesions, no arterial platelet in t-PA treated rats

Abbr: ICH, intracranial hemorrhage; MCA, middle cerebral artery; CBF, cerebral blood flow; EEG, electroencephalogram; CCA, common carotid artery; ATP, adenosine triphosphate.

untreated controls. Zivin et al. *(12)*, in a landmark 1985 *Science* study, first documented that t-PA could substantially improve neurological function after embolization with artificially made clots.

Using awake baboons, Del Zoppo et al. *(16)* studied t-PA-induced hemorrhagic transformation of ischemic brain within 3.5 h after MCA occlusion and 30 min of reperfusion. Three doses of t-PA were infused over 1 h and compared with normal saline infusion (n = 12). Peripheral (nonintracranial) hemorrhages were related to t-PA. No significant differences in the incidences or volumes of 14-d infarction-related hemorrhage occurred in any group compared with saline-treated animals, suggesting that t-PA alone does not increase the risk (incidence or volume) of hemorrhagic infarction if administered within 3.5 h after MCA occlusion and reperfusion in baboons. Five of six animals at each dose (10 of 12 total) had petechial hemorrhagic infarction at 14 d compared with 7 of 12 control animals. Their data also suggest that t-PA does not substantially decrease the infarct volume at any of the doses administered early after symptom onset.

t-PA administered later *(7)* rather than earlier *(15)*, albeit in different models, was more often associated with ICH. Lyden et al. *(17)* found no difference in the frequency of ischemic brain hemorrhagic transformation, however, when t-PA was administered 10 min, 8 h, or 24 h after injection of autologous emboli.

Vaugh et al. *(18)* demonstrated that t-PA combined with iv aspirin synergistically and markedly prolonged the template bleeding time with a significant bleeding tendency. Administering reactivated tissue plasminogen activator inhibitor-1 (t-PAI-1) can rapidly reverse this bleeding time prolongation.

Slivka and Pulsinella *(7)* investigated the hemorrhagic potential of both t-PA (200,000 units [U]; 10% bolus remainder over 4 h) and SK (10,000 U/kg bolus or 32,000 U/kg bolus, remainder over 4 h) initiated 24 h after experimental stroke in rabbits using a tandem common carotid and ipsilateral MCA occlusions with 2 h of halothane. In addition, six rabbits were administered SK (10,000 U/kg bolus) 1 h after occlusion. Microscopic hemorrhage was frequently present in infarct tissue irrespective of treatment. Gross hemorrhagic infarction did not occur in rabbits either untreated or administered SK 1 h after occlusion but did occur in the other groups of treated animals. Two of 12 animals administered SK 24 h after injection had gross hemorrhages within the infarct. Only the t-PA-treated rabbits showed a significantly greater incidence of gross ICH than controls. Their data suggest that the use of thrombolytic agents may increase the risk of microscopic hemorrhage unless the agents are administered early enough after onset of the insult.

In pioneering work that set the stage for well-conducted clinical trials, Zivin et al. *(15)* found that t-PA-induced ICH did not occur more commonly than controls when therapy was started within 4 h after the onset of vascular occlusion in rabbit emboli model of ischemic stroke. t-PA was administered at 1.0 mg/kg at 15, 30, or 60 min after small-clot embolization (24-h aged clot) and at 2 mg/kg at 45 and 60 min after small-clot embolization. t-PA was also administered 30 min or 4 h after large-clot (1 mm^3) embolization. Evaluations were performed blinded to the treatment group. The effective dose of clots required to produce a clinically apparent neurological disorder in 50% of a group of animals was significantly greater in the t-PA-treated rabbits when t-PA was administered at 15, 30, or 45 min but not at 60 min post-embolization in either the 1 mg/kg or 2 mg/kg dose. In controls, grossly apparent ICH was present in 3 of 10 (30%) animals.

When t-PA was administered 30 min after embolization, 8 of 14 rabbits had gross hemorrhage. When t-PA was delayed 4 h, 2 of 10 animals had such hemorrhages (p = NS). In the small-clot model, ICH was uncommon, visible only microscopically, and only found in association with relatively large infarcts. The presence of microscopically visible intravascular clots was a function of the time between clot injection and animal death. In the large-clot model, the microscopy of the lesions in control- and t-PA-treated rabbits was indistinguishable, and no difference was noted in neurological functions *(17,19)*.

Lyden et al. *(17)* demonstrated in the rabbit emboli stroke model that ICH rates in the t-PA (3 mg/kg or 5 mg/kg) or saline-treated group did not differ. t-PA was infused 10 min, 8 h, and 24 h after emboli were instilled. Lyden et al. *(19)* also evaluated saline, t-PA, or SK infusion in a similar rabbit embolic stroke model at various times of infusion to assess the rate of thrombolysis and ICH 24 h later. Only SK was associated with a significant increase in the rate of ICH compared with the saline controls. In animals administered 3, 5, or 10 mg/kg of t-PA, there was no clear dose–response for ICH, but there was for thrombolysis. However, only in rabbits who achieved thrombolysis was t-PA associated with double (24%) the ICH rate as saline controls (12%), whereas the hemorrhages were nearly identical in animals without thrombolysis.

Benes et al. *(20)* found that treatment with either t-PA or urokinase (UK) significantly reduced the number of emboli present in a rabbit stroke model but only t-PA significantly reduced the incidence of infarction. No animal suffered an ICH.

In summary, these studies taken together suggest that t-PA reliably opens cerebral arteries occluded with either autologous or non-autologous embolic clots. Furthermore, there is preliminary experimental data to suggest that t-PA is more effective in inducing thrombolysis within precerebral vessels than systemic vessels *(21)*.

TISSUE PLASMINOGEN ACTIVATOR ANALOGS AND OTHER THROMBOLYTIC AGENTS

In recent years, several new thrombolytic agents have been identified or synthesized and have gone into experimental and clinical studies, for both acute myocardial and cerebral ischemia. Analogs to rt-PA are available through recombinant deoxyribonucleic acid (DNA) technologies and offer the possibility of an active portion of molecule that may have better fibrin specificity and penetration and a longer in vivo half-life than t-PA *(22)*.

Tissue Plasminogen Activator Analog Fb-Fb-CF

Phillips et al. *(23,24)* investigated the effects of a t-PA analog, Fb-Fb-CF, in a rabbit embolic model. This analog consisted of the catalytic fragment of t-PA and a dimer of the B fragment of staphylococcal protein A (Fb-Fb-CF) and has a longer serum half-life (90 min) than rt-PA (3 min). When Fb-Fb-CF was given as a bolus 15 min after embolization, cerebral reperfusion occurred in 48 ± 21 min (range 30–90 min) whereas saline-treated controls did not reperfuse by 180 min ($p < 0.01$). Furthermore, reperfusion was demonstrated at 66 ± 32 min posttreatment when the treatment was delayed 90 min after embolization (control = 100 ± 25 min); two spontaneous lyses occurred in controls ($p < 0.01$). One small macroscopic hemorrhage within an infarct was observed in the Fb-Fb-CF 15-min treated group (none in controls). In the 90-min group, microscopic hemorrhage was observed in four t-PA-analog and three saline-treated animals. Plasma fibrinogen levels decreased 16% immediately after and 19% by 180 min following Fb-Fb-CF treatment. No macroscopic or microscopic ICH was observed in noninfarcted brain regions although intraventricular hemorrhages occurred on one Fb-Fb-CF and two control animals only in the 90-min group.

A t-PA analog (0.8 mg/kg, 1 mg = 500,000 IU) was given in a rabbit autologous clot cerebral embolization model, either 15 min or 90 min after embolization, in conjunction with serial angiography *(25)*. Reperfusion was documented in both the 15- and 90-min groups treated with t-PA analogs (different than controls) without a difference in median time to reperfusion in the two groups. In the 15-min group, 0 of 8 controls reperfused and in the 90-min group, 2 of 12 controls spontaneously reperfused. One small hemorrhage into a zone of infarction was observed in the 15-min t-PA analog-treated group (0 in controls) and four hemorrhages into infarcts were observed in the 90-min group (three in controls), suggesting that the risk of hemorrhage was essentially the same for t-PA analog-treated rabbits and saline-treated rabbits.

TENECTEPLASE TISSUE PLASMINOGEN ACTIVATOR

Tenecteplase (TNK), a genetically modified ("mutant") form of wild-type t-PA contains targeted mutations in three regions in the t-PA molecule designed to yield a molecule with a longer biological half-life and greater fibrin specificity (14 times that of t-PA). With these properties, TNK-t-PA could have greater safety and/or efficacy in clinical thrombolysis *(26–33)*, with more rapid *(30)* and complete thrombolysis. The longer half-life also offers the opportunity for bolus therapy over infusion therapy. As critical lysis takes place at the surface of an arterial thrombus or embolus where PAI-1 levels can be very high, mutant t-PA molecules with longer half-life and resistance to PAI-1 may be useful to reduce the contribution of PAI-1 to re-occlusion. TNK has 80-fold more resistance to PAI-1 than t-PA *(33)*.

In the rabbit embolic stroke model, Chapman et al. *(26)* found hemorrhage in 6 of 23 (26%) within the control group, 16 of 20 (80%) within the wild-type t-PA group, 12 of 21 (57%) within the 0.6 mg/kg TNK group, and 8 of 11 (73%) within the 1.5 mg/kg TNK group ($p < 0.01$, χ^2). TNK showed comparable rates of recanalization and fewer hemorrhages, compared to wild-type t-PA, although these results were not statistically significant.

In the small-clot rabbit emboli model, TNK showed a better pharmacological profile than t-PA–with more frequent lysis up to 3 h post-stroke and no increase in ICH rate *(31)*.

Intra-arterial TNK (1.5 mg/kg) reduced 48-h infarct volume when given 2 h post MCA occlusion in a rat model of focal cerebral embolic ischemia *(29)*. There was a trend ($p = 0.06$) for a reduction in lesion volume when TNK was given 4 h after occlusion ($n = 12$). There was no increase in gross ICH in either the 2-or 4-h post-occlusion treatment.

*Bat Venom Plasminogen Activator (*Desmodus *Salivary Plasminogen Activator)*

Vampire bats live on fresh blood. The saliva of the vampire bat has various factors that can maintain prolonged bleeding and preserve blood fluidity *(28)*. There are different molecular forms of *Desmodus* salivary plasminogen activator (DSPA) (all single-chain molecules) *(34–45)* that have somewhat more than 70% homology to human t-PA, including $DSPA_1$ (molecular-weight 52 kDa). They possess a relative PAI-1 resistance, greatly enhanced fibrin-selectivity and a strict requirement of polymeric fibrin as a cofactor *(28)*. Bleeding complications may also be reduced *(41)*. In humans terminal half-life for $DSPA_1$, the variant selected for clinical development, is about two orders of magnitude longer than that of t-PA. Also, $DSPA_1$ does not promote kainite- or *N*-methyl D-aspartate-mediated neurotoxicity in contrast to t-PA *(37)*. Bleeding complications may also be reduced as a result of the lack of an induced systemic lytic state *(41)*.

In a coronary thrombosis dog model of acute myocardial infarction, there was aster recanalization and less reocclusion with $DSPA_1$ than t-PA *(46)*. Clinical trials in acute ischemic stroke are currently underway with $DSPA_1$ within the 3–9 h time window. In a recently completed phase II trial, $DSPA_1$ was found to produce a dose-dependent reperfusion and clinical improvement (including the last assessment 90 d after the event), with relatively low symptomatic ICH rates at doses up to 125 μg/kg *(42)*.

Table 3
Newer Thrombolysis Agents in Development

Agents
Tenecteplase (TNK) and other t-PA "mutants"
Vampire bat saliva plasminogen activators (including Desmoteplase)
Staphylokinase
Saruplase
BB-1013
Microplasmin

GLOBAL ISCHEMIA

Moritomo et al. *(47)* studied heparin (100 U/kg) plus UK (3000 U/kg iv) given 15 min of complete *global* ischemia for 6 h in dogs. The studied group experienced up to 70% improvement in postischemic hypoperfusion cerebral blood flow with significantly improved neurological outcome, suggesting that these two drugs together might improve impaired microcirculation.

CONCLUSIONS

Data from experimental cerebral ischemia studies have consistently demonstrated the need to treat acute clinical stroke within a few hours or less to effectively reduce stroke morbidity and mortality *(48–50)*. Specifically, with reversible MCA occlusion models of focal cerebral ischemia, the animals uniformly survive without neurological deficit if the occlusion is for less than 2 to 3 h *(51)*. Similarly in primates, MCA occlusion for 3 h or less will lead to clinical improvement and a decrease in infarct size, with complete recovery generally associated with less than 2 h of MCA occlusion *(52–54)*. While it appears unlikely that ischemic brain can be salvaged if vascular occlusion persists longer than 4 to 6 h (similar to the pathophysiology of myocardial ischemia), the phase II results with Desmoteplase suggest a rethinking of this concept. If t-PA is administered immediately after experimental embolic occlusion, significant reduction in neurological damage occurs *(12)*. Newer thrombolytics (Table 3) including TNK and proteins isolated from vampire bat saliva offer the promise of more effective and safer acute pharmacological recanalization strategies, with a longer time window in selected patients.

REFERENCES

1. Del Zoppo GJ, Copeland BR, Waltz TA, et al. The beneficial effect of intracarotid urokinase on acute stroke in a baboon model. *Stroke* 1986;17:638–643.
2. Whisnant JP, Millikan CH, Seikert RG. Cerebral infarction and fibrinolytic agents. Roberts HR, Gevatz JD, eds. *Proceedings of the Conference on Thrombolytic Agents*, Chicago. 1970; pp. 235–245.

3. Centeno RS, Hackney PB, Rothsock Jr. Streptokinase clot lysis in acute occlusions of the cranial circulation: Study in rabbits. *Am J Neuroradiol* 1985;6:589–594.
4. Hirschberg M, Hofferberth B. Rapid fibrinolysis at different time intervals in a canine model of acute stroke. *Stroke* 1987;18:292 (abstr).
5. Hirschberg M, Hofferberth B. Thrombolytic therapy with urokinase and prourokinase in a canine model of acute stroke. *Neurology* 1987;37:133 (abstr).
6. Hirschberg M, Korves M, Koc I, et al. Thrombolysis of cerebral thromboembolism by urokinase in an animal model. *Schweiz Med Wochenschr* 1987;117:1811–1813.
7. Slivka A, Pulsinelli W. Hemorrhagic complications of thrombolytic therapy in experimental stroke. *Stroke* 1987;18:1148–1156.
8. DeLey G, Weyne J, Demeester G, et al. Experimental thromboembolic stroke by positron emission tomography: Immediate versus delayed reperfusion by fibrinolysis. *J Cereb Blood Flow Metab* 1988;8:539–545.
9. Lyden PD, Madden KP, Clark WM, Zivin JA, et al. Incidence of cerebral hemorrhage after treatment with tissue plasminogen activator or streptokinase following embolic stroke in rabbits. *Stroke* 1990;21:1589–1593.
10. Meyer JS, Gilroy J, Barnhart ME, et al. Therapeutic thrombolysis in cerebral thromboembolism. In:, Siekert W, Whisnant JP, eds., *Cerebral Vascular Diseases*. Grune & Stratton: Philadelphia. 1963; pp. 160–175.
11. DeLey G, Weyne I, Demeester G, et al. Streptokinase treatment versus calcium overload blockade in experimental thromboembolic stroke. *Stroke* 1989;20:357–361.
12. Zivin JA, Fisher M, DeGirolami U, et al. Tissue plasminogen activator reduces neurological damage after cerebral embolism. *Science* 1985;230:1289–1292.
13. Zivin JA. Thrombolytic therapy for stroke. In: *Current Neurosurgical Practice*, Weinstein PR, Faden AL, eds. Protection of the brain from ischemia. Williams & Wilkins: Baltimore. 1990; pp. 231–236.
14. Del Zoppo GJ, Copeland BR, Hacke W, et al. Intracerebral hemorrhage following rt-PA infusion in a primate stroke model. *Stroke* 1988;19:134,(abstr).
15. Zivin JA, Lyden PD, DeGirolami U, et al. Tissue plasminogen activator. Reduction of neurologic damage after experimental embolic stroke. *Arch Neurol* 1988;45:387–391.
17. Lyden PD, Zivin JA, Clark WA, et al. Tissue plasminogen activator-mediated thrombolysis of cerebral emboli and its effect on hemorrhagic infarction in rabbits. *Neurology* 1989;39: 703–708.
19. Lyden PD, Madden KP, Clark WM, et al. Incidence of cerebral hemorrhage after antifibrinolytic treatment for embolic stroke. *Stroke* 1990;21:1589–1593.
20. Benes V, Zabranski JM, Boston M, et al. Effect of intraarterial antifibrinolytic agents on autologous arterial emboli in the cerebral circulation of rabbits. *Stroke* 1990;21:1594–1599.
16. Del Zoppo GJ, Copeland BR, Andercheck K, et al. Hemorrhagic transformation following tissue plasminogen activator in experimental cerebral infarction. *Stroke* 1990;21:596–601.
18. Vaughn DF, DeClerck PJ, De Mol, et al. Recombinant plasminogen activator inhibitor-1 reverses the bleeding tendency associated with the combined administration of tissue-type plasminogen activator and aspirin in rabbits. *J Clin Invest* 1989;84:586–591.
21. Chehrazi BB, Seibert JA, Hein L, et al. Differential effect of tPA induced thrombolysis in the CNS and the systemic arteries. *Stroke* 1989;20:153, (abstr).
22. Fears R. Biochemical pharmacology and therapeutic aspects of thrombolytic agents. Pharmacol Rev 1990;42:202–222.
23. Phillips DA, Fisher M, Smith TW, et al. The effects of a new tissue plasminogen activator analogue Fb-Fb-CF, on cerebral reperfusion in a rabbit embolic stroke model. *Ann Neurol* 1989;25:281–285.
24. Phillips DA, Fisher M, Davis MA, et al. Delayed treatment with a tPA analogue and streptokinase in a rabbit embolic stroke model. *Stroke* 1990;21:602–605.

25. Fisher M, Phillips DA, Smith TW, et al. Early and delayed thrombolytic therapy in rabbit cerebral embolization model using a tPA analogue. In:, Ginsberg MD, Dietrich WD, eds., *Cerebrovascular Disease*. Raven: New York. 1989; pp. 29–32.
26. Chapman D, Lyden P, Lapchak A, Nunez S, Thibodeaux H, Zivin J. Comparison of TNK with wild-type tissue plasminogen activator in a rabbit embolic stroke model. *Stroke* 2001; 32:748–752.
27. Ross A. New plasminogen activators: a clinical review. *Clinical Cardiol.* 1999;22:165–171.
28. Verstraete M, Lijnen H, Collen D. Thrombolytic agents in development. *Drugs* 1995;50:29–39.
29. Zhang RL, Zhang L, Jiang A, Zhang ZG, Goussev A, Chopp M. Postischemic intracarotid treatment with TNK-tPA reduces infarct volume and improves neurological deficits in embolic stroke in the unanesthetized rat. *Brain Research* 2000;878:64–71.
30. Binbrek A, Rao N, Absher PM, Vande Werf F, Sobel B. The relative rapidity of recanalizaiton induced by recombinant tissue-type plasminogen activator (r-tPA) and TNK-tPA, assessed with enzymatic methods. *Coronary Artery Disease* 2000;11:429–435.
31. Lapchak PA, Araujo DM, Zivin JA. Comparison of Tenecteplase with Alteplase on clinical rating scores following small clot embolic strokes in rabbits. Experimental Neurology 2004;185:154–159.
32. Rabasseda X. Tenecteplase (TNK tissue plasminogen activator): a new fibrinolytic for the acute treatment of myocardial infarction. *Drugs Today* 2001;37:749–760.
33. Lapchak P. Development of thrombolytic therapy for stroke: a perspective. Expert Opin. Investig. *Drugs* 2002;11:1623–1632.
34. Bringmann P, Gruber D, Liese A, Toschi L, Krätzschmar J, Schleuning, W-D, Donner P. Structural features mediating fibrin selectivity of vampire bat plasminogen activators *J Biol Chem* 1995;270:25596–25603.
35. Toschi L, Bringmann P, Petri T, Donner P, Schleuning W-D. Fibrin selectivity of the isolated protease domains of tissue-type and vampire bat salivary gland plasminogen activators. *Eur J Biochem* 1998;252:108–112.
36. Stewart RJ, Fredenburgh§ JC, Weitz JI. Characterization of the interactions of plasminogen and tissue and vampire bat plasminogen activiators with fibrinogen, fibrin, and the complex of d-dimer noncovalently linked to fragment E. *J Biol Chem* 1998;273:18,292–18,299.
37. Liberatore GT, Samson A, Bladin C, Schleuning W-D, Medcalf R. Vampire bat salivary plasminogen activator (Desmoteplase): a unique fibrinolytic enzyme that does not promote neurodegeneration. *Stroke* 2003;34:537–543.
38. Gardell SJ, Ramjit DR, Stabilito II, Fujita T, Lynch JJ, Cuca GC, Jain D, Wang S, Tung J, Mark GE, Shebuski RJ. Effective thrombolysis without marked plasminemia after bolus intravenous administration of vampire bat salivary plasminogen activator in rabbits. *Circulation* 1991;84:244–253.
39. Montoney M, Gardell S, Marder VJ. Comparison of the bleeding potential of vampire bat salivary plasminogen activator versus tissue plasminogen activator in an experimental rabbit model. *Circulation* 1995;91:1540–1544.
40. Hare, TR, Gardell SJ. Vampire bat salivary plasminogen activator promotes robust lysis of plasma clots in a plasma milieu without causing fluid phase plasminogen activation. *Thromb Haemost* 1992;68:165–169.
41. Mellott MJ, Ramjit DR, Stabilito II, Hare TR, Senderak ET, Lynch JJ, Gardell SJ. Vampire bat salivary plasminogen activator evokes minimal bleeding relative to tissue-type plasminogen activator as assessed by a rabbit cuticle bleeding time model. *Thromb Haemost* 1994;73:478–483.
42. Hacke W, Albers G, Al-Rawi Y, et al. for The DIAS Study Group. The Desmoteplase in Acute Ischemic Stroke Trial (DIAS). *Stroke* 2005;36. In press.
43. Gardell ST. The search for the ideal thrombolytic agent: maximize the benefit and minimize the risk. *Toxicol Pathol* 1993;21:190–198.

44. Schleuning, W-D. Vampire bat plasminogen activator DSPA-Alpha-1 (Desmoteplase): a thrombolytic drug optimized by natural selection. *Heamostasis* 2001;31:118–122.
45. Sakharav DV, Barrett-Bergshoeff M, Hekkenberg RT, Rijken DC. Fibrin-specificity of a plasminogen activator affects the efficiency of fibrinolysis and responsiveness to ultrasound: comparison of nine plasminogen activators in vitro. *Thromb Haemost* 1999;81:601–12.
46. Witt W, Mass B, Baldas B, Hildebrand M, Donner P, Schleuning W-D: Coronary thrombolysis with *Desmodus* salivary plasminogen activator in dogs. *Circulation* 1995;9:91–96.
47. Morimoto N, Hashimoto H, Kosaka F. Effect of heparin-urokinase on brain damage induced by cerebral ischemia in dogs. *Stroke* 1989;20:154, (abstr).
48. Barsan WG, Brott TG, Olinger CP, et al. Identification and entry of the patient with acute cerebral infarction. *Ann Emerg Med* 1988;17:1192–1195.
49. Alexander, LF, Yamamoto Y. Ayoubi S. et al. Efficacy of tissue plasminogen activator in the lysis of thrombosis of the cerebral venous sinus. *Neurosurgery* 1990;26:559–564.
50. Segal R, Dejouny M, Nelson D, et al. Local urokinase treatment for spontaneous intracerebral hematoma. *Clin Res* 1982;30:412A, (abstr).
51. Weinstein PR, Anderson GG, Telles DA. Neurological deficit and cerebral infarction after temporary middle cerebral artery occlusion in unanesthesized cats. *Stroke* 1986;17:318–324.
52. Boisvert DP, Gelb AW, Tang C, et al. Brain tolerance to middle cerebral artery occlusion during hypotension in primates. *Surg Neurol* 1989;31:6–13.
53. Collins RC, Dobkin BH, Choi DW. Selective vulnerability of the brain: New insights into the pathophysiology of stroke. *Ann Intern Med* 1989;110:992–1000.
54. Crowell RM, Olsson Y, Klatzo I et al. Temporary occlusion of the middle cerebral artery in the monkey: Clinical and pathological observations. *Stroke* 1970;1:439–448.
55. Penar PL, Greer CA. The effect of intravenous tissue-type plasminogen activator in a rat model of embolic cerebral ischemia. *Yale J Biol Med* 1987;60:233–243.
56. Kissel P, Chchrazi B, Seibert JA, et al. Digital angiographic quantification of blood flow dynamics in embolic stroke treated with tissue-type plasminogen activator. *J Neurosurg* 1987;67:399–405.
57. Watson BD, Prado R, Dietrich W, et al. Mitigation of evolving cortical infarction in rats by recombinant tissue plasminogen activator following photochemically induced thrombosis. In: Raichle ME, Powers WJ eds. *Cerebrovascular Diseases*. New York: Raven 1987;317–330.
58. Papadopulous SM, Chandler WF, Salamat MS, et al. Recombinant human tissue-type plasminogen activator therapy in acute thromboembolic stroke. *J Neurosurg* 1987;67:394–398.
59. Chechraza BB, Seibert JA, Kissel P. Evaluation of recombinant tissue plasminogen activator in embolic stroke. *Neurosurgery* 1989;24:355–360.
60. Phillips DA, Fisher M, Smith TW, et al. The safety and angiographic efficacy of tissue plasminogen activator in a cerebral embolization model. *Ann Neurol* 1988;23:391–394.
61. Phillips DA, Davis MA, Fisher M. Selective embolization and clot dissolution with tPA in the internal carotid artery circulation of the rabbit. *Am J Neuradiol* 1988;9:899–902.
62. Bednar MM, McAuliffe M, Raymond S, et al. Tissue plasminogen activator reduces brain injury in a rabbit model of thromboembolic stroke. *Stroke* 1990;21:1705–1709.
63. Terashi A, Kobayashi Y, Katayama Y, et al. Clinical effects and basic studies of thrombolytic therapy on cerebral thrombosis. *Semin Thromb Hemost* 1990;16:236–241.

5 Combination of Thrombolytic Therapy With Neuroprotectants

James C. Grotta, MD *and Lise A. Labiche,* MD

Contents

INTRODUCTION

Thrombolysis is the first scientifically established treatment for acute ischemic stroke, but we now need to build on that success. One possible way this might be accomplished is by combining thrombolysis with neuroprotection (*see* Chapter 3). Such combination therapy might reduce complications of thrombolysis, especially hemorrhage, by protecting damaged endothelium or reducing the volume of tissue necrosis. It might also prevent secondary injury associated with reperfusion. Finally, it might augment the benefit of thrombolysis by extending the time window before irreversible damage occurs. This chapter explores the rationale behind combination therapy and describe laboratory and clinical results to date.

From: *Current Clinical Neurology: Thrombolytic Therapy for Acute Stroke, Second Edition*
Edited by: P. D. Lyden © Humana Press Inc., Totowa, NJ

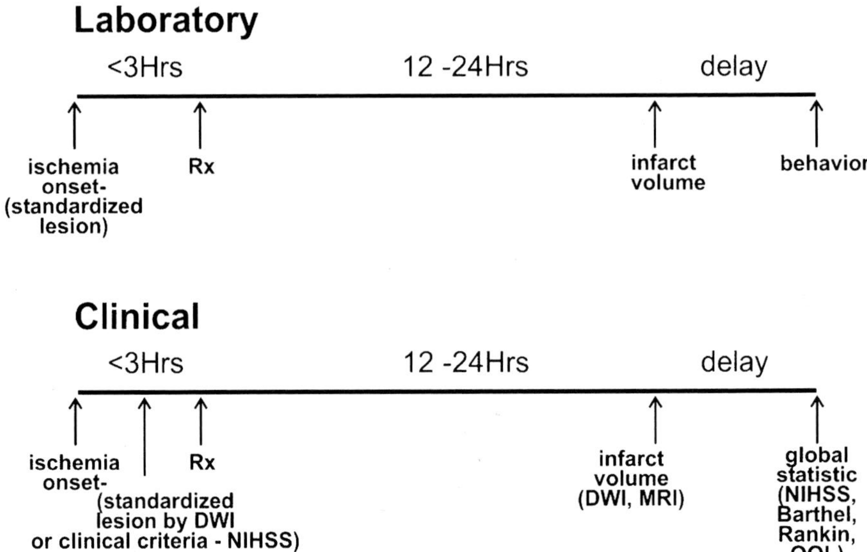

Fig. 1. Paradigm for most stroke therapy evaluations in laboratory animals *(top)* vs humans *(bottom)*.

RATIONALE FOR COMBINATION THROMBOLYSIS AND NEUROPROTECTION

Failure of Neuroprotective Drugs Alone in Clinical Trials

Despite their consistent positive effect when used in animal models of focal ischemia, when used alone in clinical trials, neuroprotective drugs have so far been ineffective. There are many explanations for these failures, the most obvious being excessive delay to starting therapy, poor selection of patients, inadequate doses, insufficient statistical power, and unfortunate selection of end points. As depicted in Fig. 1 (top), in laboratory studies of neuroprotective drugs in animal stroke models, we produce a standardized amount of injury. We start therapy within 3 h, usually within 1 h or so. We use large doses because our models may be insensitive to side effects that may limit dosing in elderly fragile stroke patients. We measure infarct volume, and then we employ a battery of behavioral outcomes. Our clinical trials should follow the same paradigm (Fig. 1, bottom), but so far have failed to do so. Let us examine these differences between the laboratory and clinical trials more closely.

The most important lesson of our attempts to model stroke in the lab and then investigate experimental therapies is the brief time window we have for effective neuronal salvage by either reperfusion or neuroprotection. The only conclusive positive clinical study of reperfusion (the National Institute of Neurological

Disorders and Stroke [NINDS] recombinant tissue plasminogen activator [rt-PA] trial) was exactly predicted by animal models; reperfusion must occur and therefore the patient must be treated within 3 h. All studies with longer time windows have failed. With regards to neuroprotection, calcium influx into neurons, as detected by its binding to calmodulin, correlates very well with ultimate cell death and functional outcome, and has been the target of many of our neuroprotective therapies. In all of our models, calcium binding to calmodulin becomes maximal within 2 h, so that the time window at least for the early events related to calcium after ischemia is very short *(1)*. Most of the various drugs we have tested in the laboratory need to be started early in order to produce neuroprotection. In the case of lubeluzole, when started 15 or 30 min after occlusion, or even up to an hour, we found some benefit. Beyond that there was no effect. With *N-tert*-butyl-α-phenylnitrone (PBN), a very effective spintrap agent, we can get some effect up to 2 h, and some combinations of neuroprotective drugs can be effective when started out to 2 h after stroke onset. There are more than 100 studies in the literature that show the efficacy of the glutamate antagonist MK-801. A random sampling of these could find none in which MK-801 could be given beyond 2 h and still reduce damage. Yet, in clinical trials of neuroprotection carried out so far, the drug been started within 4 h in only a small proportion of patients. Most trials have recruited patients 4–24 h after stroke onset.

In addition to starting our therapies earlier, we need to focus our clinical trials on those populations of patients that we think are going to respond to therapy, and then we can expand our indications beyond that point. That was the successful strategy employed by the NINDS rt-PA investigators by demonstrating efficacy in the best candidates (i.e., those treated within 3 h). In addition to those arriving in time to receive treatment early, other good candidates for neuroprotection, as in the lab, are those with a standardized amount of brain injury. Standardizing the infarct might be done through imaging, but right now, the easiest way to standardize our patient population is through putting limits on the National Institutes of Health Stroke Scale (NIHSS) that we use to allow patients into the trial, excluding those with mild strokes who are likely to recover spontaneously, and those with devastatingly severe strokes who are not likely to improve. Depending on the mechanism of action of the drug (i.e., antagonists of receptors not present in white matter), we might also try to exclude subcortical strokes.

The choice of end points is also critical. Whether infarct volume will be a surrogate measure of outcome remains to be seen. However, now that we have effective therapy, it is interesting to look back and compare the responses of rt-PA in animals to those inhumans. There are some striking similarities. Work from Zhang and colleagues *(2)* found that in a rat model, rt-PA is associated with a 56% improvement in the neurological score. In the NINDS trial in stroke patients, the drug was associated with a 62% improvement in functional outcome. In the laboratory studies, rt-PA reduced infarct volume by about 33% and

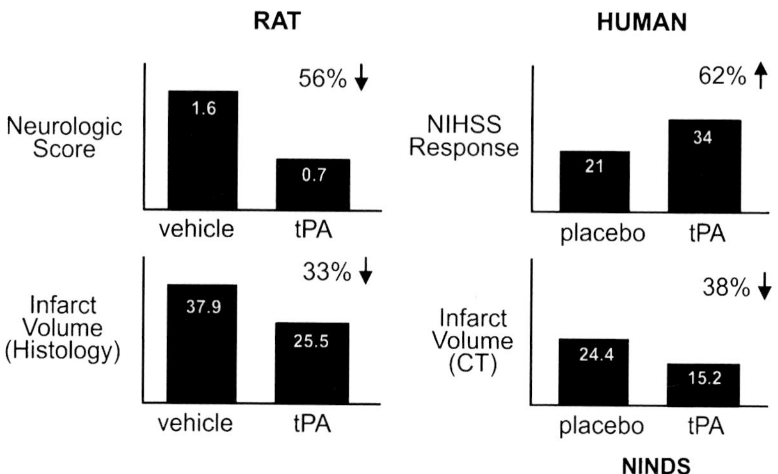

Fig. 2. Effect of t-PA in rats *(left column)* and humans *(right column)* on clinical outcome *(top row)* and infarct volume *(bottom row)*.

in the NINDS clinical trial, rt-PA reduced infarct volume by about 38% (Fig. 2). It is going to be very important, as we develop positive therapies, to look back at what our experience was in the laboratory and see what parts of the laboratory experience were most useful in deciding whether these drugs work or not. The rt-PA data suggest that our laboratory models are accurate not only in predicting the time window for effective treatment, but also for predicting the relative magnitude of effect. Furthermore, it appears that our behavioral and functional outcomes are at least as good and probably even more sensitive at detecting response to therapy than just simply measuring infarct volume.

In the laboratory, we use a battery of functional outcomes. The only trial to employ this approach was also the only positive trial (i.e., the NINDS rt-PA study). In that trial, we used the global statistic, which combines a number of different outcome measures. The global statistic is not that difficult to understand *(3)*. Consider a portrait artist; each angle gives a different perspective of the subject. One would not consider completing a portrait by painting from only one angle. Similarly, a global test that combines several different measures, each one evaluating a different but related response to therapy, is likely to give a more complete (and perhaps more sensitive) representation of the results.

Even if we take into consideration all these features of our clinical trials, and do *post-hoc* analyses of the neuroprotective trials carried out to date, it is clear that when used alone, neuroprotective drugs produce at best only a weak signal. In many of the trials with 6 h time windows (the shortest time windows yet studied with reasonably large numbers of patients), most notably the trials of aptiganel, clomethiazole, and lubeluzole, there was at best only a suggestion of benefit at the highest dose levels when imbalances in stroke severity were corrected by limiting analysis to those patients with more standardized insults. Attempting to make any extrapolations about efficacy from the phase II data in relatively small numbers of patients has proved consistently misleading when the phase III data were examined. These observations indicate that the effect of any one of these drugs alone is likely to be small, requiring a large sample size to detect a small difference between groups, and that this difference might be easily overwhelmed by small flaws in the study design or imbalances in the type of patients randomized.

An analogy would be a weak radio signal. Imagine yourself on a remote country road late at night trying to pull in a distant radio station. The music fades in and out. How might the reception be made clearer? One way of course is to drive closer to the signal. In a clinical trial, the analogy would be by moving the treatment closer to the time of onset (i.e., shortening the time window). Only as you move closer to the signal and the music gets clearer do you realize that what you had thought was reasonably good reception was really filled with interference. The other way to make the music clearer is to make the signal stronger; in that way the music may be clear at a greater distance. The clinical trial analogy would be by making the treatment more powerful. One way to do this is to combine treatments together, in this case to combine neuroprotective drugs together or with thrombolysis.

In order to justify combination therapy, the two treatments must have advantages over either one alone. There are at least three reasons why adding reperfusion might increase the effect of neuroprotection over what is achieved by neuroprotection alone. First, by increasing blood flow to threatened penumbral regions, reperfusion therapies might increase the delivery of concomitantly administered neuroprotective drugs to these target regions. Second, the fate of penumbral tissue is proportional to the depth and duration of blood-flow reduction. By limiting the depth of hypoperfusion early after the onset of ischemic injury, reperfusion therapies might reduce cellular necrosis and maintain a larger amount of ischemic brain tissue in a penumbral or salvageable state, which might be ameliorated by concomitant neuroprotective drugs. Finally, because reperfusion and neuroprotection are complementary in their mechanisms of action, adding reperfusion might produce a therapeutic effect that could not be achieved even with maximal doses of neuroprotectives.

Reperfusion Injury

Just as concomitant thrombolysis might uncover the therapeutic efficacy of neuroprotective drugs, adding neuroprotective drugs to thrombolytics might reduce side effects and secondary injury associated with reperfusion.

Although their overall effect is positive, drugs that produce reperfusion, especially thrombolytics, have well-known adverse effects. These include bleeding into ischemic regions or aggravation of infarct-related cerebral edema, both likely the result of increased hydrostatic pressure applied to a damaged blood–brain barrier (Fig. 3). Plasminogen activators themselves may also increase vascular and neuronal injury through up-regulation of matrix metalloproteinases (MMPs) *(4)*. These devastating side effects of thrombolysis might be prevented or reduced by drugs that protect the integrity of the vascular endothelium. Such drugs might include free radical scavengers or anti-adhesion molecules, which prevent leukocyte-mediated injury, or MMP inhibitors.

A less well-understood adverse consequence of reperfusion is cytotoxicity associated with reperfusion of moderately injured brain tissue. There are several explanations for this so-called reperfusion injury. First, it has been shown that reperfusion is associated with a secondary wave of glutamate and other neurotransmitter release and consequent movement of calcium intracellularly resulting in excitotoxicity *(5)*. Second, restoration of blood flow may be sufficient to allow synthesis of damaging proteins and other cytokines. Third, reperfusion may supply oxygen to ischemic regions that provides a substrate for peroxidation of lipids and free radical formation *(6)*.

We have been able to demonstrate reperfusion injury in a rat model of moderate ischemia produced by tandem occlusion of the ipsilateral common carotid and middle cerebral arteries (MCAs) (Fig. 4) *(7)*. The figure shows that opening the MCA up and allowing reperfusion following 2–5 h of MCA occlusion is associated with substantial infarction when measured after 24 h, whereas leaving the MCA permanently occluded was associated with very little damage even if histological evaluation was deferred up to 1 wk to allow for the appearance of delayed cell death. This reperfusion injury could be ameliorated by lubeluzole, but even more strikingly by the spin-trap agent PBN and the protein synthesis inhibitor cyclohexamide. These results suggest that reperfusion injury may have an inflammatory basis and suggest that combining reperfusion with appropriate neuroprotective agents, which achieve therapeutic levels by the time the artery recanalizes, might improve the outcome beyond what can be achieved by thrombolysis alone.

LABORATORY STUDIES OF COMBINED NEUROPROTECTION AND THROMBOLYSIS

One of the first studies of combination neuroprotection with reperfusion showed that calcium entry into neurons continued and actually increased upon reopening the MCA after 60 min of occlusion. The noncompetitive glutamate antagonist MK-801, which blocks the *N*-methyl D-aspartate (NMDA)-associated ion channel, partially but incompletely reduced calcium influx, and the

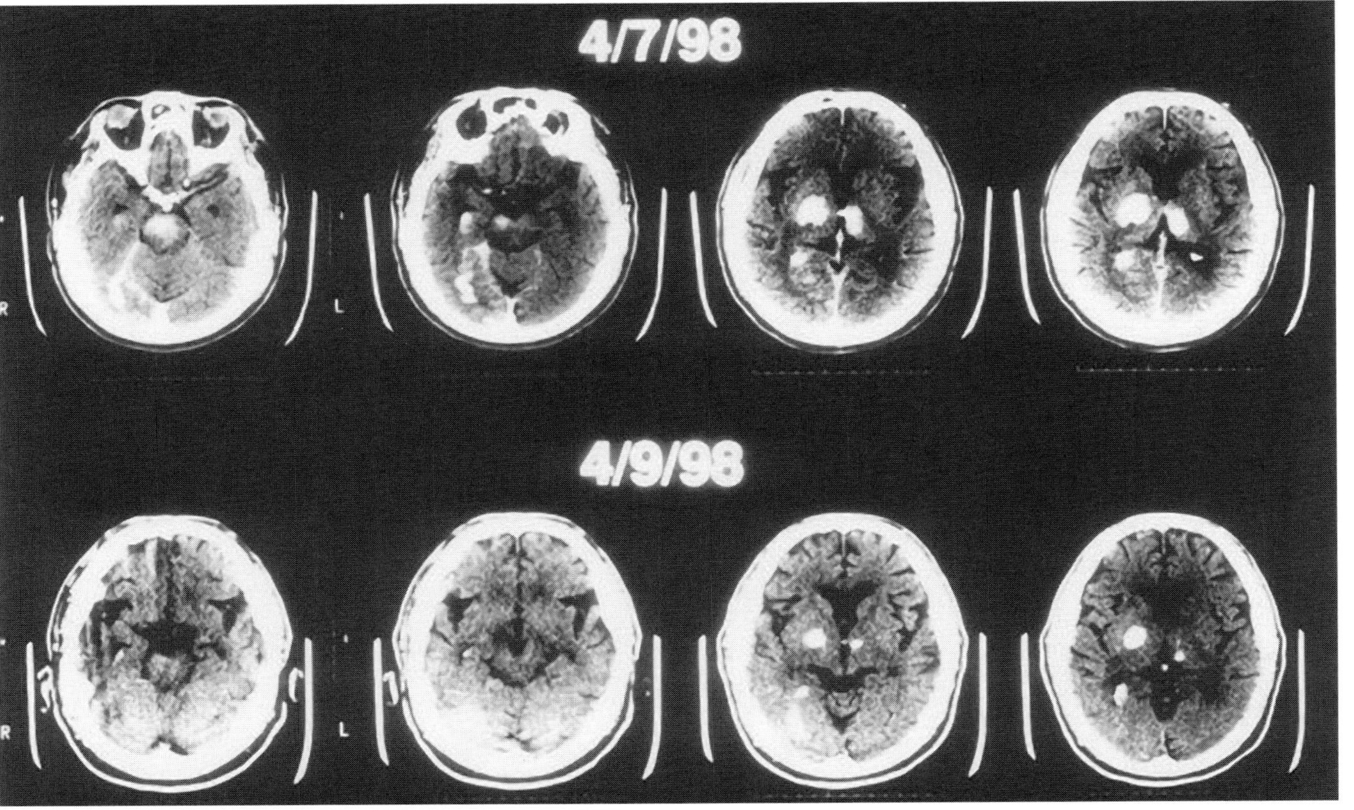

Fig. 3. *(Top)*Computed tomography (CT) scan immediately following arteriography and intra-arterial clot lysis in a patient with basilar thrombosis. Note contrast enhancement in pons, thalami, and right posterior cerebral artery territory.
(Bottom) Repeat CT 2 d later showing hemorrhagic conversion in the same areas. This is one type of reperfusion injury owing to disrupted blood–brain barrier.

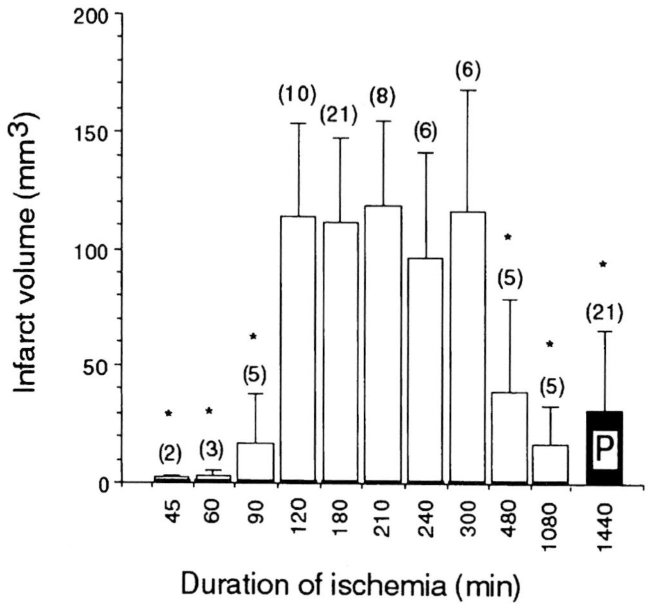

Fig, 4. Demonstration of reperfusion injury (i.e., greater damage associated with reperfusion compared to permanent occlusion), in a rat model of middle cerebral artery occlusion *(7)*. Note increasing infarct volume with increasing duration of ischemia up to 300 min. However, longer ischemia, or permanent occlusion (P), results in less damage. Numbers in parentheses = number of animals at each duration of ischemia.

combination of MK-801 and the voltage gated ion channel blocker nimodipine completely normalized the intracellular calcium signal (Fig. 5) *(8)*.

We have studied the combination of reperfusion and neuroprotection as well. In our model, reperfusion is augmented after temporary MCA occlusion by administering diaspirin crosslinked hemoglobin (DCLHb). DCLHb is an ideal hemodiluting agent. It is a stable dimer of human hemoglobin that does not dissociate and has an oxygen affinity similar to blood, but does not increase whole blood viscosity as does a comparable volume of red blood cells. It can be given as an intravenous (iv) infusion.

In our model, blood is exchanged for DCLHb to achieve a hematocrit reduction to about 30%. Treating animals with DCLHb beginning 15 min after various durations of MCA occlusion followed by reperfusion doubled the time the MCA could be occluded without resulting in ischemic damage (Fig. 6) *(9)*. Adding lubeluzole, which limits the production of nitric oxide (NO) following glutamate release, decreased the volume of infarct eventually produced, regardless of the duration of ischemia.

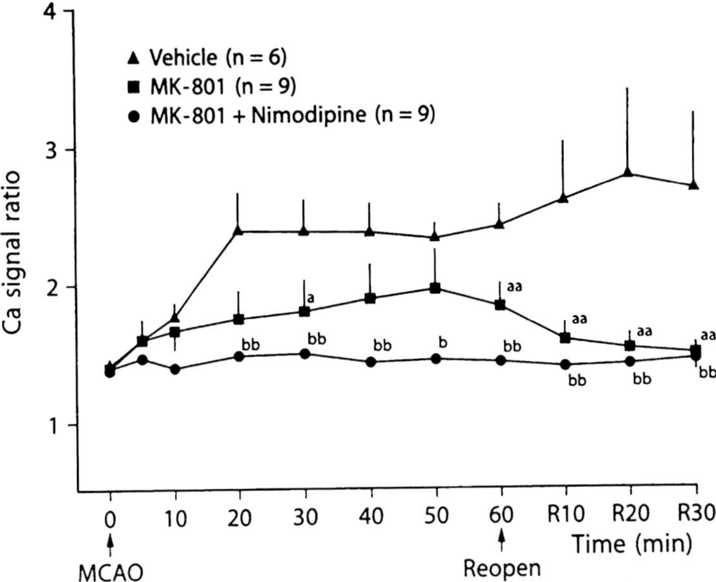

Fig. 5. Intracellular calcium, a marker of ischemic injury, in animals treated with the noncompetitive glutamate antagonist MK-801, alone or in combination with the voltage-gated calcium channel blocker Nimodipine, compared to controls *(8)*.

This experiment demonstrates the effect of adding complementary therapies. DCLHb, which increased perfusion and oxygenation after an infarct, increased the therapeutic window by maintaining injured tissue in a reversible penumbral state for a longer period of time. Lubeluzole blocked some of the key intracellular perturbations leading to irreversible injury in this penumbral region, thus reducing the ultimate volume of infarcted tissue.

Other studies have more directly examined the role of combining neuroprotection with thrombolysis. Such studies are limited by the paucity of autologous clot animal models in which to test thrombolytic drugs. One of the first such studies was carried out by Zivin and colleagues *(10,11)* in the rabbit embolism model. The rabbit model involves a simple cutdown in the neck, occlusion of the external carotid artery, and implanting a cannula in the common carotid artery to inject particles. After the surgery is complete, the animal is awake and unanesthetized, so many aspects of physiology that might influence neuroprotection, such as a blood pressure, body temperature, and blood gases, are under normal physiological regulation.

To study ischemic stroke, blood is taken from a donor animal, allowed to form clots, and injected into the carotid circulation. This produces clots in end vessels

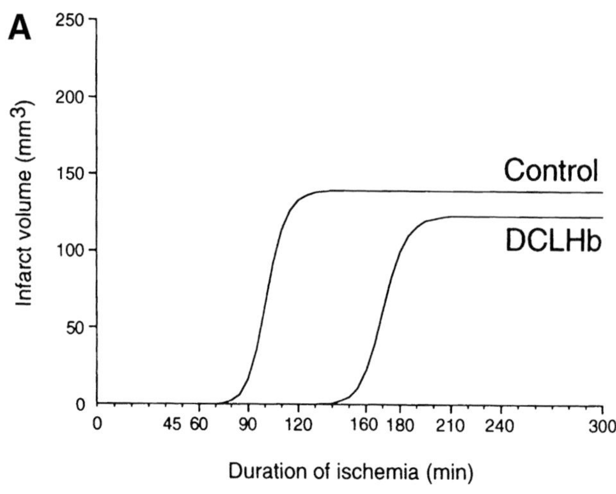
A
Infarct volume (mm3)
250
200
150
100
50
0
Control
DCLHb
0
45 60
90
120
160 180
210
240
300
Duration of ischemia (min)

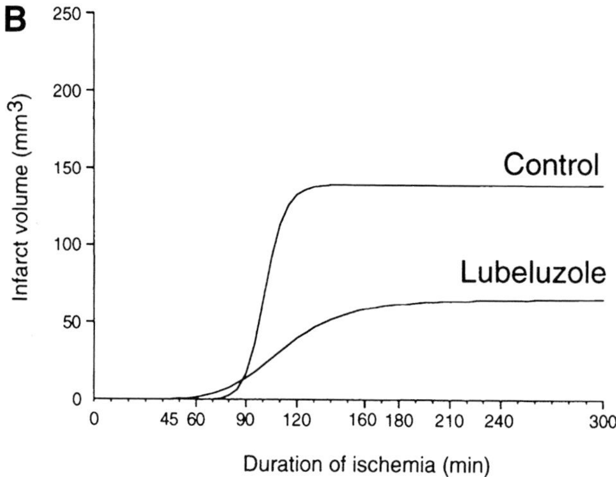
B
Infarct volume (mm3)
250
200
150
100
50
0
Control
Lubeluzole
0
45 60
90
120
160 180
210
240
300
Duration of ischemia (min)

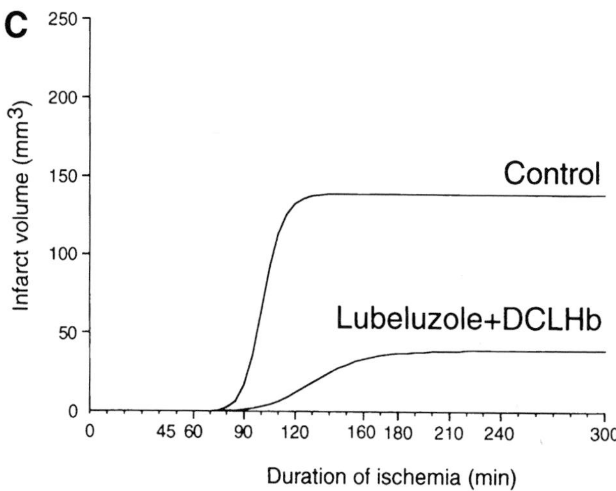
C
Infarct volume (mm3)
250
200
150
100
50
0
Control
Lubeluzole+DCLHb
0
45 60
90
120
160 180
210
240
300
Duration of ischemia (min)

in the brain. Tracer amounts of radioactive microspheres are injected with the clots and are used to measure the specific activity of the brain and to determine how many clots lodge in the brain. The result is small infarcts in random locations throughout the brain.

Data are analyzed by plotting the weight of microspheres, which is a measure of the amount of clot in the brain vs percentage of animals displaying neurological deficits (Fig. 7). There are two parameters of interest in this curve. One is the position parameter, which is the mean weight of clots the animal can tolerate. The other is the slope parameter, which is an estimate of the population variance. If the curve shifts to the right, it implies that the animals can tolerate more clots. A change in the slope of the curve means that something else has happened. Shifts in the slope typically occur when two effects are taking place at the same time. For example, a drug might provide neuroprotection but simultaneously alter blood pressure. One problem with this model is that there is a ceiling effect. Animals given high doses of clots often die before they can be treated.

Figure 7 illustrates the effect of rt-PA alone in this model *(10)*. Curve A is the control and shows that the untreated animals tolerated about 3 mg of clots. Curves B, C, and D are the results of treating with rt-PA at 15, 45, and 30 min after clots were injected. They show that the treated animals tolerated about three times more clots than the control animals. However, if treatment was delayed for 1 h, the curve was not significantly different from the control curve. This was the first demonstration in a clinically applicable model that rt-PA reduced neurological damage.

This model was used in a study of rt-PA and MK-801, which is a glutamate antagonist *(11)*. MK-801 was given at 1 mg/kg 5 min after embolization. rt-PA was given at 1 mg/kg at various later times. MK-801 alone had no significant effect. rt-PA alone at 60 min after embolization nearly doubled the amount of clots the animal could tolerate. Giving both drugs at 60 min was more effective than rt-PA alone, even though MK-801 was ineffective alone. Delaying rt-PA treatment to 90 min did not produce a therapeutic effect.

This model was also used to study combination therapy with an anti- intercellular adhesion molecule (ICAM) monoclonal antibody plus rt-PA *(12)*. Whereas the rt-PA/MK-801 study was designed to increase the amount of clot the animal could tolerate, the rt-PA/anti-ICAM study attempted to increase the window of time until start of treatment. Data showed that the combination could extend the

Fig. 6. **(A)** (*opposite page*) The blood substitute diaspirin crosslinked hemoglobin (DCLHb) prolongs the duration of ischemia (temporary middle cerebral artery occlusion) before ischemic damage occurs *(9)*. **(B)** Lubeluzole reduces the volume of infarction regardless of duration of ischemia *(9)*. **(C)** The combination of DCLHb and lubeluzole has greater effect than either one alone (**A** or **B**) *(9)*.

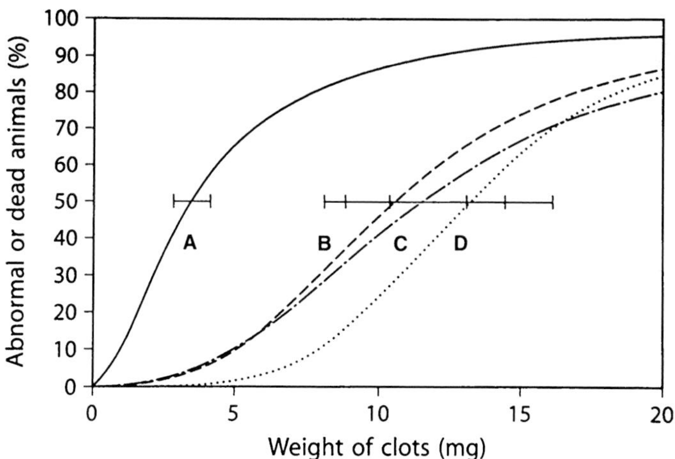

Fig. 7. Amount of injected blood clot needed to produce neurological damage in animals treated with various doses of tissue plasminogen activator (**B**, **C**, or **D**) vs controls (**A**) *(10,11)*. *See* text for details.

time window to 2 h, whereas neither drug alone was effective when treatment was initiated at 2 h. This is evidence for a positive interaction of the combination.

More recently, Zhang and colleagues *(2)* have developed an autologous clot occlusion of the MCA in rats. Treatment with rt-PA alone improved neurological deficits and reduced mean infarct volume compared to controls when the drug was started within 2 h of arterial occlusion, but had no benefit when treatment was delayed out to 4 h. The anti-CD18 antibody, which presumably prevents white blood cell adhesion to ischemic endothelium and consequent inflammatory damage to surrounding brain regions, had no effect when administered alone at either time point. However, when both rt-PA and the anti-CD18 antibody were given together, there was substantial reduction of neurological deficit even when combined treatment was delayed out to 4 h *(2)*. Thus, the synergism of this particular combination was especially notable in extending the time window of effective therapy.

CLINICAL STUDIES OF COMBINED NEUROPROTECTION AND THROMBOLYSIS

To date, only three studies specifically designed to evaluate the effect of combining thrombolysis and neuroprotection have been completed, and two were terminated prematurely. Lubeluzole was the first potentially neuroprotective agent to be evaluated in a dedicated combination trial with t-PA. Patients who qualified for and received intravenous t-PA within 3 h of symptom onset were randomly allocated 1:1 to lubeluzole (7.5 mg iv over 1 h, then continuous

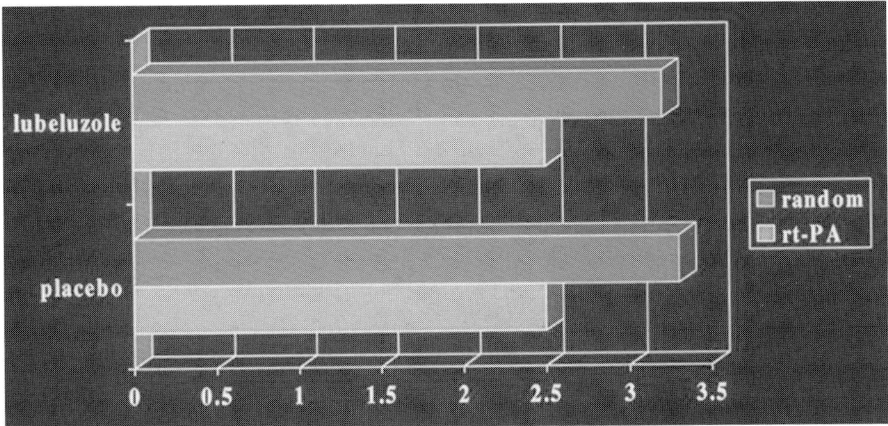

Fig. 8. Time from stroke symptom onset to treatment with lubeluzole or t-PA *(13)*.

5 d infusion of 10 mg/d) or placebo *(13)*. Lubeluzole infusion was started before the end of the 1-h t-PA infusion so that therapeutic blood levels would be achieved by the time reperfusion from the rt-PA was likely to occur. The study was designed to evaluate the safety of the combination, particularly to ensure that the incidence of hemorrhage was not increased (and perhaps decreased), and served as a companion to a larger evaluation of lubeluzole given as monotherapy 8 h following stroke onset. Eighty-nine patients were enrolled prior to the early trial termination based on the negative results of the concurrent lubeluzole phase III trial. In the enrolled patients (45% of the planned population), t-PA and study drug were administered at a mean of 2.5 and 3.2 h from symptom onset, respectively (Fig. 8). There were no significant differences in mortality (26%), intracerebral hemorrhage (ICH) (10%), serious adverse events (51%), or functional outcomes (Barthel Index) between lubeluzole and placebo. These results demonstrate the safety and feasibility of linking ultra-early neuroprotection with thrombolysis, however the premature stoppage of enrollment led to a study underpowered to detect efficacy.

The second trial to determine whether the effect of thrombolysis may be augmented by pharmacological neuroprotection evaluated the use of a γ-aminobutyric acid (GABA) agonist, clomethiazole (CLASS-T) trial *(14)*. Whereas a large study of clomethiazole monotherapy compared to placebo was conducted, this smaller pilot study was designed to test the combination of rt-PA given within 3 h, and clomethiazole given within 12 h of stroke onset. This study randomized patients in a double-blind fashion to receive t-PA and either 68 mg/kg clomethiazole or placebo over 24 h. The study included 97 patients given clomethiazole and 93 patients given placebo; all patients received t-PA first according to NINDS protocol. Overall, there was no benefit seen. In the patients with the worst strokes however, there was a possible beneficial effect. These results suggest that clomethiazole may augment the beneficial effect of t-PA in patients with large strokes. Because administration of clomethiazole was not required prior to completion of t-PA infusion, many patients received clomethiazole several hours after thrombolysis. This limitation highlights the need to require linkage of t-PA and neuroprotectant administration in future trial design of combination approaches.

The most recently completed combination trial is AMPA Receptor Antagonist Treatment in Stroke plus t-PA (ARTIST+). Enrollment has just been terminated prematurely in this trial of YM-872 and t-PA based on an interim futility analysis. This multicenter, randomized, double-blind, placebo-controlled trial was designed to compare the efficacy of YM-872 plus t-PA to that of placebo plus t-PA. Patients with acute hemispheric ischemic stroke and a moderate to severe deficit (NIHSS score from 7 to 23, LOC 0 to 1) treated with standard protocol t-PA were eligible. The planned enrollment was 600 patients and more than 400 patients were enrolled. The drug was started before the end of t-PA infusion and continued for 24 h. Primary efficacy/outcome measures include neurological function and disability scales. Although final results are not available, interim analyses showed no benefit to this combination therapy. The abandonment of this very well-designed trial is disappointing. The absence of positive results was most likely caused by a lack of a substantial magnitude of efficacy rather than trial design because linked t-PA and study drug administration was enforced.

Neuroprotective trials are now being carried out that allow treatment with rt-PA if clinically indicated, so that some patients in these studies will receive combination therapy. One example of such a trial is the Glycine Antagonist in Neuroprotection (GAIN) Americas study of gavestinel, a novel glycine site antagonist at the NMDA receptor complex *(15)*. The GAIN Americas trial randomized 1367 patients within 6 h of stroke onset and concomitant treatment with intravenous t-PA was allowed in eligible patients. Treatment consisted of an 800 mg loading dose plus five maintenance doses (200 mg every 12 h) of gavestinel or placebo. Patients were stratified at randomization by age (75 or > 75 yr) and initial stroke severity (NIHSS 2–5, 6–13, >13). Patients were well matched for baseline characteristics. Mean NIHSS was 12 and median time to treatment was 5.2 h. No statistically significant difference in mortality or 3-mo outcome measures (Barthel Index, mRS, or NIHSS score) was found between the groups. Subgroup analysis revealed a significant treatment benefit in younger patients with mild stroke (75 yr, NIHSS 2–5) that persisted even after adjustment for age, baseline NIHSS, use of t-PA, time to treat, and stroke subtype. However, no treatment effect was seen in either the t-PA treated patients (n = 333) or those treated within 4 h of onset (n = 244). However, since only a minority of stroke patients arrive in time to receive treatment within 3 h, studies like GAIN

Americas are not likely to have sufficient numbers of patients to evaluate the effect of combination treatment vs monotherapy.This can only be done if such studies are formally stratified, thereby forcing substantial numbers of patients into the combined treatment group. Other ongoing neuroprotectant trials that allow but do not require t-PA administration include hypothermia, spin-trap agents (NXY-059) and ONO-2506.

The disappointing results of combination cytoprotection/thrombolysis trials to date are extremely disappointing since these studies came closest to reproducing the experimental rat studies that consistently demonstrated benefit of neuroprotective drugs. The neutral results are likely a result of several factors including dose-limiting side effects (lubeluzole), as well as the modest efficacy of the individual cytoprotective drugs that have been tested in this fashion (YM-872, clomethiazole, gavistinel, and lubeluzole). The complexity of the ischemic cascade may necessitate pharmacological targeting of multiple levels in order to derive clinically apparent benefit. An ongoing trial of multimodal cytoprotective modalities in combination with intravenous thrombolysis is ongoing. A novel combination of combination of caffeine/ethanol (caffeinol) and hypothermia has demonstrated more robust neuroprotection than many other experimental and clinically relevant agents tested in the laboratory with a significant 83% reduction in infarct volume (Fig. 9). Extensive work has shown that combining intravenous t-PA with caffeinol imparts no increased risk of ICH in vivo, and no reduction of t-PA fibrinolytic activity in vitro *(16)*. An open-label, dose-escalation evaluation of caffeine and ethanol in acute ischemic stroke patients within 6 h of symptom onset has been completed, including patients treated with t-PA *(17)*. A dose has been identified that results in plasma levels that produce optimal therapeutic effect in animals (caffeine 5–10 mg/mL and ethanol 30–50 mg/dL) and that are clinically well tolerated by patients without any significant adverse effects. A pilot study designed to establish the feasibility and safety of administering both caffeinol and mild systemic hypothermia in acute ischemic stroke patients treated with intravenous t-PA, within 5 h of symptom onset (caffeinol within 4 h and hypothermia within 5 h) has just started. The target population includes those patients with cortical deficits with NIHSS score more than 7. The dosing schedule (caffeine 8 mg/kg and 10% ethanol 0.4 mg/kg) identified in the caffeinol dose-escalation trial will serve as the template. This trial addresses two critical factors in combination therapy trial design: forced early neuroprotectant administration linked with t-PA and application of multimodal treatment targeting multiple levels of the cascade.

CONCLUSION

Future clinical evaluation of combined neuroprotection and thrombolysis must focus on proper trial design to enhance the potential efficacy of treatment. Such

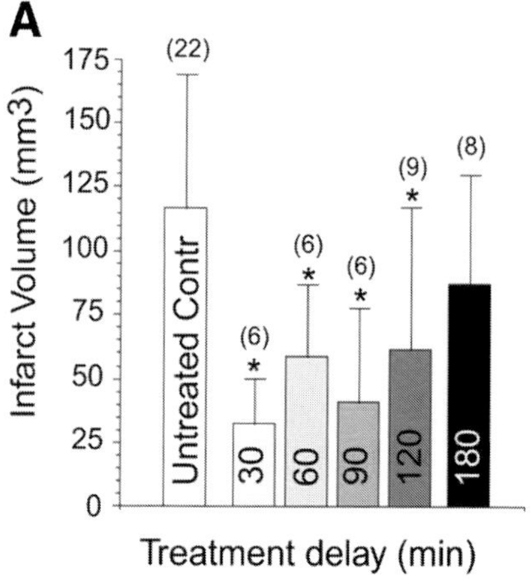

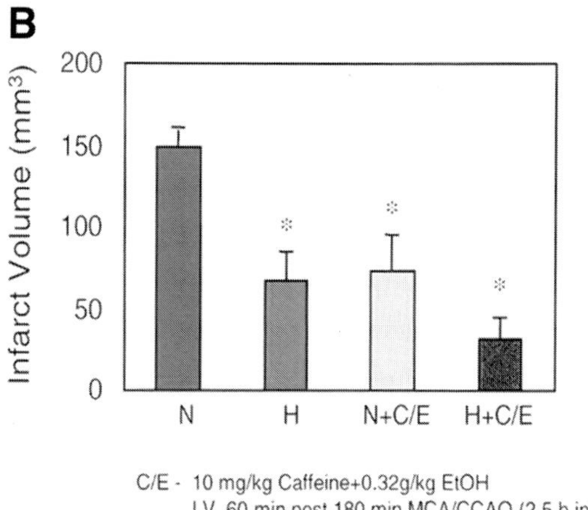

Fig. 9. **(A)** The effect of caffeinol, begun at various intervals after the onset of ischemia, on infarct volume in a rat middle cerebral artery (MCA) occlusion model. **(B)** Hypothermia to 35°. **(C)** Caffeinol, or the combination, on infarct volume in a rat MCA occlusion model *(16)*. *See* color insert following p.110.

factors include: early treatment, linkage of t-PA and neuroprotection, adequately powered sample size, homogenous populations, and multimodal approaches with synergistic agents. Additionally, neuroprotective modalities that may ameliorate the potential toxicity of t-PA should be sought, such as inhibitors of MMPs, thereby preventing both ischemic and reperfusion injury.

REFERENCES

1. DeGraba T, Ostrow P, Grotta J. Threshold of calcium disturbances after focal cerebral ischemia in rats: implications of the window of therapeutic opportunity. *Stroke* 1993;24:1212–1217.
2. Zhang RL, Zhang ZG, Chopp M. Increased therapeutic efficacy with rt-PA and anti-CD18 antibody treatment of stroke in the rat. *Neurology* 1999;52:273–279.
3. Tilley B, Marler J, Geller N, et al. for the NINDS rt-PA Stroke Trial Study Group. Use of a global test for multiple outcomes in stroke trials with application to the National Institute of Neurological Disorders and Stroke t-PA Trial. *Stroke* 1996;27:2136–2142.
4. Hosomi N, Lucero j, Heo JH, Koziol JA, Copeland BR, del Zoppo GJ. Rapid differential endogenous plasminogen activator expression after acute middle cerebral artery occlusion. *Stroke* 2001;32:1341–1348.
5. Matsumoto K, Lo EH, Pierce AR, Halpern EF, Newcomb R. Secondary elevation of extracellular neurotransmitter amino acids in the reperfusion phase following focal cerebral ischemia. *J Cereb Blood Flow Metab* 1996;16:114–124.
6. Traystman RJ, Kirsch JR, Koehler RC. Oxygen radical mechanism of brain injury following ischemia and reperfusion. *J Appl Physiol* 1991;71:1185–1195.
7. Aronowski J, Strong R, Grotta J. Reperfusion injury: demonstration of brain damage produced by reperfusion after transient focal ischemia in rats. *J Cereb Blood Flow Metab* 1997;17: 1048–1056.
8. Uematsu D, Greenberg JH, Reivich M, Karp A. In vivo measurement of cytosolic free calcium during cerebral ischemia and reperfusion. *Ann Neurol* 1988;24:420–428.
9. Aronowski J, Strong R, Grotta JC. Combined neuroprotection and reperfusion therapy for stroke: the effect of lubeluzole and diaspirin crosslinked hemoglobin in experimental focal ischemia. *Stroke* 1996;27:1571–1576.
10. Zivin JA, deGirolami U, Kochhar A, et al. A model for quantitative evaluation of embolic stroke therapy. *Brain Res* 1987;435:305–309.
11. Zivin JA, Mazzarella V. Tissue plasminogen activator plus glutamate antagonist improves outcome after embolic stroke. *Arch Neurol* 1991;48:1235–1238.
12. Bowes MP, Rothlein R, Fagan SC, et al. Monoclonal antibodies preventing leukocyte activation reduce experimental neurologic injury and enhance efficacy of thrombolytic therapy. *Neurology* 1995;45:815–819.
13. Grotta J. Combination therapy stroke trial: recombinant tissue-type plasminogen activator with/without lubeluzole. *Cerebrovasc Dis* 2001;12:258–263.
14. Lyden P, Jacoby M, Schim J, et al. The Clomethaizole Acute Stroke Study in tissue-type plasminogen activator-treated stroke (CLASS-T): final results. *Neurology* 2001;57(7): 1199–1205
15. Sacco RL, DeRosa JT, Haley C et al. for the GAIN Americas Investigators: Glycine antagonist in neuroprotection for patients with acute stroke: GAIN Americas: a randomized controlled trial. *JAMA* 2001;285:1719–1728.
16. Aronowski JA, Strong R, Shrizadi A, Grotta JC. Ethanol plus caffeine (caffeinol) for treatment of ischemic stroke: preclinical experience. *Stroke* 2003; 34:1246–1251.
17. Piriyawat P, Labiche LA, Burgin WS, Aronowski JA, Grotta JC. A pilot dose-escalation study of caffeine plus ethanol (caffeinol)in acute ischemic stroke. *Stroke* 2003; 34:1242–1245.

6 Pilot and Preliminary Studies of Thrombolytic Therapy for Stroke

Steven R. Levine, MD, *E. Clarke Haley,* MD, *and Patrick Lyden,* MD

Contents

INTRODUCTION

The demonstration that tissue plasminogen activator (t-PA) is clinically effective for acute ischemic stroke was based on many important studies over the past two decades that then led to groundbreaking preliminary clinical trials. This chapter highlights and discusses these studies and their historical significance. Thrombolytic therapy is an inherently attractive treatment for ischemic stroke based on the known pathological and angiographic substrates of ischemic cerebrovascular disease (*see* Chapters 1–3). The majority of acute ischemic strokes are the direct consequences of atherothrombosis or thromboembolism of a cerebral or precerebral artery (*see* Chapter 2). The critical event is usually the formation of an acute thrombus, so the rationale for thrombolytic treatment is to achieve arterial recanalization with a relatively safe agent soon enough to improve patient outcome.

From: *Current Clinical Neurology: Thrombolytic Therapy for Acute Stroke, Second Edition*
Edited by: P. D. Lyden © Humana Press Inc., Totowa, NJ

Timing thrombolytic therapy for stroke is key because a therapeutic window, measured in hours, is available for reperfusion-enhancing agents to maximize both efficacy and safety in the treatment (*see* Chapter 3). Correlation of the occlusive cerebral arterial lesion with clinical deficit has been noted in nearly 61 of 81 (75%) patients documented to have cerebral hemisphere infarctions studied within 6 h of symptom onset with cerebral angiography *(1)*1. Furthermore, the outcome of patients with angiographically proven middle cerebral artery (MCA) occlusions is poor when managed conservatively, as 30% die within 3 mo and an additional 38% survive with severe neurological deficits *(2)*. Clearly, aggressive strategies for the treatment of human stroke are necessary as there is a severe lack of tolerance of the brain to focal ischemia.

Although thrombolytic or fibrinolytic therapy was attempted in cerebrovascular disease three decades ago during the pre-computed tomography (CT) era, less than beneficial outcome was observed *(2,3)*. The pre-CT clinical studies of intravenous (iv) thrombolytic therapy for stroke were limited because they did not investigate truly acute ischemic stroke, assess recanalization, or assess clinical outcome independent of intracerebral hemorrhage (ICH). A brief review of these studies is presented as they are instructive for their limitations and results. More recent studies are then presented, including open label feasibility studies, followed by the preliminary controlled trials that set the stage for the definitive trials discussed in the next chapter.

INITIAL STUDIES OF THROMBOLYTIC THERAPY FOR ACUTE ISCHEMIC CEREBROVASCULAR DISEASE

Clinical Studies Without Computed Tomography

During the initial use of thrombolytic therapy for ischemic stroke *(6–8)* cerebrospinal fluid (CSF) analysis was used in most studies to exclude cerebral hemorrhage. However, CSF examination was not reliable for excluding ICH. In general, results of these trials were highly variable and frequently reported unacceptable rates of hemorrhage and death. Limitations of these pre-CT studies are summarized in Table 1. Summarizing all these trials, only 33 of 265 patients studied underwent pre- and post-treatment cerebral angiography. The size of the clot was unchanged in most patients, although only a small fraction of arteries completely recanalized. Only two of the early trials used a placebo group that would help distinguish between spontaneous and therapeutic thrombolysis *(9–10)*.

The first attempt to treat ischemic stroke using a thrombolysis was reported in 1958 by Sussman and Fitch *(11)*. They treated three patients with plasmin (fibrinolysin); one patient had moderate clinical improvement with recanalization of the MCA. The other two patients did not improve clinically despite one case of large cerebral vessel recanalization. Clifton reported a 45-yr-old woman with a hemiplegia of 3 d duration from a postoperative carotid artery thrombosis

Table 1

Thrombolytic Therapy for Presumed Ischemic Cerebrovascular Disease Pre-Computed Tomography: Major Series of Patients

Author (ref.)	*N*	*Thrombolytic agent*	*Ancillary*	*Outcome*
Herndon[a] *(13,14)*	27	Fibrinolysin over 3 d iv	Heparin, Dicoumarol	15% involved, 33% died, 4 systemic hemorrhages
Clarke *(6)*	10	Fibrinolysin up to 4 d		2 rapid complete recovery 3 rapid improvement, 2 died
Meyer[b] *(9)*	40 (randomized to thrombolytic or placebo)	Thrombolysin (iv plasmin) over 3 d	Anticoagulants	45% improved in each group 35% died in each group
Meyer[c] *(5,10)*	73 (randomized to thrombolytic or placebo, both administered heparin stroke-in-progression)	SK iv	Heparin	43% SK treated improved, 35% SK treated died
Fletcher[d] *(15)*	31	UK iv		No Improvement, SK iv Heparin, 4 with clinical ICH

[a]Duration symptoms: 2 h to 1 mo (3 treated $\leq$ 6 h).
[b]Only 1/10 treated $\leq$ 6 h, duration of symptoms = 3 h–1 mo
[c]All treated $\leq$ 72 h after symptom onset
[d]All treated $\leq$ 36 h after stroke onset (range 8–34 h)

(12). The clot was lysed after 15 min of plasmin therapy, but she died 48 h later (on Dicumarol and heparin) owing to a tracheal obstruction from a hematoma. Clifton also mentions that two cases of cerebral thrombosis were treated with plasmin (inadequate doses) without success. Two years later, Herndon et al. treated 13 patients within 3 d of presumed ischemic stroke onset (clear CSF) with bovine thrombolysin and anticoagulants*(13)*. Eight of 13 (62%) patients improved. Five patients died; however, there was no evidence for hemorrhagic infarction or ICH found at postmortem examinations.

Herndon et al. then reported 27 cases given fibrinolytic therapy for cerebral artery occlusion (CSF with more than 3000 red blood cells as a contraindication); diagnosis was confirmed by autopsy in 6 cases and by arteriography in 16 (Table 2) *(14)*. In addition, one case of retinal vein thrombosis and one case of bilateral cavernous sinus thrombosis were treated with fibrinolytic agents. Two of three patients treated died within 6 h (at 31 h and 3 d), both of whom had basilar artery thrombosis, whereas the third patient improved.

Ten patients with cerebrovascular thrombotic events treated with fibrinolytic agents (Table 2) were reported by Clark and Clifton*(6)*. Three patients treated by intra-arterial fibrinolysin all showed complete recanalization. One of these showed good clinical response but the other two died of local hematoma or a rebleeding aneurysm. Intravenous thrombolysis was performed in seven cases. Two (29%) completely recovered, three improved, and two were unchanged.

Meyer et al. used intra-arterial human thrombolysin, intravenous bovine thrombolysin, and anticoagulants in 14 patients *(4)*. Four of seven patients with internal carotid artery)–MCA distribution infarcts improved, two were unchanged, and one died. Of the five patients with vertebrobasilar disease, two improved (one then died of medical complications), and two were unchanged. Eleven of 14 patients underwent cerebral angiography; 3 showed clot dissolution, and 1 had presumed clot dissolution.

A pilot study was then reported by Meyer et al. who randomized 40 patients with occlusion of the carotid or MCA tree in a placebo-controlled trial using 200,000 U intravenous plasmin (thrombolysin) administered over 4 h daily for 3 d (Table 2)*(9)*. Thirty-four (85%) had angiography before treatment and eight (20%) had repeat arteriograms before hospital discharge. All cases were also treated with subcutaneous heparin followed by oral warfarin therapy. At 10 d there was no difference in outcome between placebo- and plasmin-treated groups when the subgroup with proven occlusive disease of the large vessels was analyzed. Of those eight patients with repeat angiography, six had no change, and two had partial recanalization (one in each treatment group). One patient who was administered plasmin and died 48 h after beginning treatment from a large hemorrhagic infarction had been given a loading dose of warfarin (30 mg) for 2 d in error.

Table 2
Thrombolytic Stroke Trials Incorporating Neuroimaging: Post-Computed Tomography Series

Author	*Year*	*n*	*Thrombolytic agent*	*Ancillary therapy*	*Outcome*
Hossmann *(38)*	1983	15	Ancrod	LMW dextran, mannitol	Improvement in neurologic deficit, no ICH, 60% 1-yr survival (47% in control group)
Fusjishima *(22)*	1988	143	iv UK for 1 to 7 d	62 also received DS	Moderate to marked improvement in 31% UK treated, in 61% UK + DS treated hemorrhagic events in 3.2% of UK + DS treated mortality 1.6%/2.5%
Del Zoppo *(25)*	1988	20	IA, UK, or SK up to 4 h	Heparin, hydroxyethyl starch in some patients	75% complete recanalization, 20% hemorrhagic transformation
Hacke *(23)*	1988	43	IA, UK, or SK up to 48 h	Heparin, hydroxyethyl starch	44% recanalized, 46% persistent occlusion, 9.3% hemorrhagic transformation
Mori *(26)*	1988	22	IA, UK	Variable: hypervolemic or isovolemic hemodilution, 10% iv glycerol, aspirin, heparin, or combination	45% immediate recanalization, 18% hemorrhagic infarction

Abbreviations: UK, urokinase; LMW, low molecular weight; ICH, intracranial hemorrhage; iv, intravenous; DS, dextran sulfate; IA, intra-arterial; SK, streptokinase.

Meyer et al. reported 73 patients with progressive stroke treated within 72 h of onset of symptoms with heparin (n = 36) or heparin plus streptokinase (SK) (n = 37) (6 h infusions, individually dosed after a dose-prediction test) in a randomized protocol (Table 2) *(5,10)*. Patients had to have a clear CSF and systolic blood pressure less than 180 mm Hg before inclusion. Arteriography was obtained on admission (demonstrating an occluded vessel in 35 patients) and repeated at 10 d if an occluded vessel was found initially. Twenty-one (58%) of 36 heparin-treated patients and (43%) of 37 SK- and heparin-treated patients improved, whereas 4 (11%) and 13 (35%) of the two groups, respectively, died. Statistical analysis was not performed. Clot lysis was demonstrated by repeat angiography or at autopsy in 10 patients (three heparin treated, seven treated with heparin plus SK). Autopsies on 13 of 17 who died (three controls, 10 in the SK group) showed 3 cerebral hemorrhages (all SK treated), 1 hemorrhagic infarction (SK treated), and 9 bland infarctions (all 3 controls and 6 SK treated).

Fletcher et al. reported results of a pilot study of intravenous urokinase (UK) in cerebral infarction involving 31 patients treated either with a single- or double-infusion period, each of 10 to 12 h (Table 2) *(15)*. Patients enrolled in the study had more severe neurological deficits than the average stroke patient observed at their institution. Angiography was performed before UK treatment in seven patients. One had no vascular lesion noted, and in two others the examination was unsatisfactory. Four patients had stenotic disease or occlusion of the MCA. One patient died from complication of a neck hematoma following traumatic carotid angiography. The investigators observed no instance of unequivocal clinical improvement attributable to treatment. Anecdotal pre-CT reports of thrombolytics for cerebrovascular disease continued as did a larger series with UK *(16)*.

In summary, arterial recanalization was shown in 31 to 100% of the patients in whom pre- and post-treatment angiography was performed. However, because of a discouraging number of ICH, enthusiasm for these agents dissipated.

EARLY POST-COMPUTED TOMOGRAPHY STUDIES

Advances in clinical and neuroimaging assessment of ischemic cerebrovascular disease combined with the expanding knowledge of the pathophysiology of human brain infarction led to a resurgence of enthusiasm for newer potentially safer thrombolytic agents and techniques in human ischemic stroke *(17)*. This renewed interest was greatly influenced by the animal studies outlined in Chapter 4. It was realized that earlier attempts initiated treatment too late (i.e., longer than 6 to 8 h and as long as beyond 2–3 d after the onset of symptoms). Beginning in the early 1980s, individual case reports documented clinical improvement from ischemic stroke following cerebral arterial recanalization with intra-arterial thrombolytic agents *(18–20)*.

Abe et al. studied stroke patients using UK (60,000 IU/d) for 7 d or placebo in a double-blind protocol. Improvement in two of three clinical outcome scales was noted in the UK-treated group *(21)*. Fujishima et al. reported on 143 patients with cerebral infarction treated with either UK (2.83×10^5 U iv over 6 h [$n = 81$] or a combination of UK-dextran sulfate [DS], 2.84×10^5 U plus 300 mg DS over 1 d [$n = 62$]) in a multicenter cooperative study*(22)*. Only 89% of the cases had head CT performed for stroke diagnosis and 30% had spinal taps. Overall, clinical improvement rate and safety was reported in 74% of UK-treated patients and 84% of the UK-dextran-treated patients.

From 1983 to May 1986, Hacke et al. treated 43 prospectively studied patients with intra-arterial UK or SK for angiographically documented vertebrobasilar artery territory thrombosis *(23)*. Heparin, 300 U/h, was routinely administered simultaneously with the thrombolytic agents and then administered at 1000 U/h intravenously with hydroxylethyl starch. All patients without recanalization died, whereas 14 (74%) of 19 who recanalized survived ($p = 0.000007$), 10 with a favorable outcome. Thrombolysis was avoided if the initial head CT showed hypodense areas in the brain stem or cerebellum. Four of the 43 cases developed hemorrhagic transformation: two of the four died. Fibrinogen, activated partial thromboplastin time , and fibrin split product measurement in the patients with hemorrhagic events were not different from the patients without ICH. Two of four with hemorrhagic infarction did not show recanalization. This study strongly suggested that recanalization of vertebrobasilar occlusions could be accomplished, and was associated with clinical salvage. Their expanded experience with 66 patients was also reported *(24)*.

Data on local intra-arterial UK or SK for acute carotid territory stroke was reported by Del Zoppo et al. from a prospective, angiographically based, two-center open-pilot study *(25)*. The longest time from symptom onset to treatment time with complete recanalization was 10 h. Seventy-five percent (15 of 20 patients) with acute stable symptoms (mean treatment onset interval 7.6 h) demonstrated complete recanalization (unblinded evaluation) with 10 of 15 exhibiting clinical improvement by the time of hospital discharge. Four patients with hemorrhagic transformation had complete recanalization and were treated 6–10 h post symptom onset (all were also treated with heparin and hydroxyethyl starch). Three of these four patients showed clinical improvement. Although these data are often cited to support a claim that patients should not receive thrombolytic therapy beyond 6 h following stroke onset, three of the four hemorrhage patients actually improved.

Mori et al. reported 22 patients who received intracarotid UK for evolving cerebral infarction resulting from angiographically documented thromboembolic occlusion of the MCA or its major branches *(26)*. Five of six with investigator-rated excellent outcome were in the recanalized group, and the volume of CT infarction was significantly less in the recanalized group (35.5 ± 55.4 mL) compared with the nonrecanalized group (172.8 ± 122.6 mL) ($p < 0.01$). Prognosis was also correlated with restoration of blood flow ($r = 0.60$, $p = 0.003$). There was no correlation between initial neurological state and recanalization. Neither interval from onset to infusion nor dose of UK correlated with prognosis.

TISSUE PLASMINOGEN ACTIVATOR PRELIMINARY TRIALS

Terashi et al. treated 364 stroke patients with either t-PA (n = 171) or UK in a double-blinded protocol *(27)*. Of the total, 36% started treatment within 24 h and 70% within 48 h. There were no statistically significant differences between the two groups at the 7-d clinical evaluation. Adverse effects were noted in approx 10% of each group, and the incidence of hemorrhagic infarction was less than 5% in each group.

Hennerici et al. reported the results of administering 70 mg alteplase intravenously over 90 min in 19 patients with ischemic stroke of less than 24-h duration *(28)*. Full-dose intravenous heparin was also administered. One patient was excluded after entry because his symptoms were later determined to be of greater than 24-h duration. Of the other 18 patients, one sustained a fatal ICH, and early arterial recanalization was achieved in only 25%. Nine additional patients died of complications of their entry strokes. The onset times of many of the patients could not be determined with certainty, and the authors proposed that delayed treatment may have contributed to the poor outcomes. They also suggested that the dose of alteplase was too low.

Later, von Kummer and associates reported on 32 patients with severe hemispheric deficits treated with a 100 mg of alteplase administered over 90 min, combined with a 5000 U bolus of intravenous heparin followed by a continuous infusion at 1000–1500 U/h, aiming to double the activated partial thromboplastin time in each patient *(29)*. All patients were treated within 6 h (mean ± SD = 3.8 ± 1.1 h) of stroke onset, and all had pretreatment CT scanning and cerebral angiography. Partial or complete recanalization of the infarct-related artery was documented angiographically in 34% immediately after the recombinant tissue plasminogen activator (rt-PA) infusion, and in an additional 19% within 12–24 h by predominantly transcranial Doppler assessment. Hemorrhagic transformation was observed in 38%, of which one-fourth (9%) was associated with neurological deterioration and death. At 4 wk, clinical outcome was classified as good (ambulatory, National Institutes of Health [NIH] Stroke Scale score <13) in 44% and poor or dead in the remainder. Good outcomes were correlated with recanalization within 24 h. Reocclusion was reported in one patient despite the heparin treatment. The authors acknowledged that their results did not show a clear benefit of concomitant heparin therapy, but suggested that it did not appear to be substantially more dangerous than t-PA alone.

Overgaard and colleagues also used a standard 100 mg dose of single-chain t-PA in 23 patients treated within 6 h of stroke onset *(30)*. Heparin was prohibited for the first 24 h. One patient died from an ICH, but that patient was also treated with heparin in violation of the protocol. Two other patients had hemorrhagic conversion without neurological worsening. Baseline and follow-up single photon emission computed tomography scans were performed in 12 patients. Ten of the 12 patients had improved blood flow at 24 h compared to baseline and had more neurological improvement, both early and late, than the two patients with persistently impaired perfusion.

In a US study sponsored by the National Institutes of Neurological Disorders and Stroke (NINDS), investigators at three centers examined the safety and clinical outcome from treatment with escalating doses of intravenous single-chain rt-PA (alteplase) in patients with very early stroke symptoms *(31)*. Eligible patients had pretreatment evaluation, including CT scanning, and treatment begun within 90 min of stroke onset. Because of the stringent time restrictions, pretreatment angiography was not a requirement. Again, systemic heparin was prohibited for 24 h.

Over the course of 32 mo, 74 patients were studied with 7 doses, ranging from 0.35 mg/kg to 1.08 mg/kg given over 60 to 90 min, with cohorts ranging from 1 to 22 patients. Hemorrhagic transformation (either hemorrhagic infarction or parenchymal hematoma) was observed in 7%, of which nearly one-half (3%) were associated with neurological worsening. Symptomatic hemorrhages occurred predominately in involved vascular territories, but also occurred in brain remote from the infarct. There was a statistically significant relationship between the incidence of symptomatic ICH and the total dose of rt-PA administered. No symptomatic hemorrhages were observed in patients receiving less than 0.95 mg/kg. No dose response with major neurological improvement, defined as a 4 or more point improvement in the NIH Stroke Scale, was observed at either 2 or 24 h. Nevertheless, the fact that 55% of patients treated with 0.85 mg/kg (with 10% of the total dose given as an initial bolus) had major neurological improvement within 24 h was viewed as an encouraging sign.

As confidence grew in the safety of intravenous alteplase administered to patients within 90 min of stroke onset, it was elected to study an additional 20 patients treated from 91 to 180 min from onset to explore the safety of expanding the potential therapeutic window *(32)*. Three doses ranging from 0.6 mg/kg to 0.95 mg/kg were tested. These 20 patients were more severely neurologically impaired at baseline than the patients treated within 90 min, and the results of treatment were not as good. Overall, hemorrhagic transformation was observed in 30% of patients, of which one-third (10%) were associated with neurological worsening and death. Whereas 25% had major neurological improvement within 2 h, only 15% were improved at 24 h. One symptomatic ICH occurred in six patients treated with 0.85 mg/kg, a dose that appeared safe in patients treated within 90 min. The investigators concluded that the results might still represent an improvement over the natural history of the disease, but concerns were raised about potential decreases in both safety and efficacy if treatment with throm-

Table 3
Pilot NINDS Dose Escalation Studies: Combined Results

Dose (mg/kg)	*Patients (n)*	*OTT[a] (n,%)*	*24 h[b] (n,%)*	*Symptomatic bleeding (n,%)*
0.35	6	3 (50%)	2 (33%)	0
0.60	19	4 (21%)	5 (26%)	0
0.85	10	4 (40%)	4 (40%)	0
0.85[c]	27	3 (11%)	13 (48%)	1 (4%)
0.95[d]	28	10 (36%)	12 (43%)	3 (11%)
0.95[c]	3	0 (0%)	1 (33%)	2 (67%)
1.05	1	0 (0%)	1 (100%)	0
Total	94	24 (26%)	38 (40%)	6 (6%)

[a]Improvement by 2 or more points on the NIH Stroke Scale at 2 h compared to baseline
[b]24-h improvement by 4 or more points on the NIHSS at 24 h compared to baseline, or return to normal
[c]10% of dose given as initial bolus
[d]90-min infusion.
OTT, "on-the-table" improvement.

bolytic therapy was delayed even beyond 90 min. Stratification by time from onset to treatment was recommended for future randomized, placebo-controlled trials of thrombolytic therapy.

Table 3 depicts the combined dose-escalation experience from the pilot NINDS studies. A dose–response relationship with symptomatic hemorrhage is suggested although the numbers are small.

Del Zoppo and colleagues employed an open-label, dose escalation design to test whether a dose–response relationship existed for two-chain form t-PA (duteplase) on cerebral artery recanalization rates *(33)*. Prospectively established safety guidelines focused on the incidence of neurological deterioration in association with hemorrhagic change, either hemorrhagic infarction or parenchymal hematoma as determined by follow-up CT scanning. The study was not designed to test the effect on clinical outcome. Eligible subjects were required to undergo pre-treatment CT scanning and selective catheter cerebral angiography and begin treatment within 8 h of the onset of stroke symptoms. Cerebral angiography was repeated immediately after the 60 min t-PA infusion. In 23 mos at 16 centers, 104 patients began treatment with study drug and 93 patients completed their infusions. Nine escalating doses ranging from 0.12 million International Units (MIU)/kg to 0.75 MIU/kg (approx 0.21 mg/kg to 1.28 mg/kg in alteplase equivalents) were examined in cohort sizes ranging from 4 to 15 patients each. Systemic heparin administration was forbidden for 24 h.

Overall, either partial or complete recanalization was observed in 34%, and no dose–response for recanalization was seen in the doses studied. However, the trial was discontinued prematurely because of withdrawal of the study drug following a patent dispute. Distal intracranial occlusions were more frequently recanalized than proximal internal carotid artery occlusions. The cumulative incidence of hemorrhagic transformation (either hemorrhagic infarction or parenchymal hematoma) was 31%, of which about one-third (10%) had associated neurological worsening. Neither hemorrhagic transformation nor associated neurological worsening were related to dose or recanalization. Patients with hemorrhagic transformation were treated 0.8 h later than patients without hemorrhage.

Yamaguchi and associates also used either 10, 20, or 30 megaunits (MU) of duteplase intravenously over 1 h to treat 58 patients with angiographically documented occlusions in the carotid territory within 6 h of the onset of symptoms *(34)*. How the patients were assigned their dose of treatment was not specified in the report. Only 18% of patients receiving 10 MU achieved complete or partial recanalization, whereas 57% and 42% were partly or completely recanalized with 20 or 30 MU, respectively. Clinical improvement appeared to be associated with recanalization, particularly if treatment was begun less than 2 h after onset. Hemorrhagic transformation was observed on follow-up CT scans in 21% of patients, but the incidence of associated neurological deterioration was not reported. The results of these preliminary open-label studies are summarized in Table 4.

INTRAVENOUS ADMINISTRATION: CONTROLLED TRIALS

The results of three small randomized, placebo-controlled trials of thrombolytic therapy were reported (Table 5). Two trials used rt-PA, whereas one employed ancrod.

Mori and colleagues recruited 31 patients with acute carotid territory ischemia and randomly assigned them to receive either placebo (12 patients), 20 MU duteplase (approx 50 mg, 9 patients), or 30 MU (approx 80 mg, 10 patients) intravenously over 60 min *(35)*. Patients were eligible for treatment within 6 h of stroke onset, and all had pre- and post-treatment angiography. Despite the small sample sizes, there was a rough balance in baseline neurological deficits. There were no apparent differences between the groups at 24 h; but by d 2, the 80 mg t-PA group showed improvement from baseline compared to the placebo group. By d 30, all three groups had improved from baseline, but the group receiving 80 mg t-PA had improved statistically significantly more than the placebo group. Parenchymal hematomas were reported in one patient in each of the treatment groups, including the placebo group. Hemorrhagic infarction was reported in 30% of the 80 mg group, 56% of the 50 mg group, and 33% of the placebo group. None of the differences were statistically significant.

Table 4
Intravenous Open Label Studies

Study	*Agent*	*n*	*Treatment window*	*Design*	*Results*
Del Zoppo *(33)*	rt-PA (duteplase)	93	0–8 h	Dose escalation Control angiography	34% recanalized, 10% worsening with hemorrhage. No dose response.
Yamaguchi *(34)*	rt-PA (duteplase)	58	0–6 h	3 doses Control angiography	Recanalization better in higher doses. 21% CT hemorrhage
Brott *(31)*	rt-PA (alteplase)	74	0–90 min	Dose escalation No angiography	Dose related risk of symptomatic hemorrhage. Safe with <0.95 mg/kg.
Haley *(32)*	rt-PA (alteplase)	20	91–180 min	Dose escalation No angiography	10% symptomatic hemorrhage; 15%sustained neurological improvement.
Hennerici *(28)*	rt-PA (alteplase)	18	0–24 h	Single 70 mg dose plus heparin; Control angiography	22% recanalization; 1 fatal hemorrhage, 9 additional deaths.
Von Kummer *(29)*	rt-PA (alteplase)	32	0–6 h	Single 100 mg dose plus heparin; Control angiography	34% immediate recanalization; 9% symptomatic hemorrhage
Overgaard *(30)*	rt-PA, (alteplase)	23	0–6 h	Single 100 mg dose; Baseline and follow up SPECT	1 symptomatic hemorrhage; reperfusion on SPECT correlated with neurological improvement

Abbreviations: CT, computed tomography; SPECT, single photon emission computed tomography.

Table 5
Randomized Trials of Intravenous Therapy

Study	*Agent*	*Dose (n)*	*Treatment window*	*Results*
Mori *(35)*	rt-PA (duteplase)	Control *(12)* 20 MIU *(9)* 30 MIU *(10)*	0–6 h	Improved arterial recanalization l and neurological scale difference scores in treated groups.
Bridging Study *(36)*	rt-PA (alteplase)	Control *(10)* 0.85 mg/kg *(10)*	0–90 min	60% early improvement in treated groups; 10% in controls.
		Control (3) 0.85 mg/kg *(4)*	91–180 min	1 fatal hemorrhage in control group, 2 with early improvement in each group
Ancrod Group *(37)* Ancrod *(64)* treated	Ancrod	Control *(68)*	0–6 h	No difference in neurological scale scores. Trends for improved mortality and functional outcome in groups.

Abbreviations: N, number of proteins; rt-PA, recombinant tissue plasminogen activator; MIU, million Internal Units.

Intended as a pilot feasibility study for a larger NINDS-sponsored trial, 27 patients were examined in the TPA Bridging Study, a randomized, double-blind, placebo-controlled trial of intravenous alteplase, 0.85 mg/kg given over 1 h with 10% of the total dose administered as an initial bolus *(36)*. Twenty patients (10 rt-PA and 10 placebo) were treated within 90 min from stroke onset, whereas 7 patients (4 rt-PA and 3 placebo) were treated from 91 to 180 min from onset. The primary end point was the proportion of patients who improved by 4 or more points on the NIH Stroke Scale as determined by a blinded evaluator at 24 h. At 24 h, 60% of t-PA-treated patients had improved by 4 or more points compared to 10% of the placebo-treated patients, a statistically significant difference ($p < 0.05$). There was no statistically significant difference in the group mean stroke scale scores at any of the follow-up time points, though, and the proportion of improvers was not statistically different at 1 wk or 3 mo. The numbers of patients in the 91–180 min group were too small to draw any meaningful conclusions, although the investigators reported the development of a fatal spontaneous hematoma in the placebo group. The investigators concluded that although the results were promising, larger studies were clearly needed, the results of which are detailed in Chapter 7.

Encouraged by results from a small pilot study performed in the late 1980s, Olinger and colleagues reported preliminary results from a larger randomized, controlled trial of ancrod in 132 patients treated within 6 h of stroke onset*(37)*. Ancrod, derived from the venom of the Malaysian pit viper, is a defibrinogenating agent that activates the thrombolytic system indirectly. The mean time to treatment was 4.6 h. While there was no statistically significant difference in the prospectively determined primary end point (Scandinavian Stroke Scale scores at 3 mo), *post-hoc* analyses suggested trends in improvement in early mortality and functional outcome at 3 mo. Further studies of ancrod in acute ischemic stroke have recently been completed (*see* Chapter 7).

CONCLUSIONS

The knowledge obtained from these earlier studies set the stage for larger, randomized clinical trials in the US and Europe by proving feasibility and safety. Given the negative experience with thrombolytic therapy for stroke in the 1960s, such stepwise, careful progression from safety, to dose-finding, to pilot feasibility studies was essential. The studies also led to the beginnings of the rapid, aggressive team approach needed to successfully treat acute ischemic stroke. Furthermore, we learned that at least one-third of ischemic stroke patients reperfuse spontaneously (and obviously too late) within 48 h of stroke onset.

REFERENCES

1. Fieschi C, Argentino C, Lenzi GL, Sacchetti ML, Toni D, Bozzao L. Clinical and instrumental evaluation of patients with ischemic stroke within the first six hours. *J Neurol Sci* 1989;91: 311–321.

2. Saito I, Segawa H, Shiokawa Y, Taniguchi M, Tsutsumi K. Middle cerebral artery occlusion: correlation of computed tomography and angiography with clinical outcome. *Stroke* 1987;18:863–868.
3. Meyer JS, Herndon R, Gotoh F, Tazaki Y, Nelson JN, Johnson J. Therapeutic Thrombolysis. In: Millikan C, Siekert RG, Whisnant JP, eds., *Cerebral Vascular Disease, Third Princeton Conference*. New York: Guren and Stratton; 1961:160–177.
4. Meyer JS, Gilroy J, Barnhart ME. Therapeutic Thrombolysis in Cerebral Thromboembolism. In: Siekert RG, Whisnant J, eds., *Cerebral Vascular Diseases*. Philadelphia: Grune & Stratton; 1963:160–175.
5. Meyer JS, Gilroy J, Barnhart ME, Johnson JF. Therapeutic thrombolysis in cerebral thromboembolism: Randomized evaluation of intravenous streptokinase. In: Millikan CH, Siekert RG, Whisnant JP, eds., *Cerebral Vascular Diseases, Fourth Princeton Conference*. New York: Grune and Stratton; 1965:200–213.
6. Clarke RL, Clifton EE. The treatment of cerebrovascular thrombosis and embolism with fibrinolytic agents. *Am J Cardiol* 1960;30:546–551.
7. Clifton EE. The use of plasmin in humans. *Ann NY Acad Sci* 1957;68:209–229.
8. Clifton EE. Early experience with fibrinolysin. *Angiology* 1959;10:244–252.
9. Meyer JS, Gilroy J, Barnhart KT, Johnson JF. Therapeutic Thrombolysis in Cerebral Thromboembolism. Double-Blind Evaluation of Intravenous Plasmin Therapy in Carotid and Middle Cerebral Arterial Occlusion. *Neurology* 1963;13:927–937.
10. Meyer JS, Gilroy J, Barnhart ME, and Johnson JF. Anticoagulants plus streptokinase therapy in progressive stroke. Journal of the American Medical Association 189, 373. 1964.
11. Sussman B, Fitch T. Thrombolysis with fibrinolysin in cerebral arterial occlusion. *JAMA* 1958;167:1705–1709.
12. Clifton EE. The use of plasmin in the treatment of intravascular thormbosis. *J Am Geriatr Soc* 1958;6:118–127.
13. Herndon R, Meyer JS, Johnson JF, Landers J. Treatment of cerebrovascular thrombosis with fibrinolysin. Preliminary report. *Am J Cardiol* 1960;6:540–545.
14. Herndon R, Meyer JS, Johnson JF. Fibrinolysin therapy in thrombotic diseases of the nervous system. *J Mich State Med Soc*.1960;59:1684–1692.
15. Fletcher AP, Alkjaersig N, Lewis M, et al. A pilot study of urokinase therapy in cerebral infarction. *Stroke* 1976;7:135–142.
16. Larcan A, Laprevote-Heully MC, Lambert H, Alexandre P, Picard L, Chrisment N. [Indications for the use of thrombolytics in cases of cerebrovascular thrombosis also treated with hyperbaric oxygenation (2 ATA)]. *Therapie* 1977;32:259–270.
17. Theron AJ, Courtheoux P, Casasco A, et al. Local intraarterial fibrinolysis in the carotid territory. *Am J Neuroradiol* 1989;10:753–756.
18. Zeumer H, Freitag H-J, Zanella F, Thise A, Arning C. Local intra-arterial thrombolytic therapy in patients with stroke: urokinase versus recombinant tissue plasminogen activator (rt-PA). *Nrad* 1993;35:159–162.
19. del Zoppo G, Zeumer H, Harker LA. Thrombolytic therapy in stroke: Possibilities and hazards. *Stroke* 1987;17:595–607.
20. del Zoppo G, Ferber A, Otis S, et al. Local intra-arterial fibrinolytic therapy in acute cartoid territory stroke. *Stroke* 1988;19:307–313.
21. Abe T, Kazawa M, Naito I, et al. Clinical effect of urokinase (60,000 units/day) on cerebral infarction—comparative study by means of multiple center double blind test. *Blood Vessel* 1981;12:342–358.
22. Fujishima M, Omae T, Tanaka K, Iino K, Matsuo O, Mihara H. Controlled trial of combined urokinase and dextran sulfate therapy in patients with acute cerebral infarction. *Angiology* 1986;37:487–498.

23. Hacke W, Zeumer H, Ferbert A, Bruckmann H, del Zoppo G. Intra-arterial thrombolytic therapy improves outcome in patients with acute vertebrobasilar occlusive disease. *Stroke* 1988;19:1216–1222.
24. Bruckmann H, Ferbert A, del Zoppo G, Hacke W, Zeumer H. The acute vertebro-basilar thrombosis. Angiological-clinical comparison and therapeutic implications. *Acta Radiol* 1987;369 (suppl):38–42.
25. del Zoppo GJ, Ferbert A, Otis S, et al. Local intra-arterial fibrinolytic therapy in acute carotid territory stroke. A pilot study. *Stroke* 1988;19:307–313.
26. Mori E, Tabuchi M, Yoshida T, Yamadori A. Intracarotid urokinase with thromboembolic occlusion of the middle cerebral artery. *Stroke* 1988;19:802–812.
27. Terashi A, Kobayashi Y, Katayama Y, Inamura K, Kazama M, Abe T. Clinical effects and basic studies of thrombolytic therapy on cerebral thrombosis. *Semin Thromb Hemost* 1990;16:236–241.
28. Hennerici, M., Hacke, W, von Kummer, R., Hornig, C. R., and Zangemeister, W. Intravenous tissue plasminogen activator for the treatment of acute thromboembolic ischemia. *Cerebrovasc Dis* 1991;Suppl 1: 124–128.
29. von Kummer R, Hacke W. Safety and efficacy of intravenous tissue plasminogen activator and heparin in acute middle cerebral artery stroke. *Stroke* 1992;23:646–652.
30. Overgaard K, Sperling B, Boysen G, et al. Thrombolytic therapy in acute ischemic stroke: A Danish pilot study. *Stroke* 1993;24:1439–1446.
31. Brott TG, Haley EC, Jr., Levy DE, et al. Urgent therapy for stroke: Part 1. Pilot study of tissue plasminogen activator administered within 90 minutes. *Stroke* 1992;23:632–640.
32. Haley EC, Jr., Levy DE, Brott TG, et al. Urgent therapy for stroke. Part II. Pilot study of tissue plasminogen activator administered 91-180 minutes from onset. *Stroke* 1992;23:641–645.
33. del Zoppo G, Poeck K, Pessin MS, et al. Recombinant tissue plasminogen activator in acute thrombotic and embolic stroke. *Ann Neurol* 1992;32:78–86.
34. Yamaguchi T, Hayakawa T, Kikuchi H, Abe T. Intravenous rt-PA in embolic and thrombotic cerebral infarction: A cooperative study. In: Hacke W, del Zoppo G.J., Hirshberg M, eds., *Thrombolytic Therapy in Acute Ischemic Stroke.* Berlin: Springer-Verlag; 1991:168–174.
35. Mori E, Yoneda Y, Tabuchi M, et al. Intravenous recombinant tissue plasminogen activator in acute carotid artery territory stroke. *Neurology* 1992;42:976–982.
36. Haley EC, Brott TG, Sheppard GL, et al. Pilot randomized trial of tissue plasminogen activator in acute ischemic stroke. *Stroke* 1993;24:1000–1004.
37. The Ancrod Stroke Study Investigators. Ancrod for the treatment of acute ischemic brain infarction. *Stroke* 1994;25:1755–1759.
38. Hossmann V, Heiss W-D, Bewermeyer H, Wiedemann G. Controlled trial of ancrod in ischemic stroke. *Arch Neurol* 1983;40:803–808.

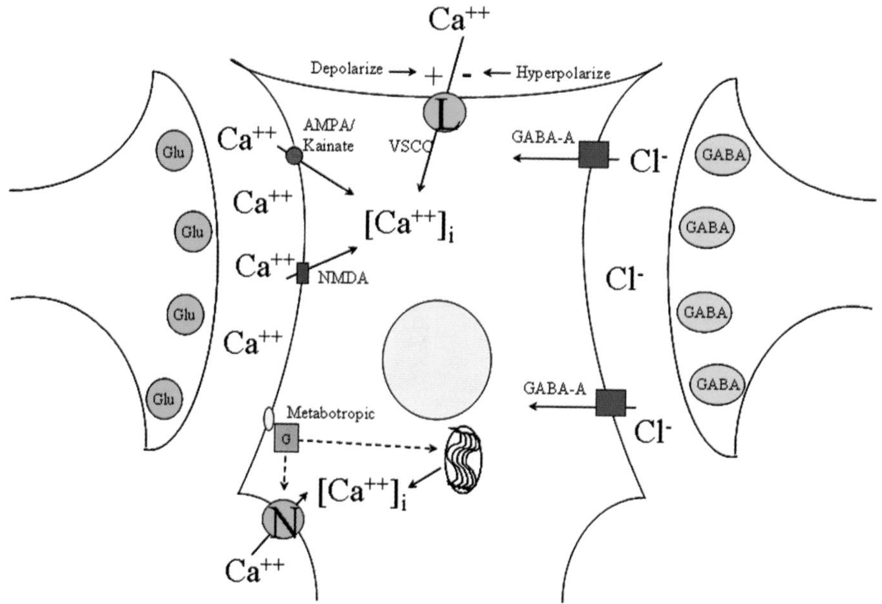

Color Plate 1, Fig. 4. γ-Aminobutyric acid-receptor activation leads to a hyperpolizing influx of chloride that blocks voltage-gated calcium influx via the L-type voltage-sensitive calcium channel. (*See* complete caption on p. 50 and discussion on pp. 49–50.)

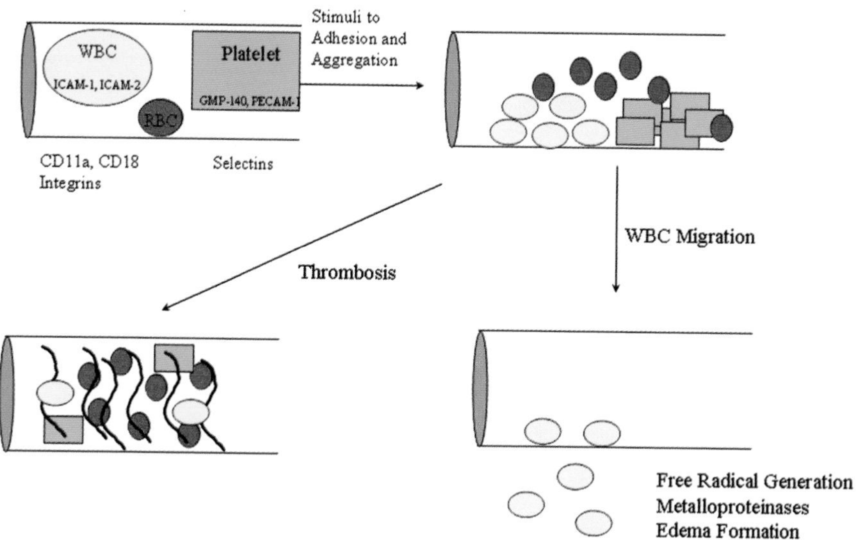

Color Plate 1, Fig. 5. Following occlusion, granulocytes leave the circulation to enter ischemic brain. (*See* complete discussion on p. 53.)

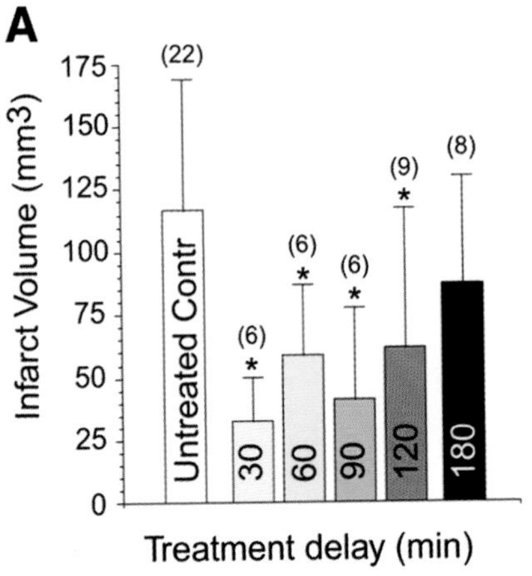

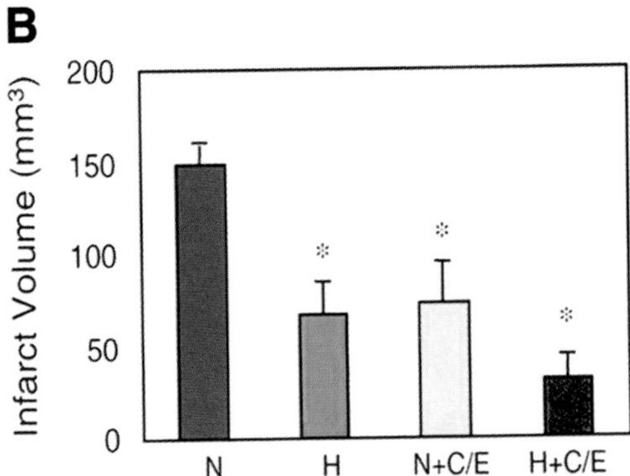

C/E - 10 mg/kg Caffeine+0.32g/kg EtOH
I.V. 60 min post 180 min MCA/CCAO (2.5 h infusion)

H - 35oC - 60 min post 180 min
MCA/CCAO for 4 hours

N - Normothermia

Color Plate 2, Fig. 9. The effect of caffeinol. (*See* complete caption on p. 92 and discussion on p. 91.)

Color Plate 3, Fig. 2. (*opposite page*) **(B)** The time-to-peak map shows an area of delayed contrast and **(D)** the cerebral blood volume is diminished within the right striatum and insular cortex. (*See* complete caption on p. 256 and discussion on pp. 253 and 256.)

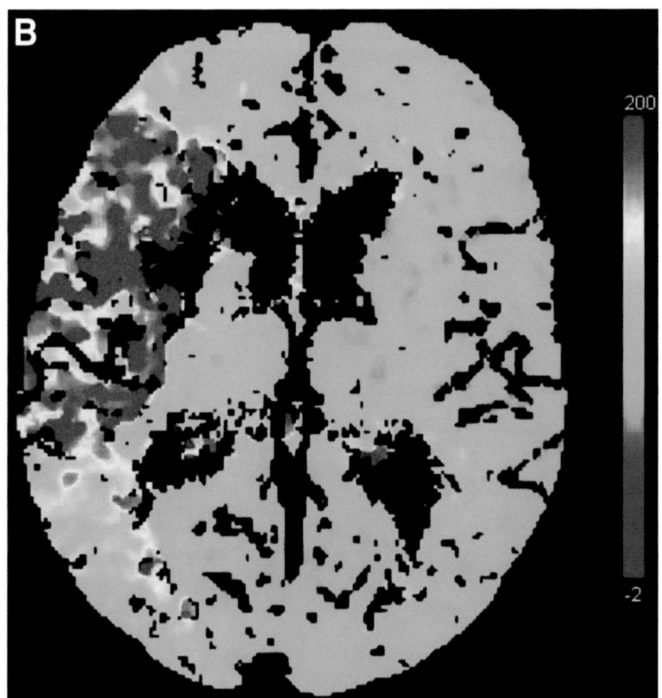
B
200
-2

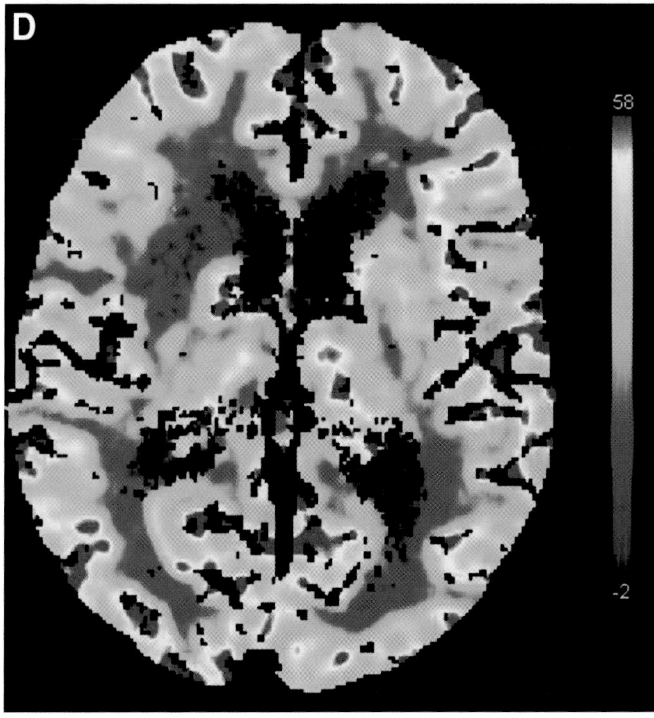
D
58
-2

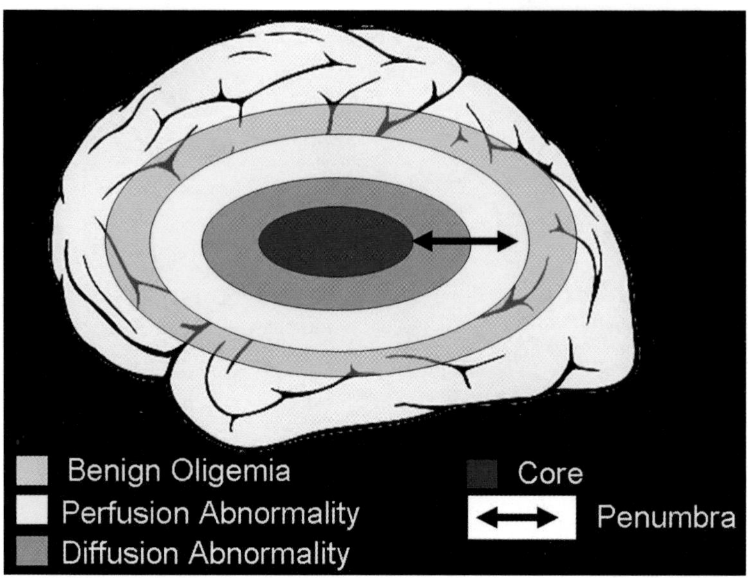

Color Plate 4, Fig. 7. Modified view of ischemic penumbra. (*See* complete caption on p. 291 and discussion on pp. 288–289.)

7 Intravenous Thrombolytic Therapy for Acute Ischemic Stroke

Results of Large, Randomized Clinical Trials

Matthew L. Flaherty, MD,
Edward C. Jauch, MD, MS,
Rashmi U. Kothari, MD,
and Joseph P. Broderick, MD

CONTENTS

INTRODUCTION

Prior to the availability of computed tomography (CT) imaging, seven case series had reported the use of various thrombolytic agents for 249 patients with ischemic strokes*(1–7)*. Mortality ranged from 20 to 50% and intracranial hemorrhage (ICH) rates from 11 to 35% in these studies (*see* Chapter 6). These discouraging results reflected the fact that patients were treated days to weeks after symptom onset and CT scanning was not yet available to appropriately exclude patients with hemorrhage.

From: *Current Clinical Neurology: Thrombolytic Therapy for Acute Stroke, Second Edition*
Edited by: P. D. Lyden © Humana Press Inc., Totowa, NJ

During the 1980s, thrombolytic therapy was investigated in the setting of acute myocardial infarction (MI), acute pulmonary embolism, and peripheral arterial disease. Subsequently, large clinical trials demonstrated that streptokinase (SK) and recombinant tissue-plasminogen activator (rt-PA) improved cardiac function and survival in patients with acute MI. Meanwhile, brain CT scanning became more widely available in the United States as successful thrombolytic treatment of acute MI became more widely dispersed. By the late 1980s there were multiple encouraging case reports and case series of thrombolytic therapy for stroke *(8–13)*. Laboratory data suggested that treatment delay time critically determined outcome, and hemorrhage rate, when using thrombolytic agents for acute ischemic stroke (*see* Chapters 4 and 7). Zivin et al. reported reduced recovery rates as the delay between the onset of ischemia and the start of thrombolytic therapy increased *(14)*. In the early 1990s several pilot clinical protocols, preludes to larger randomized trials, reported results similar to animal studies in regards to efficacy, safety, and time to treatment.

In the past decade, several large randomized trials of rt-PA and SK have provided important information regarding the safety of these thrombolytic agents, the importance of patient selection, and the time frame in which thrombolytic agents should be used. This chapter reviews the findings of these large randomized trials.

EFFICACY AND SAFETY OF RECOMBINANT TISSUE PLASMINOGEN ACTIVATOR IN STROKE

Randomized Trials of Recombinant Tissue Plasminogen Activator Given Within 0–3 h of Stroke Onset

The National Institute of Neurological Disorders and Stroke (NINDS) Recombinant Tissue Plasminogen Activator Stroke Trial was the basis for the approval of rt-PA by the Food and Drug Administration (FDA) in 1996. The NINDS rt-PA Stroke Trial was composed of two separate studies that were reported in a single publication *(15)*. The first study, a phase II-B study, enrolled 291 patients and tested whether rt-PA had early clinical activity within 24 h of symptom onset, defined as either a 4-point improvement over baseline National Institute of Heath Stroke Scale (NIHSS) or complete resolution of neurological deficit. The second study, a phase III study, enrolled 333 patients and used four outcome measures that were summarized with a combined global test statistic (Table 1) to assess whether treatment with rt-PA conveyed clinical benefit 3 mo after stroke. Both studies were randomized, double-blinded comparisons of intravenous (iv) recombinant rt-PA vs placebo in patients with acute ischemic stroke treated within 3 h of symptom onset. Both studies were based on pilot studies and dose-escalation data that suggested 0.9 mg/kg rt-PA given intrave-

Table 1
Percentages of Patients With Favorable Outcome[a] in Part 2 of the NINDS rt-PA Stroke Trial

	rt-PA (%)	*Placebo (%)*	*Odds ratio (95% CI)*	p-*value*
Global test			1.7 (1.2–2.6)	0.008
Barthel Index	50	38	1.6 (1.1–2.5)	0.026
mRS	39	26	1.7 (1.1–2.5)	0.019
GOS	44	32	1.6 (1.1–2.5)	0.025
NIHSS	31	20	1.7 (1.0–2.8)	0.033

[a]Scores of 95 to100 on the Barthel Index, 1 on the mRS and NIHSS, and 1 on the GOS were considered favorable outcomes by the investigators. mRS, modified Rankin Scale; GOS, Glasgow Outcome Scale; NIHSS, National Institutes of Health Stroke Scale. (From ref. *15*.)

nously within 3 h of stroke onset would prove beneficial while minimizing the risk of hemorrhage *(16,17)*.

Patients were randomized if they had an ischemic stroke with a clearly defined time of onset, a deficit measurable on the NIHSS, and a baseline CT showing no evidence of ICH. There were no exclusions based on CT findings of subtle early ischemia (*see* Chapter 16). Half of the patients were treated within 90 min and the other half within 91–180 min of symptom onset. The investigators emphasized careful patient selection and strict adherence to the treatment protocol; strict guidelines for blood pressure management were followed and anticoagulants and antiplatelet agents were prohibited for the first 24 h.

In the first study, no statistically significant difference was detected at 24 h between groups in the primary endpoint (a 4-point improvement on the NIHSS or complete resolution of neurologic deficit at 24 h). In a secondary, exploratory analysis, it was determined that for any other amount of improvement on the 24-h NIHSS (e.g., a 3-, 5-, 6-point, improvement), the outcome was significantly better in the rt-PA-treated than placebo-treated patients *(18)*. In addition, there was a 4-point difference in the median NIHSS at 24 h between the rt-PA and placebo group (8 vs 12, respectively) ($p < 0.02$) *(18)*. Thus, although the study was negative for its primary endpoint, there was significant treatment activity 24 h after stroke onset.

In the second (phase III) study, patients who received rt-PA were 30% more likely to have little or no disability after 3 mo when compared to controls. This was also true for the first study and a combined analysis of both NINDS studies. The benefit for rt-PA was highly significant and was found for all four measures of outcome (Table 1), with an odds ratio for a favorable outcome of 1.7 (95% confidence interval, 1.2–2.6) ($p = 0.008$) in the rt-PA group using the global test statistic. Treatment with rt-PA produced a favorable outcome regardless of the subtype of ischemic stroke (i.e., lacunar, cardioembolic) (*see* Chapter 9).

Symptomatic ICH within 36 h of stroke onset occurred in 6.4% of patients given rt-PA in the two NINDS studies but only 0.6% of the placebo group ($p < 0.001$) (Table 2). No significant difference in mortality was seen between rt-PA (17%) and placebo groups (21%, $p = 0.30$) at 3 mo. In a multivariable analysis, only stroke severity as measured by the NIHSS (five categories; odds ratio [OR] = 1.8; 95% confidence interval [CI], 1.2–2.9) and brain edema (defined as acute hypodensity) or mass effect on baseline CT (OR, 7.8; 95% CI, 2.2–27.1) were independently associated with an increased risk of symptomatic ICH *(19)*. However, even in these subgroups—patients with severe neurological deficit or CT findings of edema/mass effect—rt-PA-treated patients were more likely than placebo-treated patients to have a favorable 3-mo outcome. It was concluded that, despite a higher rate of ICH, patients with severe strokes or edema or mass effect on their baseline CT are reasonable candidates for rt-PA if administered within 3 h of stroke onset.

Randomized Trial of Recombinant Tissue Plasminogen Activator Given Within 3–5 h of Stroke Onset

Because of the narrow therapeutic window in the NINDS rt-PA Stroke Trial and the small percentage of patients presenting within this time frame, efforts were made to evaluate rt-PA beyond 3 hof stroke onset. The Alteplase ThromboLysis for Acute Noninterventional Therapy in Ischemic Stroke (ATLANTIS) study was a double blind, randomized, placebo-controlled trial evaluating the safety and efficacy of 0.9 mg/kg of IV rt-PA in patients with acute ischemic stroke *(20)*. Inclusion criteria were similar to the NINDS rt-PA Stroke Trial except for the time window studied, an age restriction (patients 80 yr of age excluded), and exclusion for subtle signs of early infarction involving more than 33% of a middle cerebral artery (MCA) territory. The ATLANTIS study was initially designed to evaluate patients treated within 0–6 h (part A). In December 1993, after enrollment of 142 patients, the time window was changed (part B) to 0 to 5 h resulting from concerns of the Data Monitoring and Safety Board (DMSB) about the 5–6 h group. Time from onset to treatment in part B was further modified to 3–5 h following FDA approval of rt-PA for patients with acute ischemic stroke treated within 3 h.

Of 142 patients enrolled in part A, 22 were entered within 3 h of stroke onset and 46 between 5 and 6 h of stroke onset. Whereas a higher percentage of patients in the rt-PA treatment group improved by 4 points on the 24-h NIHSS (21% placebo ves 40% rt-PA, $p = 0.02$), more placebo patients improved by 4 points at 30 d (75% placebo vs 60% t-PA, $p = 0.05$), and rt-PA patients had higher rates of symptomatic ICH (0% placebo ves 11% t-PA, $p < 0.01$) and mortality at 90 d (7% placebo vs 23% t-PA, $p < 0.01$) *(21)*.

Table 2
Large, Randomized Trials of Recombinant Tissue Plasminogen Activator

Study[a]	*Time to treatment*	*No. of patients*	*Dose and treatment group*	*3-mo mortality (%)*	*Intracerebral hematoma (%)*[b]
NINDS rt-PA Stroke Study (part 1) *(15)*	3 h	291	0.9 mg/kg rt-PA	NA	6
			placebo	NA	0
NINDS rt-PA Stroke Study (part 2) *(15)*	3 h	333	0.9 mg/kg rt-PA	NA	7
			placebo	NA	1
NINDS rt-PA Stroke Study (parts I & II combined) *(15)*	3 h	624	0.9 mg/kg rt-PA	17	6.4
			placebo	21	0.6
ATLANTIS part B *(20)*	3–5 h[c]	613	0.9 mg/kg rt-PA	10.9	6.7
			placebo	6.9	1.3
ECASS I*(22)*	6 h	620	1.1 mg/kg rt-PA	17.9	19.8[d]
			placebo	12.7	6.5[d]
ECASS II *(23)*	6 h	800	0.9 mg/kg rt-PA	10.3	11.8
			placebo	10.5	3.1

[a]All analyses using intent-to-treat populations.

[b]Symptomatic ICH within 36 h; p 0.001 for all values comparing placebo and rt-PA.

[c]Initially 0–5-h study; protocol amended to 3–5 h after FDA approval of rt-PA under 3 h. Results include 39 patients treated <3 h, 24 patients treated >5 h, and 3 patients never receiving study drug.

[d]Only rate of parenchymal ICH is available; no information regarding clinical deterioration is available.

NA, not available.

In part B of the ATLANTIS study, 613 patients were enrolled, including 39 patients entered within 3 h of stroke onset and 24 patients entered after 5 h. The trial was ended prematurely in July 1998 based on a DSMB analysis indicating that "treatment was unlikely to prove benficial" *(20)*. Placebo and rt-PA treated patients had median NIHSS scores of 11 and median onset-to-treatment times of 270 min and 276 min, respectively. There were no differences in the primary endpoint (the percentage of patients with a NIHSS ≤ 1 at 90 d) or any of the secondary endpoints between placebo and rt-PA-treated patients, with the exception of a more than11-point improvement on the NIHSS at 30 and 90 d ("major neurological recovery"), which favored the rt-PA group ($p = 0.02$ and $p = 0.03$, respectively). Patients treated with rt-PA had a higher rate of symptomatic ICH (1.3% placebo vs 6.7% rt-PA, $p < 0.001$) and a trend toward higher 90-d mortality (6.9 % placebo vs 10.9% rt-PA, $p = 0.08$). Analyses using only the "target population" of 547 patients—enrolled within 3–5 h of stroke onset without protocol violations—were similar to intention-to-treat analyses.

Randomized Trials of Recombinant Tissue Plasminogen Activator Given Within 0–6 h of Stroke Onset

Two large, randomized trials evaluated the safety and efficacy of rt-PA in stroke patients treated within 0–6 h, the European Cooperative Acute Stroke Study (ECASS) and ECASS II *(22,23)*. ECASS was published 2 mo before the NINDS trial results and 7 mo prior to the FDA approval of rt-PA given within 3 h. ECASS was a multi-center, double-blind, randomized trial of 1.1 mg/kg of intravenous rt-PA vs placebo in patients with acute ischemic stroke treated within 6 h of symptom onset *(22)*. Patients were eligible if they were at least 18 yr old and had a clinical diagnosis of moderate to severe hemispheric stroke. Patients with coma, hemiplegia plus fixed-eye deviation, global aphasia, vertebrobasilar stroke, or those with a CT scan showing hypodensity in more than 33% of a MCA territory were to be excluded. Primary endpoints were differences of 15 points in the median Barthel Index (BI) and one grade in the median modified Rankin Scale (mRS) at 90 d. Secondary endpoints included 30-d mortality.

In the intent-to-treat population of 620 patients, there was no difference in primary endpoints. Hemorrhagic infarction was more frequent in the placebo-treated group (30.3% placebo vs 23% rt-PA, $p < 0.001$), but parenchymal hematoma was more frequent in the rt-PA treated group (6.5% placebo vs 19.8% rt-PA, $p < 0.001$). Death associated with hemorrhage occurred in 19 of the rt-PA-treated patients and in 7 of the placebo patients. There was an overall trend toward increased 30-d mortality in the rt-PA patients (12.7% placebo vs 17.9% rt-PA, $p = 0.08$).

Neurological improvement occurred in a subset of rt-PA-treated patients, now known as the "target population." When planning the trial, the ECASS investi-

Table 3
Results of the European Cooperative Acute Stroke Study (ECASS) *(22)*

	Intent-to-treat population (n = 620)		*Target population (n = 511)*	
	rt-PA (%)	*Placebo (%)*	*rt-PA (%)*	*Placebo (%)*
30-d mortality	18	13	15	12
Parenchymal hematoma	20[a]	7[a]	19[a]	7[a]
mRS 0–1 at 3 mo	36	29	41[b]	29[b]

Abbr: mRS, modified Rankin Scale.
[a]Significant (p 0.001)
[b]Significant ($p < 0.05$)

gators anticipated that up to 20% of patients would have major protocol violations, but would be inadvertently randomized and, indeed, 109 patients were deemed major protocol violations after *post-hoc* review. The protocol violations included 66 with abnormalities on their CT scans (mainly major early infarct signs), 12 patients who received prohibited therapy (e.g., heparin in less than 24 h), 20 patients whose follow-up deviated from the 90 + 14-dtime window, and 11 others (e.g., randomized but not treated). The remaining 511 patients were prospectively defined as the target population; in this popluaion the rt-PA-treated patients showed better median 90-d mRS scores vs placebo (2 vs 3 respectively, $p = 0.035$). However, the 90-d BI scores did not differ ($p = 0.16$), nor did mortality. Overall, the total parenchymal hematoma rate in the target population was 19.4% for rt-PA and 6.8% for placebo (Table 3). In a *post-hoc* analysis of the ECASS data, application of the NINDS rt-PA Stroke Trial outcome measures to the intent-to-treat population (minus five patients who were randomized but did not receive treatment) demonstrated benefits for rt-PA patients in achieving a mRS of 0–1 at 90 d ($p = 0.044$) and a NIHSS of 0–1 at 90 d ($p = 0.001$) *(24)*.

The ECASS results sparked controversy. On the one hand, the "real-world" population might be best represented by the intent-to-treat population. For that group, no efficacy was identified in the pre-specified primary endpoints. On the other hand, proper patient selection is necessary for adequate evaluation of a given therapy; in the target population, there was evidence of benefit for patients treated with rt-PA, whereas 66 of the 109 patients excluded from the target population had CT evidence of an already established major cerebral infarction and could not be expected to benefit from thrombolysis—such patients would be excluded in future trials and in ultimate clinical practice. Additionally, the failure to show benefit in the rt-PA-treated group may have occurred because treatment was initiated more than 4 h after symptom onset in the majority of the ECASS patients: only 87 (14%) of the 620 patients were treated within 3 h of symptom onset. The controversy of ECASS clearly supported the mounting of another, confirmatory, trial.

ECASS-II was designed to address some of the issues raised by ECASS using a multicenter, double-blind, randomized, placebo controlled trial evaluating the safety and efficacy of intravenous rt-PA vs placebo within 6 h of stroke onset *(23)*. A dose of 0.9 mg/kg of IV rt-PA was used and strict blood pressure guidelines based on the NINDS trial were followed. Similar to ECASS I, but in contrast to the NINDS trial, the ECASS-II protocol excluded patients with major signs of infarction on CT (>33% the MCA distribution), patients with coma or stupor, or patients with hemiplegia plus fixed-eye deviation. The primary endpoint was the 90 d mRS, dichotomized for favorable (score 0–1) and unfavorable (score 2–6) outcome.

There were 800 patients randomized over the 14-mo study period. Despite implementation of a CT training course prior to and during the trial, there were 72 protocol violations, the majority of which were a result of CT criteria violations. There was no significant difference in the proportion of favorable outcome between the rt-PA-treated patients (40.3%) and the placebo-treated patients (36.6%, $p = 0.277$). However, a *post-hoc* analysis of the 90-d mRS, dichotomized as independent (mRS = 0–2) or not independent (mRS = 3–6) found an absolute difference of 8.3% in favor of the rt-PA-treated patients (46.0% placebo vs 54.3% rt-PA, $p = 0.024$) *(23)*.Whereas the incidence of symptomatic ICH was significantly higher in the rt-PA-treated patients (8.8%) as compared to the placebo-treated group (3.4%), there was no significant difference in 30- or 90-d mortality between the two groups.

Pooled Analysis of Recombinant Tissue Plasminogen Activator Trials

Initial published results of the NINDS rt-PA Stroke Trial did not show a difference in thrombolytic treatment effect between patients enrolled within 90 min of symptom onset compared to those enrolled between 90 and180 min (OR for a favorable outcome of 1.9 vs placebo in both groups using the global test statistic) *(15)*. This result conflicted with prior experimental evidence *(16,17)* and prompted further analysis of the study data; these further analyses showed baseline stroke severity—NIHSS at presentation—to be a confounder in the 90–180 min group *(25)*. After adjustment for this covariate, an onset-to-treatment time (OTT) interaction with treatment effect was detected, such that patients treated within 90 min of onset showed a higher odds ratio for improvement than patients treated from 90 to180 min (OR 2.11 vs 1.69) *(25)*.

Recently, an analysis of pooled data from the NINDS t-PA Stroke Trial (parts I and II), ECASS I, ECASS II, and the ATLANTIS trial (parts A and B) was performed to determine if the relation between time of treatment and stroke outcome could be confirmed *(26)*. Because endpoints differed between studies, the authors chose to focus upon 3-mo favorable outcomes as defined by mRS (0

Table 4
Pooled Analysis of NINDS, ECASS, and ATLANTIS Trials:
Odds Ratios for Favorable Outcome[a] at 3 Mo After Cerebral Infarction

Stratum	*OR*	*CI*	*Number rt-PA*	*Number placebo*
0–90	2.81	1.75–4.50	161	150
91–180	1.55	1.12–2.15	302	315
181–270	1.40	1.05–1.85	390	411
271–360	1.15	0.90–1.47	538	508

[a]Odds ratios calculated from a global statistical approach, which includes modified Rankin Scale (0–1), Barthel Index (95–100), and NIHSS (0–1). Stratum, number of min from symptom onset-to-treatment (OTT); OR, adjusted global odds ratios; CI, 95% confidence interval.

or 1), BI (95 or 100), NIHSS (0 or 1), and a global test statistic. Intention-to-treat analysis included 2775 patients with a median NIHSS of 11 and median OTT of 243 min. Of 928 patients enrolled within 3 h, 622 were from the NINDS rt-PA Stroke Trial. After stratifying OTT into quartiles (0–90 min, 91–180 min, 181–270 min, 271–360 min), a multivariate model controlling for potential confounders showed an OTT-treatment interaction with higher odds ratios for favorable recovery with earlier treatment (Table 4). A benefit for rt-PA as defined by a favorable outcome at three months was statistically significant through 270 min. For patients treated with rt-PA within 270 min, no difference in mortality was found compared to placebo, but in patients treated between 270 and 360 min, rt-PA was associated with an increased risk of death at 3 mo (hazard ratio 1.45, 95% CI 1.02–2.07). Occurrence of intracerebral hematoma (parenchymal hematoma type II) was found to be associated with rt-PA use and older age but not OTT or baseline NIHSS *(26)*.

The results of this pooled analysis lend further support to the efficacy of rt-PA when used within 3 h of ischemic stroke onset in appropriately selected patients. A possible benefit through 4.5 h was suggested, but the smaller odds ratios for favorable improvement suggest that all previous randomized studies analyzing the 3- to 4.5-h time window have been underpowered. Intravenous rt-PA administered later than 4.5 h from symptom onset may cause harm.

Post-Food and Drug Administration Approval Studies of Recombinant Tissue Plasminogen Activator for Stroke

Registries of Intravenous Recombinant Tissue Plasminogen Activator Use

Coincident to the approval of rt-PA for stroke in many countries, governmental regulatory agencies have required subsequent phase IV studies to assess the safety and clinical effectiveness in routine practice. The Standard Treatment with Alteplase to Reverse Stroke (STARS) Study was an FDA-mandated study that enrolled 389 patients at 57 medical centers *(27)*. Remarkably, even with a median time from onset to treatment of 2 h 44 min and protocol violations in 32% of patients, fewer symptomatic ICH (3.3%) occurred compared to the original NINDS study (Table 5). Despite the lack of a control group in the STARS Study and fact that clinical outcomes were assessed at 30 d rather than 90 d, it was concluded that the percentage of patients achieving good clinical outcome (35% with mRS <2) was similar to patients treated with rt-PA in the NINDS rt-PA Stroke Study. Following Canadian approval for rt-PA for stroke in 1999, the Canadian Activase for Stroke Effectiveness Study (CASES), another phase IV study, enrolled 1132 patients in 60 centers across Canada *(28)*. In a preliminary analysis of 784 patients, 45% were independent (mRS 0–2) at 90 d and fewer than 4.5% experienced symptomatic ICH.

In 2002 the European Medicines Evaluation Agency approved the use of rt-PA for ischemic stroke within 3 h from symptom onset with the condition that a registry be created to monitor rt-PA use over the subsequent 3 yr. The Safe Implementation of Thrombolysis in Stroke Monitoring Study (SITS-MOST) registry currently is evaluating symptomatic ICH, death, and 3-mo outcome. Data from SITS-MOST will aid in the decision whether to continue approval of rt-PA in Europe.

In addition to the phase IV studies noted above, a number of communities have reported the results of their experience with the use of rt-PA for stroke. These case series have been conducted in both large academic centers and community hospitals. A meta-analysis of phase IV studies and these post-FDA approval case series (n = 2639), reported an overall symptomatic hemorrhage rate of 5.2% (95% CI = 4.3 to 6.0) and a mortality rate and percent favorable outcome similar to those reported in the NINDS rt-PA Stroke Study (Table 5) *(29)*. Mortality rates across studies correlated with the rates of protocol violations. This meta-analysis suggests that the safety and efficacy of rt-PA in community use is similar to that found in the NINDS rt-PA Stroke Study, but that strict adherence to treatment protocols is essential.

Summary of Efficacy and Safety of Recombinant Tissue Plasminogen Activator in Stroke

Two randomized trials (NINDS rt-PA Stroke Trial—parts 1 and 2) evaluating the use of rt-PA within 3 h of stroke onset showed that treated patients are at least 30% more likely to have minimal or no deficits 90 d after treatment, compared to those who receive placebo. Patients treated within 90 min have improved outcome as compared to those treated between 90 and180 min. The rate of symptomatic ICH within 36 h is 6.4%, and there is no significant difference in 90-d mortality between treated and placebo groups.

There have been three large randomized trials evaluating the safety and efficacy of intravenous rt-PA beyond this 3-h window; in none was there a signifi-

Table 5
Post-FDA Approval Studies of rt-PA

Trial	*Patients (n)*	*Median baseline NIHSS*	*Sumptomatic ICH*	*Deaths (%)*	*Very favorable*	*Protocol violations (%)*
CASES *(28)*	1099	15	4.6			15.0
STARS*(27)*	389	13	3.3	13.4	34.6	32.6
Houston*(35)*	269	14	4.5	15.0		13.0
Cologne*(36)*	150	11	4.0	10.7	41.0	1.3
Berlin*(37)*	75	13	2.7	15.0	40.0	20.0
Cleveland*(38)*	70	12	15.7	15.7		50.0
Calgary*(39)*	68	15	8.8	16.2		16.2
OSF Stroke Network*(40)*	57	15	5.3	8.8	47.0	8.8
Mercy/Sacramento*(41)*	43	14	7.0	16.3	42	12
Oregon*(42)*	33	17	9.1	18.2	36.4	
tPA Stroke Survey*(43)*	189	11–15	5.8	9.5	34.0	29.6
Connecticut*(44)*	63	15	6.3	25.4		66.7
Indianapolis*(45)*	50	11	8.0	10.0		16.0
Cleveland Clinic *(46)*	47		6.4			19.1
Michigan*(47)*	37	6–10	10.8	5.4	37.9	
All studies	2639	14	5.2	13	37.1	18

CASES, Canadian Activase for Stroke Effectiveness Study, STARS, Standard Treatment with Alteplase to Reverse Stroke. (Adapted from ref. *29.*)

cant benefit for rt-PA- over placebo-treated patients on the primary endpoints and all have found significantly higher rates of ICH in the rt-PA-treated groups. A pooled analysis of randomized studies demonstrated benefit when rt-PA was administered within 4.5 h of stroke onset, but increased mortality with rt-PA administration after 4.5 h. Further adequately powered studies are needed to define the role of rt-PA beyond 3 h of symptom onset.

EFFICACY AND SAFETY OF STREPTOKINASE IN STROKE

There have been three large randomized trials of SK in the treatment of acute ischemic stroke *(30–32)*. Unfortunately, all three were halted because of increased rates of ICH and higher mortality in the SK-treated patients.

Randomized Trial of Streptokinase Given Within 0–4 h of Stroke Onset

The Australian Streptokinase Trial (ASK) was a double-blind, randomized trial comparing 1.5 million U of SK plus 325 mg aspirin to intravenous placebo and aspirin in patients with ischemic stroke who could be enrolled and treated within 4 h of symptom onset *(30–33)*. ASK was suspended based on the recommendation of the Safety and Monitoring Committee after analysis of the first 228 patients treated between 3 and 4 h of stroke onset showed increased rates of mortality and symptomatic ICH in the SK group (Table 6) *(30)*. A specific *a priori* hypothesis was that outcomes would differ between those patients treated within 0–3 h and those treated after 3 h. Subsequent analysis of the 70 patients treated within 3 h as compared to the 270 treated after 3 h found that earlier treatment was safer and associated with significantly better outcomes than later treatment ($p = 0.04$) *(33)*.

Randomized Trials of Streptokinase Given Within 0–6 h of Stroke Onset

There have been two large, randomized trials of SK given within 6 h of stroke onset *(31,32)*. The Multi-Center Acute Stroke Trial - Europe (MAST-E) was a multicenter, double-blind, randomized study of SK compared to placebo in patients with hemispheric stroke who could be randomized and treated within 6 h of stroke onset *(31)*. Patients were treated intravenously with 1.5 million U of SK or placebo given over 60 min. The study was terminated upon recommendation from the Data Monitoring and Safety Committee following the analysis of data from 270 patients (310 enrolled) *(34)*. The 10-d mortality in patients receiving SK was 34% compared to 18% in patients treated with placebo ($p = 0.002$) (Table 6). The symptomatic hemorrhage rate was 21% in the SK patients and 3% in the placebo patients ($p < 0.001$) *(31)*.

The Multi-Center Acute Stroke Trial-Italy (MAST-I) was a multicenter, randomized trial comparing treatment among four groups *(32)*. Patients within 6 h

Table 6
Randomized Trials of Streptokinase (SK)

Study[a]	*Time to treatment*	*Patients*	*Treatment group*	*Mortality (%)*	*Intracerebral hematoma (%)*
Australian Streptokinase Trial (ASK) *(33)*	4 h	340	SK + 100 mg ASA	36.2[b]	13.2[b]
			100 mg ASA	20.5[b]	3.0[b]
Multicenter Acute Stroke Trial-Europe (MAST-E) *(31)*	6 h	310	SK	34	21.2[b,c]
			Placebo	18	2.6[b,c]
Multicenter Acute Stroke Trials-Italy (MAST-I) *(32)*	6 h	622	SK + 300 mg ASA	34[b]	10[c]
			SK	19	6[c]
			300 mg ASA	10	2[c]
			Standard therapy	13[b]	0.6[c]

[a]All studies terminated prior to completion due to increased mortality in SK group.
[b]p 0.001.
[c]Symptomatic hemorrhage in hospital.SK,streptokinase; ASA, aspirin.

of symptom onset were randomized to receive either 1.5 million U of SK intravenously over 60 min, 300 mg of aspirin per day for 10 d, iv SK and aspirin, or control (standard treatment, no placebo). MAST-I was also suspended after 40% of planned recruitment *(32)*. Patients receiving both SK and aspirin had significantly greater 10-d mortality than those given neither (34 vs 13%, $p < 0.001$; *see* Table 6). There was no significant difference in mortality for those patients treated with SK alone (19 vs 13%, $p = 0.12$) *(32)*. Symptomatic ICH rates were higher in the SK-alone and SK + aspirin groups than in the group given neither (6 and 10% respectively, vs 0.6%).

Summary of Efficacy and Safety of Streptokinase in Stroke

All three studies of SK were suspended as a result of increased rates of hemorrhage and mortality in the SK-treated groups. Although pilot safety studies for SK were carried out prior to beginning the randomized trials, dose-escalation safety studies were not performed; the 1.5 million U dose used in the stroke studies is identical to that used for MI. In contrast, two dose-finding, dose-escalation trials of intravenous rt-PA preceded the larger randomized trials of rt-PA; the doses selected for the subsequent randomized trials of rt-PA were approx 60–75% of the doses used for acute MI. A lower dose of SK (e.g., 0.9–1.2 million U) may have proved effective with reasonable safety. Furthermore, safety in the SK trials may also have been improved if earlier treatment had been required. Further development of SK as intravenous therapy for acute ischemic stroke is unlikely because of the negative findings from these studies.

ONGOING STUDIES

Two large, ongoing, randomized studies are investigating the use of intravenous rt-PA for acute ischemic stroke. The Third International Stroke Trial is comparing 0.9 mg/kg of intravenous rt-PA and placebo in patients presenting within 6 h of ischemic stroke onset. A study size of 6000 patients is planned. The ECASS III trial will compare intravenous rt-PA and placebo in patients presenting with acute ischemic stroke between 3 and 4 h of onset, with a planned enrollment of 800 patients.

CONCLUSIONS

Intravenous rt-PA improves 3-mo neurological outcome if given within 3 h of symptom onset in appropriately selected patients with acute ischemic stroke. A pooled analysis of randomized trials of intravenous rt-PA suggests a potential benefit with treatment 3–4.5 h after onset, but additional data from randomized trials are needed before this can be recommended. The use of SK at a dose of 1.5 million U has not been shown to be safe or efficacious in patients with acute ischemic stroke.

REFERENCES

1. Clarke RL, Clifton E. The treatment of cerebrovascular thromboses and embolism with fibrinolytic agents. *Am J Cardiology* 1960;6:546–551.
2. Herndon RM, Meyer JS, Johnson JF. Fibrinolysin therapy in thrombotic diseases of the nervous system. *J Mich St Med Soc* 1960;59:1684–1692.
3. Meyer JS, Gilroy J, Barnhart MI, Johnson JF. Anticoagulants plus streptokinase therapy in progressive stroke. *JAMA* 1964;189:373.
4. Meyer JS, Gilroy J, Barnhart MI, Johnson JF. Therapeutic thrombolysis in cerebral thromboembolism. *Neurology* 1963;13:927–937.
5. Fletcher AP, Alkjersig N, Lewis M, et al. A pilot study of urokinase therapy in cerebral infarction. *Stroke* 1976:135–142.
6. Fears R. Biochemical pharmacology and therapeutic aspects of thrombolytic agents. *Pharmacol Rev* 1990;42:202–222.
7. Larcan A, Laprevote-Heully MC, Lambert H, Alexandre P, Picard L, Chrisment N. Indications for the use of thrombolytics in cases of cerebrovascular thrombosis also treated with hyperbaric oxygenation (2 ata). *Therapie* 1977;32:259–270.
8. Zeumer H, Hacke W, Ringelstein EB. Local intraarterial thrombolysis in vertebrobasilar thromboembolic disease. *AJNR* 1983;4:401–404.
9. Henze T, Boerr A, Tebbe U, Romatowski J. Lysis of basilar artery occlusion with tissue plasminogen activator. *Lancet* 1987;2:1391.
10. Kaufman HH, Lind TA, Clark DS. Non-penetrating trauma to the carotid artery with secondary thrombosis and embolism: Treatment by thrombolysin. *Acta Neurochirurgica* 1977; 37:219–244.
11. Nenci GG, Gresele P, Taramelli M, Agnelli G, Signorini E. Thrombolytic therapy for thromboembolism of vertebrobasilar artery. *Angiology* 1983;34:361–371.
12. Zeumer H, Ferbert A, Ringelstein EB. Local intra-arterial fibrinolytic therapy in inaccessible internal carotid occlusion. *Neuroradiology* 1984;26:315–317.
13. Jungreis CA, Wechsler LR, Horton JA. Intracranial thrombolysis via a catheter embedded in the clot. *Stroke* 1989;20:1578–1580.
14. Zivin JA, Lyden PD, DeGirolami U, et al. Tissue plasminogen activator. Reduction of neurologic damage after experimental embolic stroke. *Arch Neurol* 1988;45:387–391.
15. NINDS rt-PA Stroke Study Group. Tissue plasminogen activator for acute ischemic stroke. *NEJM* 1995;333:1581–1587.
16. Haley E, Levy D, Brott T, et al. Urgent therapy for stroke. Part II. Pilot study of tissue plasminogen activator administered 91–180 minutes from onset. *Stroke* 1992;23:641–645.
17. Brott T, Haley ECJ, Levy DE, et al. Urgent therapy for stroke. Part I. Pilot study of tissue plasminogen activator administered within 90 minutes. *Stroke* 1992:632–640.
18. Haley EJ, Lewandowski C, Tilley B, NINDS rt-PA Stroke Study Group. Myths regarding the NINDS rt-PA Stroke Trial: Setting the record straight. *Ann Emerg Med* 1997;30:676–682.
19. NINDS t-PA Stroke Study Group. Intracerebral hemorrhage after intravenous t-PA therapy for ischemic stroke. *Stroke* 1997;28:2109–2118.
20. Clark WM, Wissman S, Albers GW, Jhamandas JH, Madden KP, Hamilton S, for the ATLANTIS Study Investigators. Recombinant tissue-type plasminogen activator (alteplase) for ischemic stroke 3 to 5 hours after symptom onset. The ATLANTIS Study: A randomized controlled trial. *JAMA* 1999;282:2019–2026.
21. Clark WM, Albers GW, Madden KP, Hamilton S, for the ATLANTIS Study Investigators. The rt-PA (alteplase) 0–6 hour acute stroke trial, part a (a0276g): Results of a double-blind, placebo-controlled, multicenter study. *Stroke* 2000;31:811–816.
22. Hacke W, Kaste M, Fieschi C, et al., for the ECASS Study Group. Intravenous thrombolysis with recombinant tissue plasminogen activator for acute hemispheric stroke. The European Cooperative Acute Stroke Study. *JAMA* 1995;274:1017–1025.

23. Hacke W, Kaste M, Fieschi C, et al, for the Second European-Australasian Acute Stroke Study Investigators. Randomised double-blind placebo-controlled trial of thrombolytic therapy with intravenous alteplase in acute ischaemic stroke (ECASS II). *Lancet* 1998;352:1245–1251.
24. Hacke W, Bluhmki E, Steiner T, et al., for the ECASS Study Group. Dichotomized efficacy end points and global end-point analysis applied to the ECASS intention-to-treat data set: Post hoc analysis of ECASS I. *Stroke*. 1998;29:2073–2075.
25. Marler JR, Tilley B, Lu M, et al. Earlier treatment associated with better outcome: The NINDS t-PA Stroke Study. *Neurology* 2000;55:1649–1655.
26. ATLANTIS, ECASS, and NINDS rt-PA Study Group Investigators,. Association of outcome with early stroke treatment: Pooled analysis of the ATLANTIS, ECASS, and NINDS stroke trials. *Lancet* 2004;363:768–774..
27. Albers GW, Bates VE, Clark WM, Bell R, Verro P, Hamilton SA. Intravenous tissue-type plasminogen activator for treatment of acute stroke: The standard treatment with alteplase to reverse stroke (STARS) study. *JAMA* 2000;283:1145–1150.
28. Hill MD, Buchan AM. The Canadian Activase for Stroke Effectiveness Study (CASES): Interim results. *Stroke* 2001;32:323–a.
29. Graham GD. Tissue plasminogen activator for acute ischemic stroke in clinical practice: A meta-analysis of safety data. *Stroke* 2003;34:2847–2850.
30. Donnan GA, Davis SM, Chambers BR, Gates PC, Hankey GJ, Stewart-Wynne EG, Rosen D, Tuck RR. Trials of streptokinase in severe acute ischaemic stroke. *Lancet* 1995;345:578–579.
31. Multicentre Acute Stroke Trial-European Study Group. Thrombolytic therapy with streptokinase in acute ischemic stroke. *NEJM*. 1996;335:145–150.
32. Multicentre Acute Stroke Trial-Italy (MAST-I) Group. Randomized controlled trial of streptokinase, aspirin, and combination of both in treatment of acute ischemic stroke. *Lancet* 1995;346:1509–1514.
33. Donnan GA, Davis SM, Chambers BR, et al., for the Australian Streptokinase (ASK) Trial Study Group. Streptokinase for acute ischemic stroke with relationship to time of administration. *JAMA* 1996;276:961–966.
34. Hommel M, Boissel JP, Comu C, et al., for the MAST Study Group. Termination of trial of streptokinase in severe acute ischaemic stroke. *Lancet* 1994;315:57.
35. Grotta JC, Burgin WS, El-Mitwalli A, et al. Intravenous tissue-type plasminogen activator therapy for ischemic stroke: Houston experience 1996 to 2000. *Arch Neurol* 2001;58: 2009–2013.
36. Schmulling S, Grond M, Rudolf J, Heiss WD. One-year follow-up in acute stroke patients treated with rt-PA in clinical routine. *Stroke* 2000;31:1552–1554.
37. Koennecke HC, Nohr R, Leistner S, Marx P. Intravenous t-PA for ischemic stroke team performance over time, safety, and efficacy in a single-center, 2-year experience. *Stroke* 2001;32:1074–1078.
38. Katzan IL, Furlan AJ, Lloyd LE, et al. Use of tissue-type plasminogen activator for acute ischemic stroke: The Cleveland area experience. *JAMA* 2000;283:1151–1158.
39. Buchan AM, Barber PA, Newcommon N, et al. Effectiveness of t-PA in acute ischemic stroke: Outcome relates to appropriateness. *Neurology* 2000;54:679–684.
40. Wang DZ, Rose JA, Honings DS, Garwacki DJ, Milbrandt JC. Treating acute stroke patients with intravenous t-PA. The OSF stroke network experience. *Stroke* 2000;31:77–81.
41. Akins PT, Delemos C, Wentworth D, Byer J, Schorer SJ, Atkinson RP. Can emergency department physicians safely and effectively initiate thrombolysis for acute ischemic stroke? *Neurology* 2000;55:1801–1805.
42. Egan R, Lutsep HL, Clark WM, et al. Open label tissue plasminogen activator for stroke: The Oregon experience. *J Stroke Cerebrovasc Dis* 1999;8:287–290.

43. Tanne D, Bates VE, Verro P, et al. Initial clinical experience with IV tissue plasminogen activator for acute ischemic stroke: A multicenter survey. The t-PA Stroke Survey Group. *Neurology* 1999;53:424–427.
44. Bravata DM, Kim N, Concato J, Krumholz HM, Brass LM. Thrombolysis for acute stroke in routine clinical practice. *Arch Intern Med* 2002;162:1994–2001.
45. Lopez-Yunez AM, Bruno A, Williams LS, Yilmaz E, Zurru C, Biller J. Protocol violations in community-based rt-PA stroke treatment are associated with symptomatic intracerebral hemorrhage. *Stroke* 2001;32:12–16.
46. Katzan IL, Hammer MD, Furlan AJ, Hixson ED, Nadzam DM. Quality improvement and tissue-type plasminogen activator for acute ischemic stroke: A Cleveland update. *Stroke* 2003;34:799–800.
47. Smith RW, Scott PA, Grant RJ, Chudnofsky CR, Frederiksen SM. Emergency physician treatment of acute stroke with recombinant tissue plasminogen activator: A retrospective analysis. *Acad Emerg Med* 1999;6:618–625.

8 Further Analysis of NINDS Study

Long-Term Outcome, Subgroups, and Cost Effectiveness

Susan C. Fagan, PharmD,
Thomas Kwiatkowski, MD,
and Patrick D. Lyden, MD

CONTENTS

INTRODUCTION

Following the initial publication of the National Institute of Neurological Disorders and Stroke (NINDS) tissue-plasminogen activator (t-PA) Stroke Trial results, the NINDS investigators published a series of additional data and analyses. These analyses were necessary because not all the relevant data could be included in the primary report, and to answer criticisms of the original article. Some of these analyses are summarized in other chapters, including Chapters 9 and 18. This chapter focuses on three important issues: cost effectiveness, subgroup selection, and long-term follow-up. The cost-effectiveness issue is critical because thrombolytic drugs are expensive. To show that the drug cost is worthwhile, the costs of stroke care absent treatment, including how costs might increase or decrease with successful treatment, were examined. Subgroup selection is addressed because some have advocated such analysis to help select

From: *Current Clinical Neurology: Thrombolytic Therapy for Acute Stroke, Second Edition*
Edited by: P. D. Lyden © Humana Press Inc., Totowa, NJ

patients at particular risk or susceptibility of benefit. Regression modeling was used to rigorously identify any subgroups that could be preferred for treatment. To ensure that the benefits of thrombolysis were sustained over the long term, the original cohort of patients up to 1 yr after stroke was followed. The essentials of these three follow-up analyses, cost effectiveness, subgroup selection, and long-term follow-up, have been published, so only brief descriptions of the methods are given here *(1–3)*. The aim of this chapter is to put the results of these analyses into perspective for the practicing clinician.

COST EFFECTIVENESS

The cost effectiveness of t-PA was demonstrated in 1998 *(2)*. A rigorous methodology to estimate the cost savings and any additional costs associated with thrombolytic stroke therapy was used. Certain assumptions about stroke costs and outcomes were based on data from the literature and from the original study (Table 1). Then, to account for possible errors in the assumptions, a simulation method was used to vary the values of those assumptions.

Methods

Health and economic outcomes from the NINDS Recombinant Tissue Plasminogen Activator (rt-PA)Stroke trial, comparing t-PA and placebo, were estimated using a Markov modeling approach. A Markov model allows decision analysis of problems that are ongoing. Over time, a patient can be in any one of a set of states and can transition between states based on probabilities defined by empirical data or assumptions. To illustrate, a patient may transition from no disability to moderate disability because of a recurrent stroke, the rate of which may be predicted to be 5% per year. For the purpose of this study, a Markov model was particularly appropriate because it allowed us to focus on the impact of stroke over the lifetime of the patient.

Sensitivity analyses was used (one-way and multi-way) to assess the probability that the model accurately estimated costs and outcomes. The number of quality-adjusted-life-years (QALYs) was saved as the health outcome summary measure. This measure is standard for these sorts of studies, in which no effect on mortality is expected. It was therefore predicted that the main impact of t-PA would be an increase in the quality of the patients' life (through decreased disability) rather than the quantity of life (no decreased mortality). The economic outcome summary measure of the model is the difference in estimated health care costs between the two treatment alternatives.

Assumptions

It was desired to model outcome for 30 yr following stroke, and since data from the NINDS rt-PA Stroke Study was only available for 1 yr, certain assump-

Table 1
Assumptions Used to Estimate Cost Effectiveness of Thrombolytic Therapy for Stroke

Epidemiological assumptions	*Low*	*Best*	*High*
Stroke recurrence rate per year	0.03	0.052	0.08
Recurrent stroke mortality	0.1	0.19	0.3
Multiplier for age specific mortality[a]	1.25	2.67	4
Discharge to NH from rehab—age 65 to 75	0.13	0.18	0.21
Discharge to NH from rehab—age >75	0.24	0.32	0.34
Disability distribution (utilities)			
Rankin 0—No Symptoms	0.85	0.90	0.95
Rankin 1—No Disability Despite Symptoms	0.70	0.80	0.9
Rankin 2—Slight Disability	0.35	0.46	0.65
Rankin 3—Moderate Disability	0.20	0.34	0.5
Rankin 4—Moderate/Severe Disability	0.12	0.30	0.45
Rankin 5—Severe Disability	–0.20	–0.02	0.2
Dead	0.00	0.00	0.00
Cost assumptions			
Cost/day of hosp	$1000	$1200	$1400
Average t-PA acquisition cost	$2100	$2230	$2400
Preparation and administration of t-PA	$10	$20	$30
Physician cost for administration of t-PA	$200	$300	$400
ICU additional cost for t-PA patients	$600	$775	$1000
ICH additional cost	$3000	$4500	$6000
Inpatient Rehabilitation	$10,000	$21,233	$40,000
Outpatient Rehabilitation	$1200	$2236	$2500
Nursing home cost per year	$20,000	$39,996	$50,000

[a]Inflates US age-specific mortality rate to account for the increase in mortality observed in patients who have had a stroke. NH, nursing home; ICU, intensive care unit; ICH, intracerebral hemorrhage.

tions had to be made, as listed in Table 1. Stroke recurrence rate and age-adjusted mortality could be estimated from natural history studies available in the literature. It was assumed that among survivors after a recurrent stroke there was an equal chance of categories of equal or greater disability. Each of the disability categories was assigned a utility value based on the results of a published patient preference survey for stroke outcomes *(4)*. For cost assumptions, no published accepted estimate existed and wide extrapolations were required in many situations. In assumptions with greater uncertainty, the ranges of values used in the sensitivity analyses were broadened.

Table 2
Actual Distribution of Patients
by Modified Rankin Disability Scores and Deaths by Time From Randomization

	10 Days		*3 Months*		*6 Months*		*1 Year*	
Disability category	*PLA*	*t-PA*	*PLA*	*t-PA*	*PLA*	*t-PA*	*PLA*	*t-PA*
Rankin 0	23	49	33	57	33	59	32	61
Rankin 1	31	52	50	74	56	68	50	66
Rankin 2	29	26	36	23	32	25	36	23
Rankin 3	29	29	44	40	50	42	38	39
Rankin 4	87	68	60	42	42	30	34	19
Rankin 5	77	63	20	19	18	14	17	14
Dead	31	23	64	54	72	65	87	76
Total patients with data	307	310	307	309	303	303	294	298

Data is from patients in the NINDS rt-PA Stroke Trial. $N = 312$ per t-PA and placebo groups. Patients with missing values were excluded. PLA, placebo.

Table 3
Disposition Results From the NINDS rt-PA Stroke Trial

Discharge destination	*Number (%) t-PA*	*Number (%) Placebo*
Home	151 (48)	112 (36)
Rehabilitation unit	91 (29)	115 (37)
Nursing home	22 (7)	39 (13)
Dead	35 (11)	40 (13)
Other facility	13 (4)	6 (2)

Compared home to all other dispositions, chi-square test $p < 0.01$

Results

NINDS rt-PA Stroke Trial Data

The initial hospital stay was 12.4 ± 11 d for t-PA-treated patients, compared to 10.9 ± 10 d for placebo-treated patients in the trial ($p = 0.02$ Wilcoxon Rank Sum Test). The difference was attributable to the treatment, and not to other confounding factors such as stroke subtype. Disability status over the first year after a stroke is listed in Table 2. Discharge disposition data for 535 of the 572 patients alive at discharge are summarized in Table 3. More patients treated with t-PA were discharged to their own home (or that of a relative or friend) and fewer required inpatient rehabilitation and nursing home care (Table 3) ($p = 0.002, \chi^2$).

SENSITIVITY ANALYSES

The health and economic outcomes, calculated per 1000 patients potentially eligible for early thrombolytic therapy, are shown in Table 4. For every 1000 patients treated with t-PA, the model predicts 55 more intracerebral hemorrhages (ICH) and 116 more patients discharged home, compared to placebo. Discounted costs for hospitalization are about $1.7 million greater owing to treatment. However, costs for nursing home care and rehabilitation, are significantly reduced by t-PA treatment by about $4.8 and $1.3 million, respectively. The increase in acute care costs represents an incremental cost of $15,000 for each additional patient discharged home rather than to a rehabilitation facility or nursing home. The overall impact on both acute and long-term costs (90% certainty) is a net decrease of over $4 million ($13 to $0.5 million) to the health care system for every 1000 patients treated. The estimated impact on long-term health outcomes is 751 QALYs saved over 30 yr for 1000 patients. The variables with the largest impact on health outcome were the t-PA hemorrhage rate and the overall mortality factor. As the hemorrhage rate was varied from 6 to 20%, the number of QALYs saved decreased from 765 to 335. As the overall mortality factor was varied from 1.25 to 4, the number of QALYs saved decreased from 1129 to 575. The variables with the largest impact on cost were initial length of stay and annual nursing home cost. In order to eliminate the overall cost savings, the t-PA group length of stay would have to exceed the placebo group by 2.1 d or the annual nursing home cost would have to be less than $4700 per year. The t-PA drug cost had minimal impact.

Implications for Clinicians

The decision to administer t-PA to an eligible patient should be based on the proven health benefits alone, as detailed in Chapters 6 and 7. The cost-effectiveness analysis becomes important only when forecasting budget costs at a macro-level for a health care system. Also, the costs of interventions designed to increase the number of eligible patients should be compared to the predicted cost savings. In a recent investigation, the cost of implementing an "NINDS-compliant" protocol for administering rt-PA to ischemic stroke patients was shown to be "cost effective" by increasing the numbers of treatable patients *(5)*. It was estimated that the cost of such a strategy would be $434 per patient and the proportion of treated patients could be nearly tripled.

Since the publication of the cost analysis of the NINDS rt-PA Stroke Trial, two separate Canadian groups and a UK group have also reported "cost savings," using different cost estimates and different methodology in a similar, but different health care system *(6–8)*. Thus, thrombolytic stroke therapy joins a very small number of therapies that not only reduces disability, but also saves dollars. To put

Table 4
One-Way Sensitivity Analysis of Health and Economic Outcomes Per 1000 Patients Eligible To Be Treated with t-PA

Health outcomes	*Placebo*	*t-PA*	*Difference*	*5th and 95th Percentiles*[a]
Life years by Rankin category				
Rankin 0—No Symptoms	826	1520	694	257 to 1072
Rankin 1—No Disability Despite Symptoms	1394	1866	472	–244 to 1017
Rankin 2—Slight Disability	1101	776	–325	–719 to –59
Rankin 3—Moderate Disability	1268	1322	54	–357 to 393
Rankin 4—Moderate/ Severe Disability	1366	959	–407	–863 to –133
Rankin 5—Severe Disability	1179	1054	–125	–514 to 147
Total Life Years (30 yr)	7135	7498	363	–985 to 982
QALYs	3183	3934	751	–15 to 1142
Economic outcomes				
(discounted[b], $ thousands)				
t-PA acquisition cost	0	2250	2250	2135 to 2406
Physician cost for t-PA administration	0	300	300	206 to 389
Initial hospitalization	14,923	14,121	(803)	–2282 to 1236
Future hospitalization for stroke	5222	5493	271	–861 to 813
Nursing home	32,975	28,157	(4818)	–12,195 to –1002
Rehabilitation	11,146	9768	(1378)	–3970 to –398
Total cost (acute plus long-term care)	62,716	58,461	(4255)	–13,022 to 531
Cost at 1 year	29,810	29,207	(604)	–3481 to 2004
Cost-effectiveness ($1000)				
Hospitalization cost per additional patient discharged home			15	1.9 to 80
Cost per QALY gained			(8)	–76 to 17

[a]Represents the estimated 5th and 95th percentiles for the distribution of possible values of the difference based on the Monte Carlo one-way sensitivity analysis using the ranges specified and 10,000 iterations.

[b]Discounted at 5% per year

QALYs, Quality adjusted life years.

these results in perspective, note that few other therapies result in net cost savings to the health care system; two traditional examples are prenatal care and early childhood vaccinations *(9–12)*. These therapies cost money to administer, but overall there is a net cost reduction owing to lower disease incidence. Actual cost savings are realized to the health system when reduced disability at discharge translates into a significant reduction in the utilization of subacute and long-term care facilities. In this analysis, t-PA for eligible stroke patients appears to represent a win–win situation: improved patient outcomes are associated with a net cost savings to the health care system.

SUBGROUP ANALYSIS

The inclusion and exclusion criteria used in the original study are now used to select eligible patients for thrombolytic therapy. In applying the selection criteria to individual patients (*see* Chapter 18), it would be useful to know if there are any particular subgroups of patients with increased likelihood to benefit or suffer harm from t-PA. Indeed, some critics of the original work have noted the lack of such subgroup data in the literature *(13)*. To address these concerns, the outcome in t-PA- and placebo-treated patients with pretreatment information to identify subgroups that may or may not particularly benefit from t-PA treatment was compared *(1)*.

Methods

The original report found that odds of a good outcome were associated with age, race, gender, smoking, problem drinking, diabetes, hypertension, atherosclerosis, atrial fibrillation, other cardiac disease, stroke subtype, baseline National Institute of Heath Stroke Scale (NIHSS), presence of thrombus or early signs of infarction (hypodensity or midline shift) on baseline computed tomography (CT) scan, admission and baseline blood pressure (Table 5). None of the findings, however, could be used to subselect patients because the odds ratios were calculated using univariate models. That is, corrections were not made for the fact that some of these variables interact with each other; such an interaction could erroneously indicate a subgroup of patients susceptible to increased benefit or harm. A multivariable modeling method was used and it was found that race, diabetes, hypertension, baseline mean arterial pressure (MAP), and baseline systolic blood pressure showed a significant interaction with t-PA treatment. The selected variables and interactions were then included in a multivariable model, and interactions among confounding variables were identified.

Results

To illustrate the preliminary univariate results, the effect of age on outcome is shown in Fig. 1. In each decile the proportion of responders was greater in the

Table 5
Relationship Between Baseline Covariates and Outcome (Global Odds Ratio): Univariate Analyses and Treatment Interactions

Variable	*Global odds ratio*	*95% Confidence limits*	*p-value*[a]	*Treatment Interaction p-value*[b]
t-PA treatment	1.86	1.38–2.5	<0.001	
Age	0.97	0.95–0.98	<0.001	0.49
Race				
Hispanic vs black	1.05	0.49–2.21		
Hispanic vs white	1.34	0.65	0.31	0.13
Gender	1.29	0.95–1.75	0.10	0.83
Cigaret smoking in previous year	1.54	1.13–2.10	0.007	0.78
Drinking problems	1.48	1.10–2.00	0.01	0.98
History of diabetes	0.57	0.39–0.84	0.004	0.05
History of hypertension	0.55	0.41–0.75	<0.001	0.19
History of atherosclerosis	0.69	0.49–0.98	0.04	0.34
History of atrial fibrillation	0.57	0.38–0.86	0.008	0.96
History of other cardiac disease	0.82	0.61–1.10	0.18	0.66
Prior stroke	0.96	0.70–1.31	0.79	0.99
Aspirin (NSAID)	0.96	0.70–1.31	0.78	0.68
Baseline stroke subtypes[c]			0.008	0.78
Small vs cardioembolic	0.44	0.28–0.69		
Small vs large	0.45	0.29–0.71		
Small vs other	0.69	0.27–1.71		
Baseline NIH Stoke Scale	0.86	0.84–0.88	0.0001	0.78
Early CT findings with thrombus	0.43	0.28–0.66	0.0001	0.53
Early CT findings without thrombus	0.65	0.33–1.26	0.20	0.42
Weight (actual, ranked)	1.00	1.00–1.00	0.87	0.69
Percent of correct dose (ranked)	1.00	1.00–1.00	0.30	0.80
Admission blood pressure (MAP)	0.99	0.99–1.00	0.12	0.18
Admission systolic blood pressure	1.00	0.99–1.00	0.14	0.53
Admission diastolic blood pressure	0.99	0.99–1.00	0.22	0.89
Baseline blood pressure (MAP)	0.99	0.98–1.00	0.22	0.64
Baseline systolic blood pressure	0.99	0.99–1.00	0.13	0.14
Baseline diastolic blood pressure	0.99	0.98	0.27	0.33
Centers	1.01	0.94–1.08	0.82	0.23
Time from stroke onset to treatment	1.00	1.00–1.01	0.62	0.28
Admission temperature	1.15	1.003–1.33	0.046	0.83

[a]Association of specified variable with outcome (global) including treatment effect.

[b]Association of specified treatment interaction with outcome (global) in model including the interaction and effects for treatment and the other variable in the interaction. [c]Stroke subtype was diagnosed based on all information available to the treating physician prior to starting t-PA therapy. Small, small vessel (lacunar), large, large vessel.

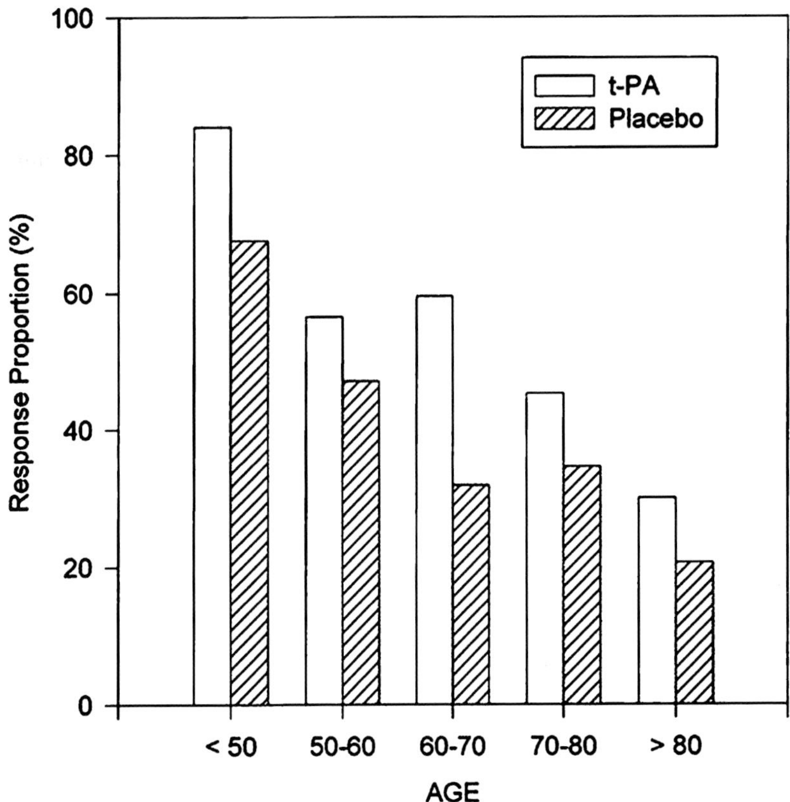

Fig. 1. Effect of age on likelihood of favorable response.

t-PA group. Similarly, the effect of stroke subtype is illustrated in Fig. 2. Again, the benefit of thrombolysis was apparent in each subtype of ischemic stroke. During the multivariable analysis, however, significant confounding interactions among several variables was found. Age-by-baseline NIHSS and age-by-MAP interactions were significant (i.e., patients with older age and higher baseline stroke scale scores or older age and higher admission mean arterial blood pressure were less likely to have a favorable outcome). None of the two-way interactions significantly interacted with treatment, however, suggesting that none of these confounds influenced patient responsiveness to treatment. This concept is illustrated in Fig. 3. The proportion of patients who achieve a favorable outcome declines markedly with increasing levels of severity. In each severity quartile, however, the proportion of favorable responders is always greater in the thrombolysis group, and the relative benefit is always positive, ranging from 20 to 40%. Thus, although many variables adversely affect outcome, none reduce the chances of favorable response to thrombolysis.

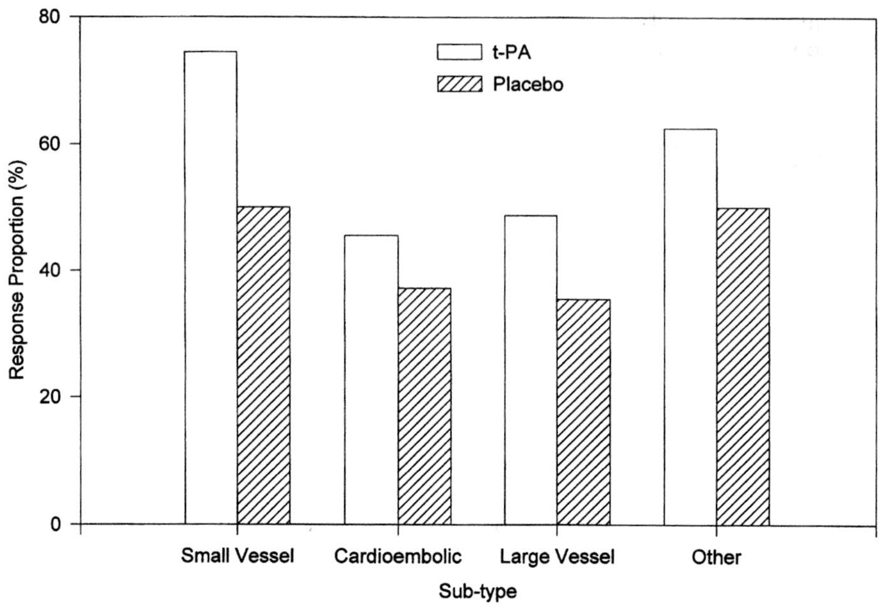

Fig. 2. Effect of stroke subtype on likelihood of favorable response.

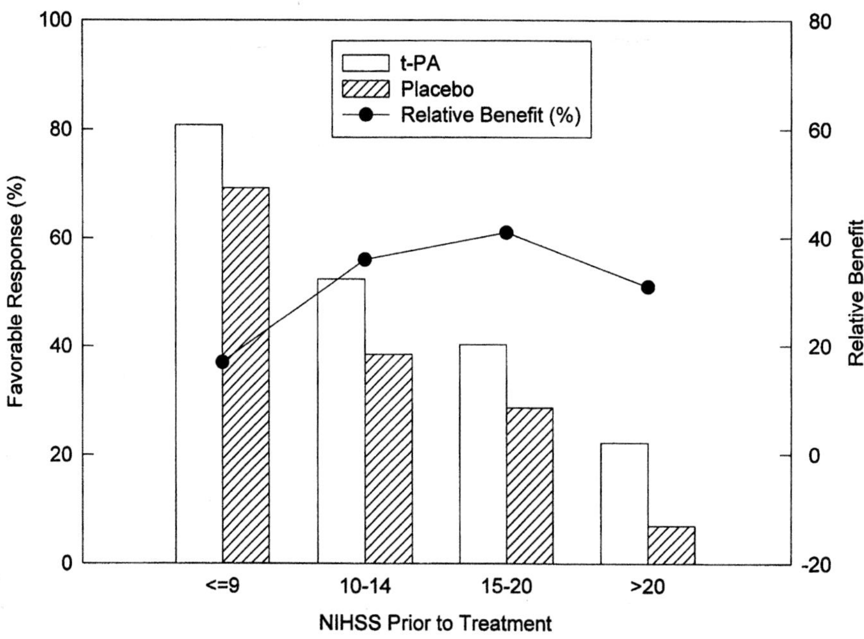

Fig. 3. Effect of stroke severity (NIHSS) on likelihood of favorable response.

Table 6 shows the final results of the multivariable model process. Treatment with t-PA remained strongly and independently associated with favorable outcome (global odds ratio 1.96, $p < 0.0001$). The only terms that remained important predictors of outcome, after correcting for the influences of all other confounding variables, were the age-by-NIHSS interaction term, diabetes, admission MAP-by-age interaction, and thrombus or hypodensity/mass effect on baseline CT scan (i.e., for all randomized patients, global odds ratios <1). None of these terms, however, had a significant interaction with t-PA treatment. That is, each of the variables and interactions in Table 6 significantly influenced outcome, but none of them influenced the likelihood of differential response to t-PA. In nearly all subgroups, the proportion of patients with favorable outcome is greater in the t-PA treated group. Furthermore, in the 49 patients older than 75 years and admission NIHSS of more than 20 there appeared to be no favorable response to treatment. However, closer evaluation of this subgroup, including analysis of outcome categories such as mild or moderate, suggested a treatment benefit, as shown in Fig. 4. The proportion of patients who achieved a nearly normal score on the NIHSS was zero, suggesting no benefit. In the mild category, however, with NIHSS scores between 2 and 8, there was a significant benefit in the treated group. Similarly in this most severe patient cohort, the treated group was significantly more likely to show independence in Activities of Daily Living, as shown in Fig. 4 by the proportion with Barthel Index (BI) scores of 50 or more.

Implications for Clinicians

Despite rigorous procedures, and a liberal *p*-value cut-off of 0.1, no pretreatment information that predicted a differential response to t-PA treatment was identified. Thrombolytic treatment was independently and strongly associated with increased likelihood of favorable outcome 3 mo after stroke *(14)*. After other confounding variables were included in the multivariable model, the absence of any interactions with treatment suggests a persistent beneficial effect of t-PA treatment across all subgroups tested. Although tempting, it is fallacious to select a subgroup from univariate data, such as Table 5, and conclude that t-PA is not beneficial for that subgroup *(15)*. The broader trend of t-PA benefit demonstrable across all subgroups, using rigorous statistical methods, makes the single isolated subgroup aberration more likely to be a random occurrence related to small sample size in the subgroup than a clinically meaningful, biological trend. That is, no evidence to justify withholding t-PA from any of the subgroups studied was found.

There are a few limitations to the analysis presented here. The original trial included enough patients to address the primary hypothesis, not the subgroup analyses. Nevertheless, power analyses showed that significant treatment interactions with a power greater than 90% could have been detected: if an important

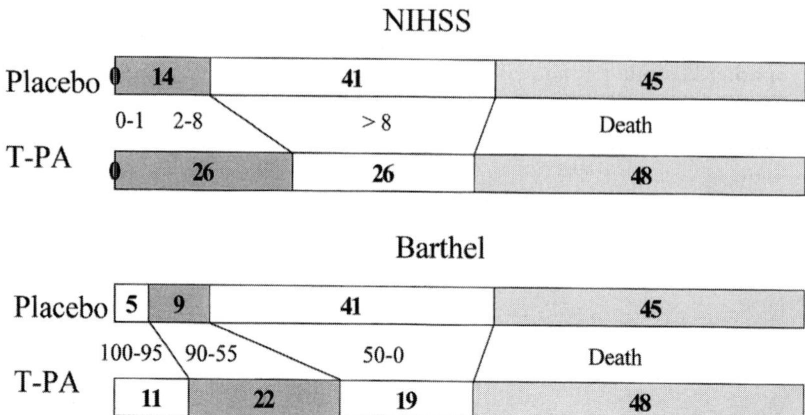

Fig. 4. Effect of t-PA on outcome (Barthel and NIHSS) in 49 patients with age >75 and baseline severity >20. Note the beneficial effect in mild and moderate categories. *See* text for explanation.

interaction was present, there is a greater than 90% probability that it would have been found. Another limitation is the selection of variables for the analysis. Twenty-seven baseline data items were chosen that were likely to be related to either outcome or differential treatment response. There could be other variables but no literature supporting inclusion of such was found. In prior studies, the variables usually associated with long-term stroke outcome included age, severity, smoking, diabetes, heart disease, and hypertension *(16–21)*. These same variables appeared in our analyses, suggesting that there are probably not other important variables missing.

Some of the predictor variables show important effects on long-term outcome. Patients with more severe baseline deficits, or who are older, do poorly over the long term, but t-PA was effective in such patients (Figs. 1 and 3). There was no threshold value for age, NIHSS score, or any particular stroke subtype that precluded t-PA treatment. Thus, t-PA offers some benefit for older, sicker patients, even if the overall likelihood of a good outcome is less (Fig. 4). The careful clinician will note, however, that the t-PA package insert cautions that use in patients with an NIHSS score greater than 22 may be hazardous. The analyses reported here were not available to the US Food and Drug Administration at the time the drug was approved for stroke. Since then, it has become clear that no single value of the NIHSS can be used rigidly for selecting patients; the clinician must exercise judgment in each case.

LONG-TERM OUTCOME

In the original report, benefit of thrombolysis was demonstrated using follow-up data obtained 3 mo after stroke. Although the 3-mo outcome of patients

Table 6
Final Multivariate Model
Comparing Possible Predictor Variables to Outcome Using 3-Mo Outcome Data

Variable	*Global odds ratio*	*95% Confidence limits*	*p-value*
t-PA treatment	2.02	1.45, 2.81	0.0001
Age X NIHSS[a]	0.993	0.993,0.998	0.0001
History of diabetes	0.47	0.31, 0.72	0.0004
Age × admission map	1.0009[a]	1.000, 1.0016	0.026
Early CT findings with thrombus	0.49	0.29, 0.80	0.0046

*Age, NIH Stroke Scale and admission Mean arterial pressure (MAP) are also included individually in the model. Their odds ratios are not shown, as they cannot be interpreted directly in the presence of the interaction.

treated with t-PA for acute ischemic stroke is compelling, showing a long-term benefit would solidify the case for the use of t-PA in similar patients. Any short-term risk would be offset by a long period of disease-free survival, long-term independence, and reduced long-term supportive care costs. If a long-term benefit could not be demonstrated, however, the argument in favor of thrombolytic stroke therapy weakens. The decision to use thrombolysis for stroke would depend on the short-term benefits and risks only.

To address these important issues, the 1-yr outcome data for patients enrolled in the NINDS t-PA stroke study are presented *(3)*. These data may allow clinicians to understand the true benefit of t-PA for patients with acute ischemic stroke, especially with regard to long-term quality-of-life issues.

Methods

All patients enrolled in the original trial were followed for 1 yr and outcome data were collected at 24 h and 3, 6, and 12 mo following stroke. Telephone contact was made at 6 and 12 mo to determine the patient's status (alive or dead); their ability to perform daily activities (BI) *(22)* and assessment of functional disability (Modified Rankin Scale [mRS]) *(23)* and Glasgow Outcome Scales (GOS) *(24)*. Data were also collected for serious medical events including ICH and recurrent stroke. During the entire follow-up period, telephone evaluators (certified nurse coordinators or study physicians), patients, and their caregivers remained blinded to treatment allocation. Several studies have validated telephone assessment of stroke outcome *(25–27)*. Using an intention-to-treat analysis, patients who died before follow-up or those for whom follow-up was unavailable, were assigned the most unfavorable scores for all outcome measures.

A total of 624 patients were randomized into the NINDS t-PA Stroke Trial: 291 in part 1 and 333 in part 2. Only 15 patients (2.4% : 7 t-PA, 8 placebo) were not available for 6-mo follow-up and 26 patients (4.1% : 14 t-PA, 8 placebo) were

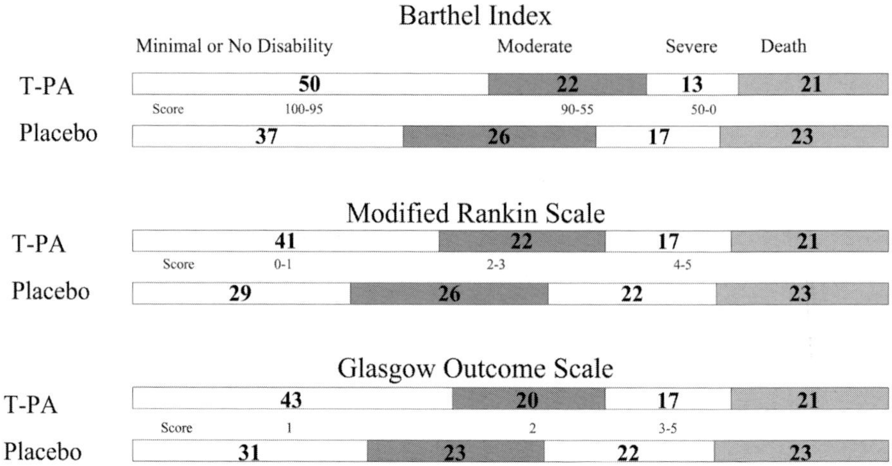

Barthel Index

Minimal or No Disability | Moderate | Severe | Death

	Minimal or No Disability	Moderate	Severe	Death
T-PA	50	22	13	21
Score	100-95	90-55	50-0	
Placebo	37	26	17	23

Modified Rankin Scale

T-PA	41	22	17	21
Score	0-1	2-3	4-5	
Placebo	29	26	22	23

Glasgow Outcome Scale

T-PA	43	20	17	21
Score	1	2	3-5	
Placebo	31	23	22	23

Fig. 5. Effect of t-PA on outcome 6 mo following stroke. *See* text for explanation.

unavailable for follow-up at 1 yr for all the three scales. Under the intent-to-treat analysis, these patients were considered to have an unfavorable outcome in each scale. By assigning an unfavorable outcome to these patients, a worst-case scenario for treatment with t-PA is created (i.e., all of these patients are assumed to have done poorly, therefore, biasing the results against treatment). If any of these patients had a good outcome, the actual benefit of t-PA will be underestimated in the analyses.

Results

A favorable outcome at 6 and 12 mo occurred more often in t-PA compared to placebo-treated patients. The odds ratio (95% confidence intervals) for favorable outcome at 6 mo was 1.7 (1.3, 2.3) and for 1 yr 1.7 (1.2, 2.3). A similar pattern is seen in the univariate tests for BI, mRS, and GOS. The distributions of outcome scores for the three scales are summarized in Fig. 5. For each scale, the proportion of patients improved to minimal or no disability was greater in the t-PA group. The proportions of patients suffering moderate or severe disability, or death, were reduced by t-PA on all three scales. At 1 yr, the range of absolute improvement was from 11 to 13% and relative improvement from 32 to 46% for the three outcome scales. The distributions are summarized in Fig. 6. These results are very similar to those seen at 3 mo: t-PA treated patients were at least 30% more likely to be independent of their stroke symptoms at 1 yr compared to placebo patients (relative risk 1.3–1.5 for the individual scales at 1 yr). Importantly, the favorable outcomes were not accompanied by an increase in severe disability or mortality.

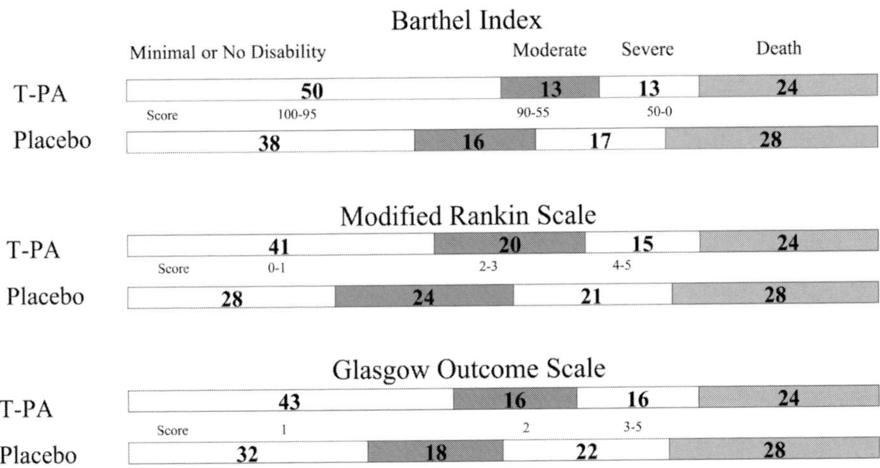

Fig. 6. Effect of t-PA on outcome 1 yr following stroke. *See* text for explanation.

In the treatment group, there were 23 symptomatic hemorrhages during the first 3 mo of which 20 occurred within the first 36 h. Six (26%) of these patients were alive at 1 yr. In the placebo group, four symptomatic hemorrhages occurred within 3 mo, two of which occurred within 36 h. One (25%) of these four patients was alive at 12 mo. Between 3 mo and 1 yr there were two additional symptomatic hemorrhages in the treatment group, of which one survived to 1 yr. In the placebo group, there was one additional symptomatic hemorrhage between 3 mo and 1 yr, and this patient did not survive.

The proportion of patients surviving between 3 and 12 mo after stroke was consistently higher in the t-PA group compared to placebo, illustrated in Fig. 7. However, there were no statistically significant differences in mortality between the two groups at 6 mo ($p = 0.31$) and 1 yr ($p = 0.29$). Recurrent stroke in 1 yr occurred in 34 of 624 patients, including two patients with two recurrences. Recurrent stroke in the first 3 mo occurred in 24 of these 34 patients (12 t-PA, 12 placebo). The recurrence rate difference between treatment groups was not significant, using the log-rank test ($p = 0.89$ at 6 mo and 0.96 at 1 yr).

Using the subgroup analysis methods described here, a multivariable model to identify baseline variables associated with a favorable outcome or death at 6 mo and 1 yr was also fit. The final multivariable models are presented in Table 7 for the 12-mo outcomes. Variables included in the 6-mo final model were diabetes, age, NIHSS score at baseline, age by NIHSS score interaction, early CT findings including hyperdense artery sign, time (from stroke onset to treatment), and time-by-treatment interaction. The variables remaining in the final 12-mo model were diabetes, age, NIHSSS, and age-by-NIHSSS interaction. There was

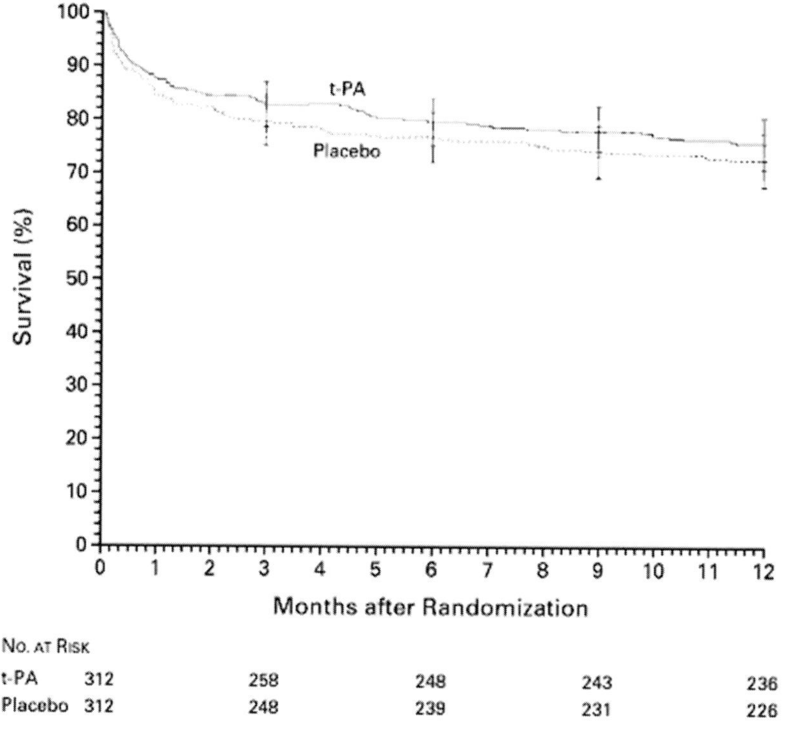

Fig. 7. One-year survival in the NINDS t-PA Stroke Trial.

Table 7
Final Multivariate Model
Comparing Possible Predictor Variables to Outcome Using 1-Yr Outcome Data

Variable	*Global odds ratio*	*95% Confidence limits*	*p-value*
t-PA treatment	1.81	1.27, 2.57	0.001
Age × NIHSS*	0.996	0.993, 0.999	0.002
History of diabetes	0.39	0.25, 0.62	0.001

no interaction between treatment response and presumed stroke subtype at 6 and 12 mo, confirming that no particular subgroup was more likely to benefit from thrombolysis.

The baseline variables that were predictors of death at 12 mo were age, NIHSS score, diabetes, and diabetes-by-age interaction. After adjusting for these variables identified as prognostic for death at 12 mo, treatment with t-PA remained significant. Patients with higher baseline NIHSS score have a lower chance of survival than patients with lower NIHSS scores.

Implications for Clinicians

Consistent benefit of t-PA at 3 mo, 6 mo, and 1 yr indicate that the beneficial effect of t-PA is durable over the long term. The data strongly argue in favor of the use of t-PA for acute ischemic stroke when patients can be treated within 3 h of symptom onset. The long-term follow-up of patients enrolled in the NINDS t-PA Stroke Study demonstrates that the magnitude of benefit associated with t-PA 3 mo after stroke was sustained at 6 mo and 1 yr. Patients treated with t-PA were at least 30% more likely than placebo-treated patients to have minimal or no disability at 6 mo and 1 yr after treatment. In addition, t-PA-treated patients at 1 yr were less likely to be severely disabled or to have died from their stroke. These figures demonstrate an overall improvement for t-PA treated patients. Treated patients were also more likely to have lesser degrees of disability with fewer moderately or severely disabled patients.

Multivariable analysis revealed similar results to that reported for the 3 mo favorable outcome (*see* above) where associated baseline characteristics included age interacting with baseline NIHSS, age interacting with admission blood pressure, early CT findings, and diabetes. Consistent with the 3-mo model, age interacting with baseline NIHSS and diabetes remained in both the 6- and 12-mo models. This data suggests that for any age, patients with a higher NIHSS at baseline have less chance of having a favorable outcome compared to the patients with a lower NIHSS. As of 3 mo, however, none of the identified variables associated with 6- or 12-mo favorable outcome interacted with treatment: patients cannot be selected for treatment a priori based on the presence or absence of these features (*see* Fig. 4). In addition, after adjusting for other baseline variables, an association between presumed stroke subtype and favorable outcome over the long term could not be detected. This suggests that patients should not be selected for or excluded from treatment with t-PA based solely on stroke mechanism.

SUMMARY

In this chapter much of the data presented in the NINDS t-PA for stroke trial was amplified to show three points: thrombolytic therapy for stroke is cost effective; there are no particular subgroups to be preferred or avoided for treatment; and the benefits are sustained over the long term. These data could not be included in the original report, but the main points have now all been subjected to peer review and are published. Taken together with the initial report, these analyses show that in the NINDS trial, thrombolytic therapy was effective.

REFERENCES

1. NINDS rt-PA Stroke Study Group. Generalized Efficacy of t-PA for Acute Stroke. *Stroke* 1997; 28:2119–2125.
2. Fagan SC, Morgenstern LB, Petitta A, et al. Cost-effectiveness of tissue plasminogen activator for acute ischemic stroke. *Neurology* 1998; 50:883–890.
3. Kwiatkowski TG, Libman RB, Frankel M, et al. Effects of tissue plasminogen activator for acute ischemic stroke at one year. *N Engl J Med* 1999; 340:1781–1787.
4. Solomon NA, Russo CJ, Lee J, Schulman KA. Patient preferences for stroke outcome. *Stroke* 1994; 25:1721–1725.
5. Stahl JE, Furie KL, Gleason S, Gazelle GS. Stroke: Effect of implementing an evaluation and treatment protocol compliant with NINDS recommendations. *Radiology* 2003; 228(3): 659–668.
6. Sandercock P, Berge E, Dennis M, et al. Cost-effectiveness of thrombolysis with recombinant tissue plasminogen activator for acute ischemic stroke assessed by a model based on UK NHS costs. *Stroke* 2004; 35(6):1490–1497.
7. Sinclair SE, Frighetto L, Loewen PS, et al. Cost-Utility analysis of tissue plasminogen activator therapy for acute ischaemic stroke: a Canadian healthcare perspective. *Pharmacoeconomics* 2001; 19(9):927–936.
8. Nadareishvili Z, Oh P, Smurawska LT, Tran C, Norris JW. Cost-effectiveness of tissue plasminogen activator for acute ischemic stroke. *Neurology* 1999; 52(4):895–896.
9. Avruch S, Cackley AP. Savings achieved by giving WIC benefits to women prenatally. *Public Health Rep* 1995; 110:27–34.
10. Koplan JP, Schoenbaum SC, Weinstein MC, Fraser DW. Pertussis vaccine—an analysis of benefits, risks and costs. *N Engl J Med* 1979; 301:906–911.
11. Koplan JP, Preblud SR. A benefit-cost analysis of mumps vaccine. *Am J Dis Child* 1982; 136:362–364.
12. Cutting WA. Cost-benefit evaluations of vaccination programmes. *Lancet* 1980; 8195 pt 1:634–635.
13. Furlan A, Kanoti G. When Is Thrombolysis Justified in Patients with Acute Ischemic Stroke? A Bioethical Perspective. *Stroke* 1997;(28):214–218.
14. NINDS rt-PA Stroke Study Group. Tissue plasminogen activator for acute ischemic stroke. *N Engl J Med* 1995; 333(24):1581–1587.
15. Yusuf S, Wittes J, Probstfield J, Tyroler H. Analysis and Interpretation of Treatment Effects in Subgroups of Patients in Randomized Clinical Trials. *JAMA* 1991; 266:93–98.
16. Prescott RJ, Garraway MB, Akhtar AJ. Predicting functional outcome following acute stroke using a standard clinical examination. *Stroke* 1982; 13:641–647.
17. Olsen TS. Arm and leg paresis as outcome predictors in stroke rehabilitation. *Stroke* 1990; 21:247–251.
18. Loewen SC, Anderson BA. Predictors of stroke outcome using objective measurement scales. *Stroke* 1990; 21:78–81.
19. Demchuk AM, Buchan AM. Predictors of stroke outcome. Neurologic Clinics 2001; 18: 455–473.
20. Allen CMC. Predicting the outcome of acute stroke: a prognostic scorex. *J Neurol Neurosurg Psych* 1984; 47:475–480.
21. Katz S, Ford AB, Chinn AB, Newill VA. Prognosis after strokes: II. Long-course of 159 patients. *Medicine* 1966; 454:236–246.
22. Mahoney FT, Barthel DW. Functional evaluation: Barthel Index. *Md State Med J* 1965; 14:61–65.
23. Rankin J. Cerebral vascular accidents in patients over the age of 60: Prognosis. *Scott Med J* 1957; 2:200–215.

24. Jennett B, Bond M. Assessment of outcome after severe brain damage. A practical scale. *Lancet* 1975;480–484.
25. Candelise L, Pinardi G, Aritzu E, Musicco M. Telephone interview for stroke outcome assessment. *Cerebrovasc Dis* 1994; 4:341–343.
26. Lyden P, Broderick J, Mascha E, NINDS rt-PA Stroke Study Group. Reliability of the Barthel Index Outcome Measure selected for the NINDS t-PA Stroke Trial. In: Yamaguchi T, Mori E, Minematsu K, del Zoppo G, editors. *Thrombolytic Therapy in Acute Ischemic Stroke III*. Tokyo: Springer-Verlag, 1995: 327–333.
27. Shinar D, Gross CR, Bronstein KS, et al. Reliability of the activities of daily living scale and its use in the telephone interview. *Arch Phys Med Rehabil* 1987; 68:723–728.

9 Community Experience With Intravenous Thrombolysis for Acute Stroke

Lama Al-Khoury, MD *and Christy M. Jackson,* MD

Contents

INTRODUCTION

The US Food and Drug Administration (FDA) approved intravenous tissue plasminogen activator (t-PA) as treatment for acute ischemic stroke in June 1996, based on the results of the National Institute of Neurological Disorders and Stroke (NINDS) study (*see* Chapter 7). The next important question was whether t-PA treatment could be applied in nonstudy community medical centers with a feasibility, safety, and efficacy comparable to that of NINDS trial. This question was answered by many community studies, which evaluated t-PA therapy in acute ischemic stroke. This chapter discusses community experience with intravenous t-PA in stroke treatment from 1996 to the present. Those studies are discussed in chronological order, highlighting the outcome and complication rates of each. Table 1 summarizes the results.

From: *Current Clinical Neurology: Thrombolytic Therapy for Acute Stroke, Second Edition*
Edited by: P. D. Lyden © Humana Press Inc., Totowa, NJ

Table 1
Community Experience With Thrombolysis

Year	*Series*	*n (t-PA)*	*t-PA mg/kg*	*sICH*	*tICH*	*Outcome*
1998	Houston, 3 h *(1)*	30	0.9	7%	10%	30%[a]
1998	Cologne, 3 h *(2)*	100	0.9	5%	11%	40%[b]
2000	t-PA Stroke Survey study, 3 h *(3)*,	189	0.9	6%	–	34%[c]
1998	Lyon, 7 h *(15)*	100	0.8	–	7%	45%[d]
1999	Oregon, 3 h *(4)*	33	0.9	9.1%	–	36.4%[e]
2000	Illinois (OSFSN) *(7)*	57	0.9	5%	9%	47%[f]
2000	Cleveland, 3 *(5)*	70	0.9	15.7%	–	Increased death[g]
2000	STARS, 3 h *(8)*	389	0.9	3.3%	11.5%	35%[h]
2000	Vancouver, 3 h *(9)*	46	0.9	2.2%(36h)	–	43%[i]
2001	Berlin, 3 *(13)*	75	0.9	–	2.7%	40%[j]
2001	Indianapolis, 3 h *(12)*	50	0.9	10%	14%	34%[k]
2001	Calgary, 3 h *(10)*	84	0.9	7.1%	–	54%[l]
2001	Houston, 3 h *(14)*	269	0.9	5.6% m	–	–
2002	CASES, 3 h *(11)*	1099	0.9	4.6%	–	46%[n]
2003	Cleveland Update, 3 h *(6)*	47	0.9	6.4%	–	–
In press	Lyon, 7 h *(17)*	200	0.8	5.5%		35%[o]

[a]mRS<=1 on follow-up in Dec 1996. Enrollment was between Dec. 1995 and Dec. 1996.
[b]mRS<=1 at 3 mo.
[c]mRS<=1 at 90 d.
[d]mRS<=1 at 90 d.
[e]mRS<=1 at 3 mo.
[f]mRS<=1 on discharge from the hospital.
[g]Increased protocol violations and deaths. Only 1.8% were treated with t-PA.
[h]mRS<=1 at 30 d.
[i]mRS<=1 at 13 mo.
[j]mRS<=1 at 3 mo.
[k]NIHSS<=or central nervous system (CNS) >11 on discharge.
[l]mRS<=2 at 3 mo.
[m]Mean baseline NIHSS 14.4 (± 6.1). At 24 h mean NIHSS 10 (±8). Mean discharge NIHSS 7 (±7).
[n]mRS<=2 (Independence) at 90 d.
[o]mRS<=1 at 3 mo.

FIRST RESULTS

In 1998, Chiu et al. published the results of the first experience with recombinant tissue plasminogen activator (rt-PA) for acute stroke outside of a clinical trial. The study evaluated 30 patients with acute ischemic strokes enrolled in three community hospitals and one academic medical center in Houston, Texas, between December 1995 and December 1996. The rate of symptomatic intracranial hemorrhage (sICH) was 7% and the rate of fatal ICH was 3%. Thirty-seven percent of patients recovered to fully independent function, defined as a score on the Barthel Index (BI) of 95 to 100. Thirty percent of patients had no disability, defined as a modified Rankin Score (mRS) of 0 to 1 upon follow-up in December 1996. Mortality was 20% at 3 mo compared with 17% in the NINDS study. There was no difference in outcome or safety measures between the community and the academic medical centers in this study *(1)*.

The Cologne community experience was described by Grond et al. in 1998 *(2)*. The authors studied 100 patients (22% of 453 patients with a presumed diagnosis of acute stroke) who received t-PA: 26% were treated within 90 min from stroke onset. The average time from emergency department (ED) arrival to treatment (door-to-needle time) was 48 min, and the average arrival time from stroke onset was 78 min. At 3 mo post-t-PA, 53% of patients recovered with fully independent function (BI 95–100), 40% had no disability (mRS 0–1), and 42% had a National Institute of Heath Stroke Scale (NIHSS) score, of 0 to 1. sICH occurred in 5%, fatal ICH in 1%, and total ICH in 11%. The mortality rate was 12%. It was concluded that thrombolysis was effectively applied in acute stroke treatment with outcome and complication rates comparable to the NINDS studies.

Taken together, the Houston and Cologne results showed that rt-PA could be used for acute stroke with results comparable to the NINDS trials. However, these were single-center reports; a multicenter survey was needed. The t-PA Stroke Survey *(3)* was a multicenter study that included 13 study centers (5 university and 8 community hospitals) where a standardized retrospective survey was performed to collect 189 patients who received intravenous rt-PA for acute ischemic stroke. Three months after treatment, 34% of patients had an mRS of 0–1, and 32% had an mRS of 2–3. Forty-six percent of patients were discharged home, 47% to rehabilitation, and 12% to nursing homes. The incidence of sICH was 6%, similar to the NINDS trial. Deviations from the NINDS protocol guidelines were identified in 30% of patients (56 of 189). Those deviations included use of heparin within the first 24 h in 15%, initiation of t-PA infusion beyond 3 h in 8%, excessively elevated blood pressure in 3%, and abnormal baseline coagulation in 4%. The incidence of sICH was 11% among patients with protocol deviations as compared with 4% in patients who were treated according to the NINDS protocol guidelines, suggesting that adherence to the protocol guidelines is mandatory *(3)*.

A multicenter experience from Oregon was described in 1999*(4)*. Thirty-three patients with acute ischemic strokes received t-PA within the 3-h window from stroke onset at six hospitals. The NINDS exclusion criteria were followed in addition to a new criterion of excluding patients with computed tomography (CT) ischemic changes of more than one-third of the middle cerebral artery

(MCA) territory. The mean baseline NIHSS was 16.6 (compared to 14 in the NINDS study). Full or near-full clinical recovery (mRS of 0–1) was found in 36.4% of the patients, comparable to 39% in the NINDS trial. Symptomatic ICH occurred in 9.1% of patients, mostly associated with severe strokes of NIHSS greater than 20. Mortality was 18.2% and mortality secondary to ICH was 6.1% (17% and 3%, respectively in NINDS). In conclusion, t-PA was found to be a feasible and efficacious treatment after comparison to the NINDS results *(4)*.

Published in 2000, the initial Cleveland multicenter experience with t-PA was disappointing *(5)*. This retrospective chart survey showed a higher ICH rate and a smaller responder rate than the NINDS study. End points measured were the rate of t-PA use in the community, the outcomes of t-PA treatment, and the incidence of ICH. The study evaluated 3948 ischemic stroke patients from 29 hospitals in the metropolitan areas of Cleveland, Ohio. An attempt was made to collect cases prospectively, however most cases were included through retrospective chart review, using the so-called "omniscient" approach: all data in the chart, whether or not it would have been available at the time of the treatment decision, were used to judge the appropriateness of the treatment. The omniscient review method will obviously lead to a higher rate of protocol violations, since critical information may become available well after the time the thrombolytic decision was made. Of these patients with acute ischemic strokes presenting between 1997 and 1998, 17% were admitted within 3 h of onset, of these patients only 1.8% received intravenous t-PA treatment. Protocol violations occurred in 50% of patients who received t-PA; sICH occurred in 15.7% of the t-PA patients. Protocol violations included use of antiplatelet agents or anticoagulants within 24 h from treatment with t-PA, treatment beyond the 3-h-window, and deviation from the blood pressure guidelines. Moreover, in-hospital mortality and the length of hospital stay were significantly higher in the t-PA group.

The differences between the results of the initial Cleveland community survey and the results of the rest of the community studies are, in part, the result of differences in methodology. In this initial Cleveland community survey, nurse abstractors used retrospective chart review that may have led to case-ascertainment bias. This bias causes a drift toward difficult cases with memorable adverse outcomes. In the other community series, stroke team physicians used prospective collection of acute ischemic stroke patients to avoid this bias.

Most recently, the Cleveland group published an update of the Cleveland community experience with intravenous t-PA *(6)*. The method used was a retrospective chart review of all ischemic stroke patients who presented to the Cleveland Clinic Health System between June 2000 and June 2001. The omniscient review approach was used again, as in the first Cleveland area study. This survey followed implementation of a stroke quality improvement program that started in 1999, consisting of very frequent review of acute stroke data, performance monitoring, implementation of a stroke protocol in the emergency rooms, the use of a 24-h stroke beeper, and medical education about acute stroke management and intravenous t-PA use. As a result, intravenous t-PA was given in 18.8% of patients who arrived within the 3-h time window. Protocol deviations were significantly fewer, occurring in 19.1% of those patients who received t-PA. The symptomatic ICH rate was 6.4%, similar to that of the NINDS study. The authors concluded that intravenous t-PA could be given safely to eligible stroke patients at the community hospital level with appropriate education and training.

To summarize, the difference between the two different Cleveland community experiences lies in the higher rate of protocol violations in the initial Cleveland community experience, which led to the higher frequency of adverse events. Moreover, extensive stroke education and continuous training played an important role in decreasing the protocol deviations and therefore the symptomatic ICH rate in Cleveland.

In January 2000, the results of the Illinois multicenter community experience were published *(7)*. This study consisted of 57 consecutive acute stroke patients treated with intravenous t-PA. The majority of the patients were treated within 3 h of onset and only 5 patients were treated between 3 and 6 h of onset. Treatment centers consisted of different hospitals belonging to a stroke network in Illinois known as "The Sisters of the Third Order of Saint Francis Stroke Network" (OSFSN). Patients were followed between June 1996 and December 1998. In 35% of the patients, the ED or primary care physician administered t-PA in consultation with a neurologist. On discharge, 47% of the patients had minimal or no disability measured by a mRS ≤1, 44% had an NIHSS ≤1, 54% were discharged home, 25% were transferred to in-patient rehabilitation, 12% were discharged to a nursing home or skilled care facility, and 9% died. The total ICH rate was 9% and the sICH rate was 5%. The OSFSN study showed that t-PA therapy for ischemic stroke following the NINDS guidelines is safe and efficacious even when a neurologist is not physically available; the drug was successfully administered by the ED or primary care physicians *(7)*. The results of The Standard Treatment with Alteplase to Reverse Stroke (STARS) study were published in March 2000; the study evaluated 389 consecutive acute ischemic stroke patients who presented within 3 h of onset during the time interval between February 1997 and December 1998. The study sites included 57 academic and community hospitals in the United States. Median NIHSS was 13. Protocol violations, including anticoagulant use, treatment out of the recommended time period and nonadherence to blood pressure guidelines, occurred in 127 patients (32.6%). Outcome measures of recovery were mRS at 30 d post-t-PA treatment. Complete or near-complete recovery with a mRS ,â§1 occurred in 35% of patients and partial recovery with mRS ,â§2 (independence) occurred in 43% of patients.

The rate of sICH was 3.3% and that of asymptomatic ICH 8.2%. In summary, STARS showed favorable clinical outcome with intravenous t-PA treatment in community as well as academic centers, and a relatively low rate of symptomatic hemorrhage *(8)*.

THE CANADIAN EXPERIENCE

The Canadian health system uses a centralized approach, and thrombolytic therapy for stroke did not receive government approval for several years after the US FDA approval. Once the drug was approved, however, the provincial governments were directed to implement stroke systems. Coincidentally, the Canadian Stroke Consortium—a voluntary confederation of stroke researchers throughout Canada—were organizing educational programs to assure widespread familiarity with advanced stroke care. As a result of the government mandates and the Stroke Consortium efforts, stroke care is more centralized in Canada than in the United States. Stroke victims are transported efficiently to specialized stroke centers with expertise available all hours; this does not happen in the United States. On the other hand, the population density in Canada is less, resulting in longer travel times for many patients in Canada. Several reports from Canada reveal the significant benefits of regionalized stroke care.

The Vancouver experience was published in December 2000. This combined retrospective and prospective study evaluated 46 consecutive ischemic stroke patients who received intravenous t-PA within the 3-h time window using the NINDS protocol. The sICH rate at 36 h was 2.2%. Upon follow-up at 13 mo, 22% of patients were dead (comparable to NINDS), 43% had a favorable outcome with mRS of 0–1 and 48% had BI of 95–100 *(9)*.

The Calgary study, published in 2001, evaluated 2165 consecutive acute stroke patients between October 1996 and December 1999. Of these patients, 1168 (53.9%) were diagnosed to have ischemic strokes, 31.8% to have hemorrhagic stroke, and 13.9% to have transient ischemic attacks. Among the 1168 ischemic strokes, 73.1% were excluded a result of delayed presentation. The causes for delay included uncertain time of onset in 24.2%, patients waiting at home with symptoms in 29%, transfer from another hospital in 8.9%, and poor accessibility to the treating hospital (long distance from treating hospital or patient transferred from outlying hospital) in 5.7% of patients. Twenty-seven percent of the patients with ischemic stroke were admitted to the hospital within 3 h; 26.7% of those received intravenous t-PA. Exclusion of those patients who were time-eligible resulted from mild strokes in 13.1%, clinical improvement in 18.2%, other protocol exclusions in 13.6%, ED referral delay in 8.9%, and significant morbidity in 8.3% *(10)*. On 3-mo follow-up, 54% of t-PA patients had mRS 0 or 1 and 7.1% had sICH. Overall, 4.7% of all patients who presented with acute stroke within this time period were treated with t-PA; the majority of t-PA exclusions were related to delay in presentation. Of the patients who were excluded because of a mild neurological deficit or because of rapid improvement, 32% were dependent on hospital discharge or died during hospital admission. This raises the issue of whether patients with rapid improvement or mild deficits should be treated with t-PA rather than be exluded *(10)*. A large, multicenter Canadian experience, called Canadian Activase for Stroke Effectiveness Study (CASES) was published in May 2002. The authors evaluated 1099 patients with acute ischemic stroke who were treated with intravenous t-PA during the period between February 1999 and June 2001 in 49 Canadian hospitals. Median baseline NIHSS was 15 (range 2–40). At 90 d following stroke, 30% of these patients had minimal or no residual neurological deficit (mRS 0–1), and 46% were independent (mRS 0–2). ICH occurred in 4.6% of patients, and protocol violations in 15%. Further analysis revealed that predictors of outcome were baseline NIHSS, baseline ASPECT score (a score that evaluates the radiological changes of stroke on brain CT), patient's age, atrial fibrillation, and the patient's baseline serum sugar. Predictors of ICH were mean arterial blood pressure and baseline serum glucose. The investigators concluded that intravenous t-PA is safe and efficacious in Canada *(11)*.

MOST RECENT EXPERIENCE

In January 2001, the results of the Indianapolis community experience were reported. This study was a retrospective evaluation of the medical records of 50 stroke patients treated with intravenous t-PA in 10 community hospitals in Indianapolis from July 1996 to February 1998. Seventy percent of the patients were treated by neurologists 24% by stroke neurologists, and 6% by ED physicians. In-hospital mortality rate was 10%. Good outcome with NIHSS (0 or 1) or Canadian Neurologic scale >11 was present in 34% of patients upon discharge. Protocol deviations occurred in 16% of patients. Complications were more frequent among patients with protocol violations compared to those without. Protocol violations were uncontrolled blood pressure, prolonged prothrombin time of more than 15 s, severe head trauma within the last 3 wk prior to stroke presentation, prior stroke within the last 2 wk prior to current stroke, pre-infusion heparin with a prolonged partial prothrombin time, and heparin administration immediately after t-PA. The total hemorrhage rate was 75% in patients with protocol violations vs 12% in those without ($p < 0.001$), sICH rate 38% vs 5% respectively ($p < 0.02$), and the rate of ICH attributable to t-PA (occurring within 36 h within t-PA treatment) 38% vs 2.4% respectively ($p < 0.01$). Therefore, it can be concluded that when the NINDS protocol is adhered to, complication rates are comparable to those of NINDS *(12)*.

Results of the Berlin study were published in May 2001. This study evaluated patients with acute ischemic stroke enrolled over a period of 2 yr: 9.4% received intravenous t-PA; median baseline NIHSS was 13 ± 6. The average time for thrombolysis was 144 min from onset of stroke. Treatment beyond the 3 h was given to 17% of patients; 2.7% of t-PA patients had ICH. Outcome was good with mRS of 0–1 at 3 mo in 40% of t-PA patients, moderate with mRS of 2–3 in 32%, and poor with mRS of 4–5 in 13%; the death rate was 15%. Moreover, this study showed that with time, the median door-to-CT time and door-to-needle time shortened, whereas the number of patients treated per month increased from 2 to 4. Therefore, the Berlin experience was an additional study to demonstrate that intravenous t-PA is safe, feasible, and efficacious *(13)*. It also provided proof that with time and experience, the performance and activity of the stroke team improves.

In December 2001, Grotta et al. updated the Houston community experience with t-PA in 269 patients with acute ischemic stroke. The design was a prospective inception cohort registry of acute ischemic stroke patients seen by the stroke team at the University of Texas-Houston Medical School and three community hospitals, added to a retrospective medical record review of all patients treated with t-PA all within the time period between January 1996 and June 2000. The rate of t-PA administration for ischemic stroke was 15% within this study period. Twenty-eight percent were treated within 2 h of onset. Mean door-to-needle time was 70 min. sICH occurred in 4.5%. Protocol violations occurred in 13% of all treated patients, with an ICH rate of 15% in the protocol violation population. The mean NIHSS before treatment was 14.4 ± 6.1, at 24 h 10 ± 8, and on discharge 7 ± 7. In-hospital death rate was 15%. In summary, this community experience proved that intravenous t-PA could be given in up to 15% of patients with acute ischemic stroke with a low risk for intracerebral bleeding, noting that successful therapy with t-PA treatment depends on the experience and organization of the treating team and on adhering to the treatment protocol *(14)*.

The Lyon stroke group adopted a thrombolysis protocol different from the NINDS trial *(15)*. The t-PA dose was 0.8 mg/kg (10% of the dose given as an intravenous bolus and the remaining 90% given as intravenous drip over 1 h after the bolus) and the window of t-PA administration was 7 h with the majority of patients receiving the t-PA within the 3-to 6-h window. Moreover, the patients also received heparin or low-molecular-weight heparin (LMWH). The results of the first 100 patients were published in 1998 *(15)*. On follow-up at 90 d, 45% of the patients had good outcome with mRS of 0–1, 18% had moderate outcome with mRS of 2–3, and 31% of patients had serious neurological outcome with mRS of 4–5. Death occurred in 6% of the patients. Of the 11 patients treated within the 6- to 7-h window, 45% had good results, which included 2 patients with intracerebral hematoma after having received intravenous heparin within the first 24 h. The intracerebral hematoma rate was 7%. An update of the results was further published in a poster abstract in 2002 *(16)* showing a rate of good outcome (i.e., mRS 0 or 1 at 5 yr of 37.4% and a mortality rate of 23.9%). Follow-up data and results, currently in press, showed that among the 200 patients enrolled so far in the Lyon trial, the rate of good outcome with mRS of 0–1 was 35% at 3 mo, the rate of parenchymatous anatomical hematoma within 7 d 9% and the rate of sICH 5.5%. The mortality rate at 3 mo was 11.5%. Independent predictors of bad outcome were the following variables: presence of a hypodensity on the initial baseline brain CT, hyperdense MCA sign on the initial baseline brain CT, internal carotid artery thrombosis, poor distinction of the gray–white matter junction, nonuse of intravenous heparin within 24 h or after 24 h, use of LMWH, and use of intravenous Mannitol *(17)*.

CONCLUSIONS

In summary, the above community experiences provide supportive evidence that intravenous t-PA therapy given within the 3-h window in the treatment of acute ischemic stroke is feasible, safe, and efficacious with similar success rates and complication rates to those of original NINDS and European Cooperative Acute Stroke Study trials. Moreover, these studies show the importance of adhering to the NINDS protocol in selecting and managing patients eligible for such therapy (detailed in Chapter 18). Furthermore, few of these trials emphasize the favorable yet underutilized role of training physicians and emergency services. Utilization of such resources improves the number of patients treated with t-PA and therefore favorably affects the outcome of these patients. Moreover, such training reduces the protocol violation rate and therefore decreases the complication rates associated with t-PA therapy. Concentrating stroke care in a few specialized, regional centers, as in Canada, appears to improve the outcomes and reduce the complication rates.

REFERENCES

1. Chiu D, Krieger D, Villar-Cordova C, et al. Intravenous tissue plasminogen activator for acute ischemic stroke feasibility, safety, and efficacy in the first year of clinical practice. *Stroke* 1998; 29:18–22.
2. Grond M, Stenzel C, Schmulling S, et al. Early intravenous thrombolysis for acute ischemic stroke in a community-based approach. *Stroke* 1998; 29:1544–1549.
3. Tanne D, Bates V, Verro P, et al. Initial clinical experience with IV tissue plasminogen activator for acute ischemic stroke: a multicenter survey. *Neurology* 1999; 53:424–427.
4. Egan R, Lutsep HL, Clark WM, et al. Open label tissue plasminogen activator for stroke: The Oregon experience. *J Stroke Cerebrovasc Dis* 1999; 8(5):287–290.
5. Katzan I, Furlan A, Lloyd L, et al. Use of tissue-type plasminogen activator for acute ischemic stroke: the Cleveland area experience. *JAMA* 2000; 283:1151–1158.
6. Katzan I, Hammer M, Furlan A. Quality improvement and tissue-type plasminogen activator for acute ischemic stroke. A Cleveland update. *Stroke* 2003; 34:799–800.
7. Wang D, Rose JA, Honings DR, Garwacki DJ, Milbrandt JC. Treating acute stroke patients with intravenous t-PA: the OSF Stroke Network experience. *Stroke* 2000; 31:77–81.

8. Albers GW, Bates V, Clark W, et al. Intravenous tissue-type plasminogen activator for treatment of acute stroke: the Standard Treatment with Alteplase to Reverse Stroke (STARS) study. *JAMA* 2000; 283:1145–1150.
9. Chapman KM, Woolfenden AR, Graeb D, et al. Intravenous tissue plasminogen activator for acute ischemic stroke. *Stroke* 2000; 31(12):2920–2924.
10. Barber PA, Zhang J, Demchuk A, Hill M, Buchan A. Why are stroke patients excluded from TPA therapy? *Neurology* 2001; 56:1015–1020.
11. Teal P, Hill MD, Buchan AM. *Canadian Aactivase for Stroke Effectiveness Study (CASES).* Available at http://www.thrombolysis-acute-stroke-therapy.org/pdf/78.pdf, 77. Accessed May 5, 2002.
12. Lopez-Yunez AM, Bruno A, Willliams LS, et al. Protocol violations in community-based rt-PA stroke treatment are associated with symptomatic intracerebral hemorrhage. *Stroke* 2001; 32(12):16.
13. Hans-Christian Koennecke, Nohr R, Leistner S, Marx P. Intravenous tPA for ischemic stroke team. Performance over time, safety and efficacy in a single center-2-year experience. *Stroke* 1 A.D.; 32(5):1074–1078.
14. Grotta J, Burgin WS, El-Mitwalli A, et al. Intravenous tissue-type plasminogen activator therapy for ischemic stroke. *Arch of Neurology* 2001; 58(12):2009–2013.
15. Trouillas P, et al. Thrombolysis with intravenous rt-PA in a series of 100 cases of acute carotid territory stroke. *Stroke* 1998; 29:2529–2540.
16. Trouillas P, Nighoghossian N, Derex L, Honnorat J. Prognosis at 5 years of acute cerebral infarcts of the carotid territory treated by intravenous rt-PA: data from the Lyon thrombolysis registry. *Stroke* 2002; 33(1):395. (Abstract)
17. Trouillas P, Nighoghosian N, Derex L, et al. *Final Resultsof the Lyon rtPA Protocol (200 cases): Effect of intravenous rtPA within 7 hours without radiological and clinical exclusions in carotid territory acute cerebral infarcts.* Letter, 2003.

10 Intra-Arterial Thrombolysis in Acute Ischemic Stroke

Anthony J. Furlan, MD, *Randall Higashida,* MD, *Irene Katzan,* MD, *Alex Abou-Chebl* MD, *and Andrew N. Russman,* DO

CONTENTS

INTRODUCTION

Intra-arterial (IA) thrombolysis provides an alternative to intravenous (iv) thrombolysis in selected patients with acute ischemic

From: *Current Clinical Neurology: Thrombolytic Therapy for Acute Stroke, Second Edition*
Edited by: P. D. Lyden © Humana Press Inc., Totowa, NJ

stroke. Recent advances in the field of neuro-interventional radiology, with the development of extremely soft, compliant microcatheters and steerable microguidewires, along with high-resolution fluoroscopy and digital imaging, and nonionic contrast agents, have made it feasible and safe to access the major intracranial blood vessels around the circle of Willis from a percutaneous transfemoral approach under local anesthesia. Rapid local delivery of fibrinolytic agents is now feasible using these techniques and is performed at many major medical centers in selected patients with acute cerebral ischemia.

INITIAL PATIENT SELECTION FOR DIRECT INTRA-ARTERIAL THROMBOLYSIS

The initial clinical and computed tomography (CT) scan selection criteria for IA thrombolysis are similar to those for intravenous tissue plasminogen activator (t-PA)*(1)*. Intra-arterial thrombolysis has been used most successfully in patients with acute middle cerebral artery (MCA) occlusion. There is evidence that the treatment window for IA thrombolysis extends to at least 6 h from stroke onset in patients with MCA occlusion. Other potential candidates for IA thrombolysis include patients with extracranial internal carotid artery (ICA) occlusion, ICA "T" occlusions that involve the distal carotid and proximal MCA, and basilar artery occlusion.

Patients who present with an acute stroke within 6 h of symptom onset should initially be examined by a neurologist familiar with the intravenous t-PA selection criteria. The baseline National Institutes of Health Stroke Scale Score (NIHSS) in most patients considered for IA thrombolysis is greater than10. Baseline laboratory evaluation should include a complete blood count with platelets and differential, coagulation studies, including thrombin time, activated partial thromboplastin time (aPTT), international normalization ratio (INR), activated clotting time (ACT), fibrinogen, plasminogen, and α2- antiplasmin levels, serum electrolytes, random blood glucose, troponins, creatine kinase, creatine kinase MB fraction, and an electrocardiogram. Additionally, laboratory studies to determine reversible stroke risk factors may be drawn at this time, in order to limit the number of posttreatment blood draws. These additional laboratory investigations may include a super sensitive C-reactive protein, plasma homocysteine level, and a lipid panel if the patient has not eaten in at least 8 h.

A CT scan is performed to exclude hemorrhage and major early signs of infarction, which would preclude thrombolytic therapy. The precise site of arterial occlusion in patients with acute ischemic stroke of less than 6 h duration cannot be determined solely on the basis of a neurological examination (NIHSS) and CT scan *(2)*. In about 33% of patients with acute stroke caused by occlusion of the MCA, the CT scan will demonstrate a hyperdense MCA sign signifying thrombus in the MCA (Fig. 1) *(3)*. In addition, visualization of a hyperdense

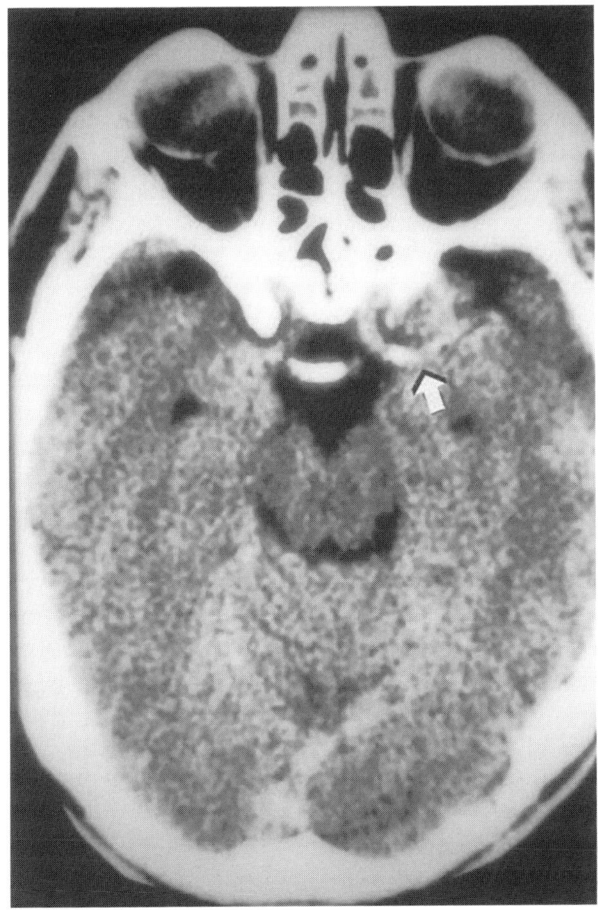

Fig. 1. Hyperdense middle cerebral artery sign or computed tomography indicating thrombus in LMCA.

circle in the sylvian fissure or MCA "dot" sign is 38% sensitive and 100% specific for an M2 or M3 occlusion *(4)*. Patients with an appropriate clinical picture and a hyperdense MCA sign or MCA "dot" sign on CT scanning should be considered for immediate angiography and IA thrombolysis. If quickly available, noninvasive testing with carotid duplex and transcranial Doppler, CT angiography (CTA), or magnetic resonance angiography (MRA) can be used to screen for major vessel occlusions treatable with IA thrombolysis. Moreover, availability of rapid perfusion imaging using either CT perfusion (PWCT) or magnetic resonance perfusion-weighted (PWI) and diffusion-weighted imaging (DWI) may assist in the identification of at-risk, but salvageable ischemic brain tissue. Mismatch between a PWI deficit and a smaller area of restriction on DWI may predict the final infarct volume after thrombolysis *(5)*. Also, pretreatment PWCT lesion volumes may predict both the final infarct volume on CT and clinical outcome after thrombolysis *(6)*.

GENERAL TECHNIQUE OF INTRA-ARTERIAL THROMBOLYSIS

In patients with appropriate clinical and CT criteria, a complete four-vessel cerebral angiogram, from a transfemoral approach, should be performed to evaluate the site of vessel occlusion, extent of thrombus, number of territories involved, and collateral circulation. A diagnostic catheter is guided into the high cervical segment of the vascular territory to be treated, followed by the introduction of a 2.3 French coaxial Rapid Transit Microcatheter with an 0.016 inch Instinct steerable microguidewire (Cordis Endovascular Systems). Under direct fluoroscopic visualization, the microcatheter is gently navigated through the intracranial circulation until the tip is embedded within or through the central portion of the thrombus.

Many variations in catheter design and delivery technique have been described *(7)*. Two types of microcatheters are being used most often for local cerebral thrombolysis, depending on the extent of clot formation. For the majority of intra-arterial cases, a single end-hole microcatheter is used, whereas for longer segments of clot formation, multiple side-hole infusion microcatheters are used. Superselective angiography through the microcatheter is performed at regular intervals to assess for degree of clot lysis and to adjust the dosage and volume of the thrombolytic agent.

A superselective angiogram is performed and if there is partial clot dissolution, the catheter is advanced into the remaining thrombus where additional thrombolysis is performed. As the thrombus is dissolved, the catheter is advanced into more distal branches of the intracranial circulation, so that the majority of the thrombolytic agent enters the occluded vessel and is not washed preferentially into adjacent open blood vessels. Recanalization can be achieved up to 2 h after the procedure begins, although a successful procedure is unlikely if the vessel is at least not partially recanalized before 1 h. The goal is to achieve rapid recanalization with as little thrombolytic agent as possible to limit the extent of brain infarction and to reduce the risk of hemorrhage.

THROMBOLYTIC AGENT

The agent preferred by most neuro-interventionalists for IA thrombolysis had been urokinase (UK) (Abbokinase®; Abbott Laboratories) in the dose range of 25–50,000 units (U) over 5–10 min intervals, at the rate of 250–500,000 U/h. Recombinant prourokinase (r-proUK) is a fibrin-selective pro-enzyme that is converted to UK at the clot surface by fibrin-associated plasmin. The recanalization efficacy, safety, and clinical efficacy of r-proUK in patients with acute ischemic stroke resulting from MCA occlusion were demonstrated in the Prolyse in Acute Cerebral Thromboembolism Trials (PROACT I and PROACT II) *(8,9)*. However, r-proUK is not yet approved by the US Food and Drug Administration (FDA) and is not currently available for general use. Alteplase (Activase®; Genentech) is a serine protease made by recombinant techniques that cleaves the same peptide bond as UK to activate plasminogen. Alteplase attaches preferentially to a formed thrombus, and its fibrin specificity allows it to lyse this thrombus without significant systemic activation. Doses of 20–50 mg of IA alteplase over 1 h have been used by various investigators, but there is considerable uncertainty about the effective dose range and safety of IA alteplase in the cerebral circulation. Reteplase (Retavase; Boehringer Mannheim) is a recombinantly produced, fibrin-selective, human plasminogen activator consisting of the kringle-2 and protease domains of human t-PA. It has a longer half-life than alteplase. IA doses of up to 8 U have been reported by one group of investigators. Safety and efficacy of IA reteplase for acute ischemic stroke has not been established. Desmoteplase (DSPA) (PAION; Aachen, Germany) is a recombinantly produced form of t-PA originally isolated as an extract from the saliva of the common vampire bat, *Desmodus rotundus*. DSPA is highly fibrin specific. DSPA-specific activity is 105,000 higher in the presence of fibrin compared to 550 for t-PA. DSPA is not activated by β-amyloid and is not neurotoxic in animal stroke models *(10)*. Intravenous DSPA appears promising in phase II clinical trials (DIAS/DEDAS) but has not been tested for IA use. Tenecteplase (TNKase; Genentech) is a t-PA molecule with three amino acid substitutions that confer several advantages. TNKase has a longer half-life than eitherdesmoteplase, reteplase, or alteplase. TNKase is highly fibrin selective and is structurally resistant to plasminogen activator inhibitor-1 (PAI-1) that is the primary inactivator of t-PA in the circulation. These properties make TNKase an intriguing thrombolytic for IA use, although no efficacy or safety data are currently available for its use in acute stroke management.

Adjunctive Therapy Once a site of vascular occlusion is angiographically confirmed that corresponds to the patient's neurological deficit, intravenous heparin is given by most neuro-interventionalists. Systemic anticoagulation with heparin reduces the risk of catheter-related embolism. Also, the thrombolytic effect of some agents such as r-proUK is augmented by heparin. Another rationale for anti-thrombotic therapy is prevention of acute re-occlusion, which is more common with atherothrombosis than with cerebral embolism. These indications are counterbalanced by the potentially increased risk of brain hemorrhage when heparin is combined with a thrombolytic agent.

There is no standard heparin regimen established for IA thrombolysis in acute stroke. Some neuro-interventionalists employ weight-adjusted heparin keeping the ACT between 200 and 300. PROACT I *(8)* reported a 27% rate of symptomatic brain hemorrhage when a conventional heparin regimen (100 U/kg bolus, 1000 U/hfor 4 h) was employed with IA r-proUK. Subsequently, a standard low-dose heparin regimen was used (2000 U bolus, 500 U/hfor 4 h), which reduced the symptomatic brain hemorrhage rate with IA r-proUK to 7% in PROACT I and 10% in PROACT II. This dose of heparin does not prolong the aPTT in most patients. Based on the PROACT trials, many neuro-interventionalists now use the low-dose heparin regimen during IA thrombolysis.

The potent IIb/IIIa platelet inhibitor abciximab (Reopro®, Centocor, Malvern, Pennsylvania) has been used successfully instead of heparin in patients undergoing acute or elective cerebrovascular interventions *(11–13)*. Coronary doses of abciximab appear to be safe in patients with acute ischemic stroke up to 24 h after onset *(14)*. IIb/IIIa agents may be most efficacious when the risk of acute re-occlusion is great such as with basilar artery atherothrombosis. The safety and efficacy of IIb/IIIa agents in patients with embolic occlusion of cerebral vessels, which is the usual cause of MCA occlusion, is less clear.

RATIONALE FOR INTRA-ARTERIAL THROMBOLYSIS

The recanalization efficacy of thrombolysis varies with the site of arterial occlusion *(15)*. Patients with ischemic stroke of less than 6 h duration have a wide variety of arterial occlusion sites, and 20% have no visible occlusion, despite similar neurological presentations *(2)*. In the intravenous thrombolysis stroke trials, neither the sites of arterial occlusion nor the recanalization rates are known. Intra-arterial thrombolysis permits documentation of both the site of arterial occlusion and recanalization rates.

Recanalization rates with IA thrombolysis are superior to intravenous thrombolysis for major cerebrovascular occlusions. Recanalization rates for major cerebrovascular occlusions average 70% for IA thrombolysis compared to 34% for intravenous thrombolysis *(15)*. The differences in recanalization rates are most apparent with large vessel occlusions such as the ICA, which is the most difficult vessel to achieve any thrombolysis, the carotid T-segment (supraclinoid carotid artery and proximal middle and anterior cerebral artery) and the proximal (M1) segment of the MCA *(15,16)*. Recanalization has been linked with improved clinical outcome, especially in patients with good collateral blood flow and no major early signs of infarction on CT.

The time window for IA thrombolysis appears to be at least 6 h for MCA occlusion, and may be even longer in the vertebrobasilar circulation with some reports of successful therapy up to 48 h after stroke onset *(17)*. The possibly longer time window in posterior circulation occlusions may be a result of greater collateral blood flow in that region (*see* below) *(18)*.

SELECTED CASE SERIES OF INTRA-ARTERIAL THROMBOLYSIS: CAROTID ARTERY (FIG. 2)

Early attempts at IA thrombolysis for carotid artery territory occlusions include the reports of Sussman et al. *(19)*, Atkin et al. *(20)*, and Labauge et al. *(21)*. Zeumer *(22)* is often credited with ushering in the modern era of IA stroke thrombolysis in 1983 with a series of case reports describing IA thrombolysis for ICA occlusion using either UK or streptokinase (SK).

In 1988, del Zoppo et al. *(23)* reported 20 patients treated with either IA SK or UK. Complete recanalization occurred in 15 cases (75%) and 10 patients (50%) had improvement of neurological symptoms. There were three deaths (15%) and three patients (15%) with embolic strokes in his series.

Also in 1988, Mori et al. *(24)* reported a series of 22 patients treated for acute occlusion of the MCA with IA UK, in doses ranging between 0.8 and 1.32 million U. Recanalization occurred in 10 cases (45%), of which 4 were complete and 6 had residual stenosis. There was symptomatic improvement in 8 of the 10 (80%) cases with recanalization. In addition, there was a significant correlation between recanalization and improved clinical outcome in his series.

Theron et al. *(25)* reported 12 patients with carotid territory occlusions treated with local IA SK or UK. Most patients were treated within 10 h of stroke onset, although in one case symptoms had recurred over 5 wk. Theron et al. speculated that occlusions involving the lenticulostriate vessels carry the highest risk of hemorrhage since the two symptomatic brain hemorrhages in this series both occurred among the five patients with occlusions at this level.

Zeumer et al. *(26)* reported their experience with local IA UK (750,000 IU) or t-PA (20 mg) given over 2 h in 31 patients with acute carotid territory and 28 patients with acute vertebrobasilar occlusion. All patients received a bolus injection of 5000 U heparin, followed by a 1000 U/h intravenous heparin infusion during the procedure. In carotid territory patients, treatment had to be finished 6 h after stroke onset. Assuming a very bad prognosis, no time limit was placed on vertebrobasilar cases and the average delay to treatment was 8 h. In the carotid territory, recanalization was achieved in 94% of patients (complete 38%). Five types of carotid territory occlusions were identified: (1) carotid siphon $C^1/_2$ segment only, (2) MCA M1, (3) MCA M1 plus M2, (4) MCA M2 or M3, and (5) multiple occlusions or multiple emboli beyond M1 and A1. Optimal recanalization and clinical results were obtained only in type 1 and type 4 occlusions. The neurological deficit was minimal or mild in 32%. In the vertebrobasilar territory, a 100% recanalization rate was achieved (complete 75%). The mortality rate was 65%; 7 patients (25%) had a minimal or mild deficit. There were no brain hemorrhages with clinical neurological deterioration, and no apparent difference in efficacy between IA UK and t-PA.

Higashida et al. *(27)* in 1994 also reported their results of 27 cases who were treated for an acute arterial occlusion in 45 vascular territories. Clinically there

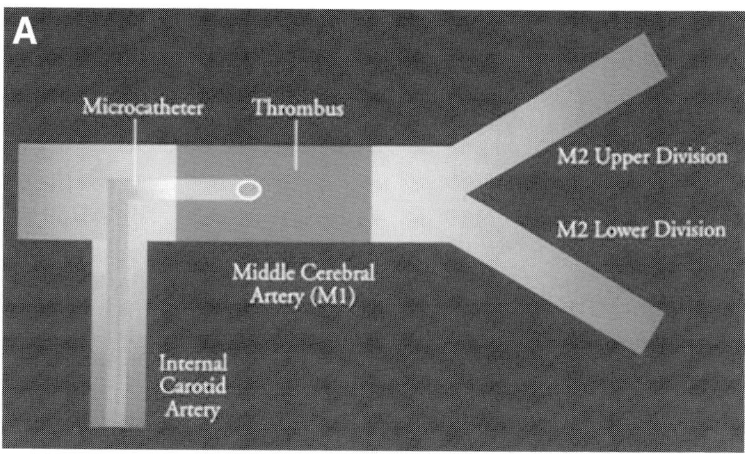
A
Microcatheter
Thrombus
M2 Upper Division
M2 Lower Division
Middle Cerebral
Artery (M1)
Internal
Carotid
Artery

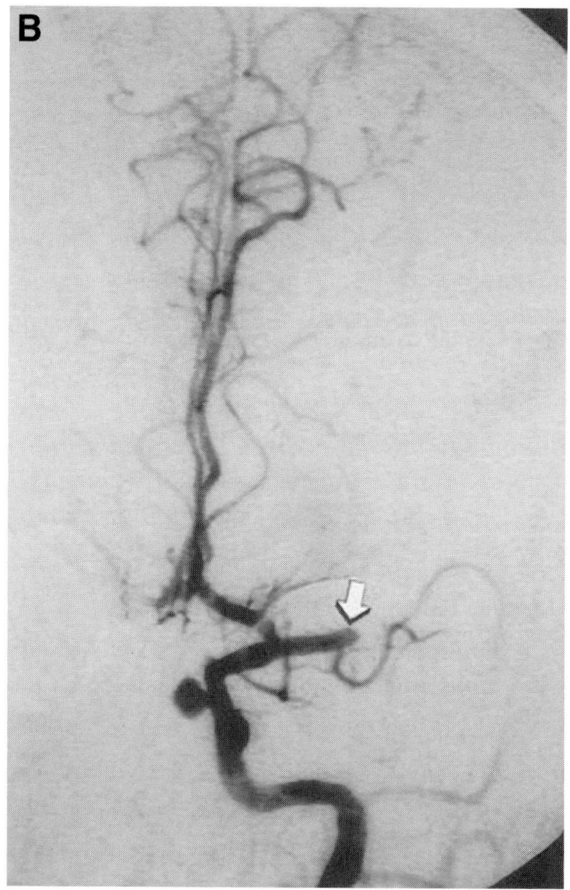
B

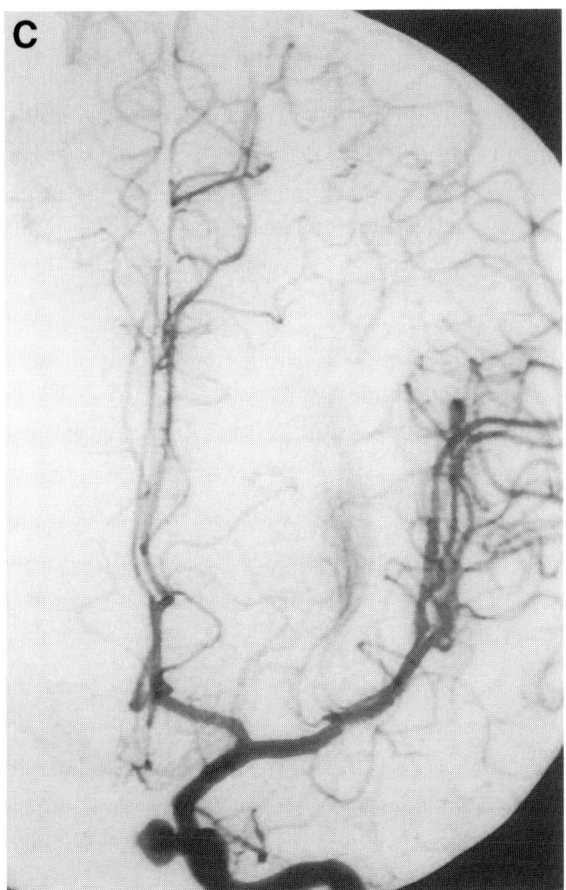

Fig. 2. (A) Illustration of microcatheter placement into an MCA clot. **(B)** Angiogram demonstrating acute occlusion of the M1 segment of the MCA (*arrow*). **(C)** Recanalized MCA after 600,000 U IA UK.

was neurological improvement in 18 (66.7%) cases. Complications directly related to therapy included symptomatic intracranial hemorrhage in 3 cases (11.1%). In 8 (29.6%) patients, there was no evidence of clinical improvement and in long-term follow up there were 9 (33.3%) patient deaths.

In an attempt to speed the time to recanalization, Freitag et al. *(28)* compared 40 patients with carotid territory stroke treated with IA UK or IA t-PA, to 15 patients treated with up to 30 mg IA t-PA plus lys-plasminogen (PG). Only 1 patient (2%) experienced brain hemorrhage with clinical neurological deterioration. Forty percent of the UK-t-PA patients had a Barthel index (BI) score higher than 90 at 3 mo compared to 60% in the lys-PG/t-PA group. For vertebrobasilar patients, long-term survival was 50% in the UK–t-PA group ($n = 20$), and 58% in the lys-PG–t-PA group ($n = 12$).

Matsumoto and Satoh *(29)* have studied IA thrombolysis in 93 patients (1995). This series is atypical in that a 24h entry window was used. Fifty-seven patients received regional IA UK with a maximal does of 1,200,000 IU. Nineteen patients received local IA UK, and 18 patients received local IA t-PA. Among the 36 patients with ICA occlusions, none completely recanalized with regional UK ($n = 21$), whereas 33% recanalized with local IA UK (3 of 8) or IA t-PA (2 of 7). Outcome was said to be good or excellent in 8 patients (22%); the mortality rate was 44% (16 of 36). Forty-one patients had MCA occlusions. The MCA complete recanalization rates were: regional UK, 62% (13 of 21); local UK, 64% (7 of 11); local t-PA, 78% (7 of 9). Clinical outcome was good or excellent in 37% of all MCA patients, and 50% for patients treated with local thrombolysis. Overall MCA mortality was 22% (9 of 41). The parenchymal hematoma rate for ICA occlusion was 6% (2 of 36), and for MCA occlusion 10% (4 of 41). Fourteen of 16 patients with basilar artery occlusion received regional UK (2 local t-PA). Forty-four percent of basilar artery cases had a good or excellent outcome, whereas 31% died. There was 1 parenchymal hematoma (6%) in the basilar artery group. Gotoh and Ogata *(30)* reported a 93% recanalization rate in 14 patients (12 MCA) treated with local IA UK starting at the distal clot interface. There were no complications.

Sasaki et al. *(31)* retrospectively reviewed 95 cases of thrombolysis for acute stroke at their institution between 1983 and 1992 to determine whether the location of infusion affected the results. Forty-four patients were given either IA UK or t-PA to the local area of vascular occlusion, whereas 18 patients were given intra-carotid infusion of UK. Only 2 of 18 patients receiving intra-carotid UK for M1 occlusion experienced even partial recanalization; the other 16 patients demonstrated no change. In the local fibrinolytic group, complete recanalization occurred in 52% of patients and partial recanalization was achieved in another 32% of patients. The highest rates of recanalization were seen in M1 and basilar artery occlusions, whereas the lowest rate of recanalization was seen in patients with ICA siphon occlusions. The reduction in infarction size and outcome were good in patients with complete recanalization. No differences were observed between IA UK and IA t-PA in achieving recanalization. Patients were given an intra-procedural infusion of up to 5000 U of heparin which was stopped at the conclusion of the procedure. Hemorrhagic infarction was seen in 22% of patients at 24 h post-IA thrombolysis, although the number of symptomatic hemorrhages was not identified.

Gönner et al. *(32)* retrospectively analyzed a series of 43 consecutive patients treated with IA thrombolysis and found that there was a statistically significant improvement in the success of recanalization if therapy was initiated within 4 h of stroke onset compared to patients treated after 4 h. Lansberg and colleagues *(33)* reported a 73-yr-old patient who received IA t-PA into three occluded left hemispheric vessels. On DWI there was no abnormality in the region of the vessel successfully recanalized under 3 h from onset, but there were DWI abnormalities in the region of the artery recanalized at 3.5 h and in the territory of the vessel that failed to reopen.

Qureshi and Suri et al. *(34)* studied eight consecutive patients given IA t-PA to determine the most efficacious dosing regimen. Interval from presentation to treatment ranged from 1 to 8 h. Patients were given escalating doses of local IA t-PA beginning with 10 mg and incrementally grading reperfusion using a modified Thrombolysis in Myocardial Infarction (TIMI) scale to a total possible dose of 40 mg. The infusion was stopped if recanalization was achieved. Increasing mean perfusion grades were seen with higher doses of t-PA. Four of the eight patients (50%) experienced neurological improvement after IA t-PA. No anticoagulation was given as part of the procedure. Two of the eight (25%) patients exhibited an asymptomatic hemorrhage at 24 h post-infusion.

Qureshi and Ali et al. *(35)* prospectively treated 16 consecutive patients with an acute stroke with an NIHSS 10–26 between 2 and 9 h from the time of onset. Patients were given up to 8 U of IA reteplase. Seven of 16 patients received adjunctive angioplasty of the occluded vessel. Modified TIMI grade 3 or 4 was achieved in 88% of patients and modified TIMI 2 in 1 more patient. Only 1 patient did not achieve at least partial recanalization. Forty-four percent experienced a 4-point or better improvement in the NIHSS. Four of the 16 (25%) patients experienced an intracerebral hemorrhage (ICH) seen on CT at 24 h post-thrombolysis. Only 1 of the 16 (6%) patients had a symptomatic hemorrhage. The overall mortality was 56% largely owing to massive ischemic strokes.

Embolic occlusions of the intracranial vasculature may result as a complication of neuroendovascular procedures. Hähnel et al.· *(36)* retrospectively reported 9 of 723 patients who underwent a neuroendovascular procedure that was complicated by thromboembolism. Time from detection of embolic occlusion until the start of IA t-PA infusion was between 10 and 90 min. Despite successful recanalization in 4 of the 9 patients, and the relatively short duration from onset to drug infusion, all patients suffered infarcts and were at least moderately disabled at 3 mo.

The relationship between recanalization, t-PA dose, and occlusion type has been examined by Eckert et al. *(37)* One hundred and thirty-seven patients with angiographic occlusion of the anterior circulation within 6 h of symptom onset received either UK, low- (10–20 mg) or high-dose (40–90 mg) t-PA, or t-PA plus lys-plasminogen. Fifty-seven percent of patients with good neurological outcome (BI score >90) were recanalized, whereas only 10% of nonrecanalized patients had a good outcome. Occlusion type had a significant impact on neurological outcome. Patients with proximal M1 occlusions had higher rates of recanalization (70%) and a higher rate of moderate to good outcomes (80% with BI score >50) at 3 mo. Recanalization rates were slightly better with high-dose t-PA vs lose-dose t-PA (50 vs 32%, respectively), but were highest with the combination of t-PA and lys-plasminogen (83%) with similar rates of hemorrhage. Among 35 patients with occlusion of the carotid-T, a poor neurological outcome (BI index score >50) was seen in 49% of patients, and the mortality rate was 43% of patients at 3 mo. In addition, Arnold et al. *(38)* demonstrated that the sufficiency of leptomeningeal collaterals is a predictor of favorable outcome in patients with carotid-T occlusions

SELECTED CASE SERIES INTRA-ARTERIAL THROMBOLYSIS: VERTEBROBASILAR TERRITORY (FIG. 3)

The natural history of basilar occlusion is extremely poor with mortality ranging from 83 to 91% *(39)*. Because of this poor natural history, IA thrombolysis has been preferred in patients with acute basilar artery occlusion. Approximately 278 cases have been reported with an overall basilar artery recanalization rate of 60% *(40)*. Basilar artery occlusions are usually a result of atherothrombosis. There is a high incidence of residual stenosis after basilar artery recanalization which often requires adjuvant therapies including angioplasty and/or stenting, antithrombotic, and antiplatelet agents.

In a compilation of reported cases of vertebrobasilar IA thrombolysis, the mortality in patients failing recanalization was 90% compared to 31% mortality in patients achieving at least partial reperfusion *(40)*. Good outcomes are strongly associated with recanalization after thrombolytic therapy Hacke et al. *(41)* described 65 consecutive patients with vertebrobasilar occlusion treated either with local IA UK, or IA SK plus heparin (n = 43), or conventional antiplatelet/anticoagulation therapy (n = 22). The recanalization rate among thrombolysis cases was 44% (19 of 43). All patients without recanalization died, whereas 14 of 19 with recanalization survived, 10 with a favorable outcome. The mortality rate with conventional therapy was 86% compared to 67% with thrombolysis. The rate of brain hemorrhage with clinical neurological deterioration was 7% in thrombolysis patients. Schumacher et al. *(42)* reported 29 patients with vertebrobasilar occlusion of less than 6 h duration treated with up to 1.5 million IU local UK plus iv heparin. Recanalization was achieved in 66%. There was no or minimal deficit in 45%. The mortality rate was 45%. Eckert et al. *(43)* performed IA thromboly-

Fig. 3. *(opposite page)* **(A)** Angiogram demonstrating acute thrombosis of the junction of the distal left vertebral and basilar artery *(arrow)*. **(B)** Microcatheter placement within proximal basilar artery. Thrombus partially recanalized after 200,000 U IA UK *(arrow)*. **(C)** Further recanalization of basilar artery thrombus. **(D)** Final basilar artery recanalization *(arrow)* after 600,000 U IA urokinase.

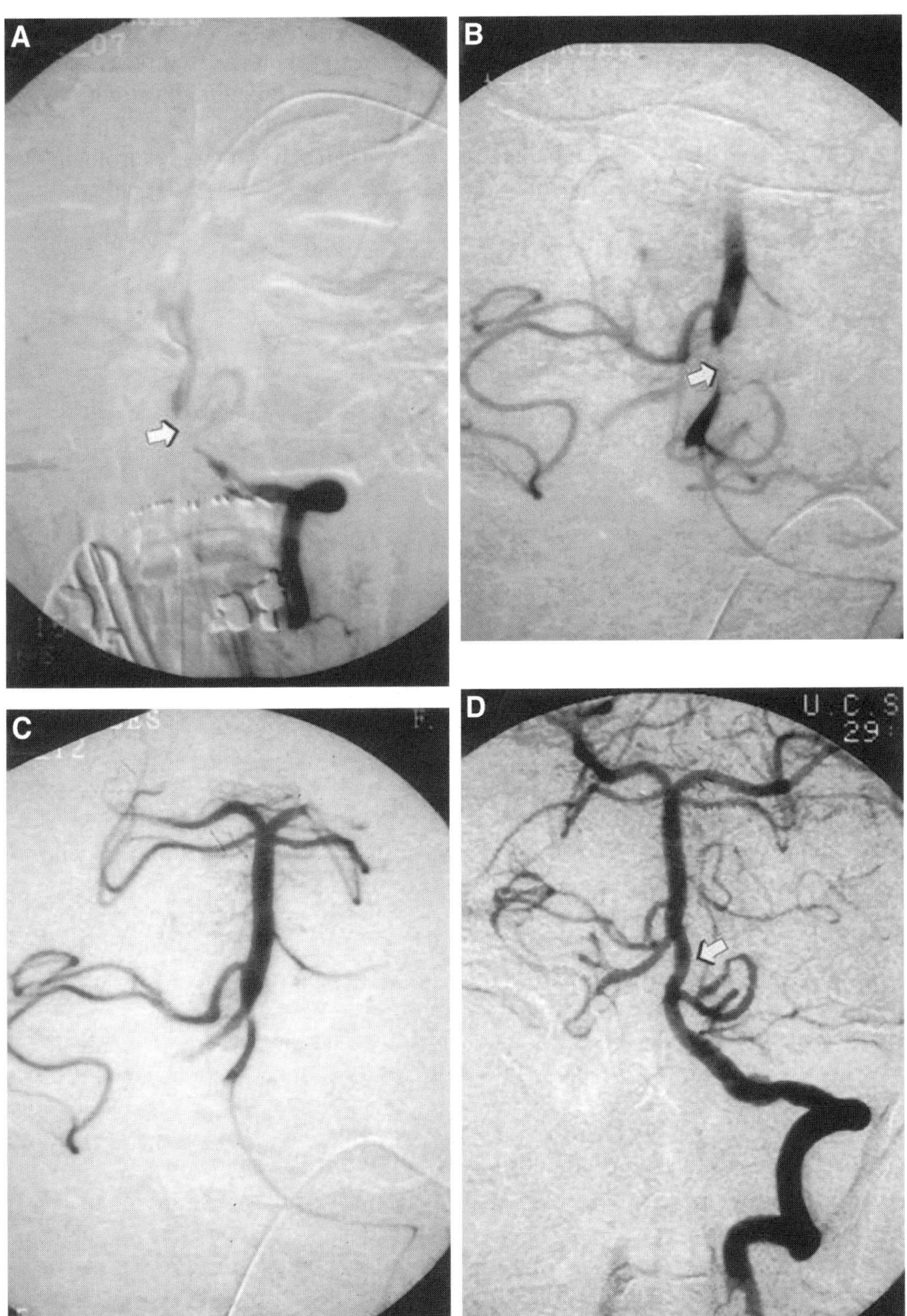
A
B
C
D
U.C.S
29

sis using 30 mg of t-PA given over 2 h in combination with 12 h of iv abciximab therapy (0.25 mg/kg bolus followed by 0.125 μg/kg/min infusion) in three patients. Recanalization occurred in two of three patients, both of whom achieved clinical independence at 3 mo post-thrombolysis.

Recanalization rates depend on the location of the vertebrobasilar occlusion. Distal basilar occlusions have higher recanalization rates than proximal occlusions. Emboli often lodge in the distal basilar artery and are easier to lyse than atherosclerosis-related thrombi, the usual cause of proximal basilar occlusions *(44)*. Short-segment occlusions are easier to lyse than longer segment occlusions *(45)*. Younger patients have higher recanalization rates *(46)*, probably because of the increased incidence of embolic occlusions seen in this age group.

The timing of IA vertebrobasilar thrombolysis is often a difficult decision. The presence of coma or tetraparesis for several hours portends a poor prognosis, despite recanalization *(41,44,46)*. Such symptoms do not preclude survival, however, and recovery has been documented after successful recanalization in such patients *(44,45,47)*.

The time window for thrombolysis may be longer in the vertebrobasilar circulation. Many series have included patients up 24 h, *(41)* 48 h *(44,48)*, and even 72 h *(41,45)* after symptom onset in patients with stuttering courses. An association between time to treatment and outcome has been suggested *(49)* but many series do not support this *(44,50,51)*. In fact, in some studies, the time to treatment was actually longer in patients who survived or had good outcomes *(44,50)*. A longer time window may result from higher ischemic tolerance or improved collateralization in the posterior circulation. Cross and colleagues *(45)*, reporting on 20 patients with basilar artery thrombosis who received IA thrombolysis, found that better collateral blood flow was correlated with improved responses to thrombolysis and with longer tolerance of ischemia. Patients with proximal basilar artery thrombosis did not seem to have the same benefit.

Patients with vertebrobasilar ischemia often have chronic atherosclerotic disease, which allows collaterals to develop over time. As hypothesized by Cross et al. *(45)*, there may be two distinct populations of patients with vertebrobasilar occlusion. Patients with a progressive stuttering course may have better collateral circulation and have better outcomes despite later treatment than patients with the sudden onset of severe deficits caused by poor collaterals who may be brought to treatment earlier.

Although some authors believe that patients with brainstem infarction on CT are not candidates for thrombolytic therapy *(41,44)* others have found no correlation with neurological outcome *(44,50)*. In two separate series, none of the patients who had CT evidence for brainstem ischemia developed a hemorrhage. However, because of the experience in the anterior circulation, caution should be used when considering thrombolysis in patients with early infarct signs.

THE PROLYSE IN ACUTE CEREBRAL THROMBOEMBOLISM TRIALS (PROACT I AND PROACT II)

The only randomized, controlled, multicenter trials of IA thrombolysis in acute ischemic stroke are PROACT I *(8)* and PROACT II *(9)*. In PROACT I, the safety and recanalization efficacy of 6 mg r-proUK was examined in 40 patients with acute ischemic stroke of less than 6 h duration owing to occlusion of the MCA. The control group received IA saline placebo. The recanalization rate was 57.7% in the r-proUK group and only 14.3% in the placebo group. Two doses of heparin were used in PROACT I. In the high-heparin group (5000 U bolus followed by 1000 U/h infusion) the recanalization rate was 80% but the symptomatic ICH rate was 27%. In the low-heparin group, the recanalization rate was 47% but the ICH rate was decreased to 6%. Although not a clinical efficacy trial, there appeared to be a 10–12% increase in excellent outcomes in the IA r-proUK group.

The follow-up clinical efficacy trial, PROACT II *(9)* was launched in February 1996 and completed in August 1998. The results were first reported in February 1999. PROACT II used an open design with blinded neurological follow-up. Patients were screened with conventional angiography for occlusion of the MCA and had to have a NIHSS score between 4 and 30. The patients in PROACT II had a very high baseline stroke severity score with a median NIHSS of 17. Patients with early signs of an infarct in greater than one third of the MCA territory (European Cooperative Acute Stroke Study [ECASS] criteria) on the baseline CT scan were excluded from the study. One hundred and eighty patients were then randomized to receive either 9 mg of IA r-proUK plus low-dose intravenous heparin or low-dose intravenous heparin alone. The primary outcome measure was the percent of patients who achieved a modified Rankin score of no more than 2 at 90 d, which signified slight or no neurological disability. Secondary measures included the percentage of patients who had a NIHSS of no more than 1 at 90 d, angiographic recanalization, symptomatic ICH, and mortality. The median time from onset of symptoms to initiation of IA thrombolysis was 5.3 h.

In the r-proUK-treated group there was a 15% absolute benefit in the number of patients who achieved a modified Rankin score of no more than 2 at 90 d ($p = 0.043$). Therefore, on average, seven patients with MCA occlusion would require IA r-proUK for one to benefit. The benefit was most noticeable in patients with a baseline NIHSS between 11 and 20. Recanalization rates were 66% at 2 h for the treatment group and 18% for the placebo group ($p < 0.001$). Symptomatic brain hemorrhage occurred in 10% of the r-proUK group and 2% of the control group. In PROACT II, as in the NINDS trial, despite the higher early symptomatic brain hemorrhage rate, patients overall benefited from the therapy and there was no excess mortality (r-proUK 24%, control 27%).

BRAIN HEMORRHAGE IN INTRA-ARTERIAL THROMBOLYSIS

Aggregate data indicates an 8.3% risk of symptomatic brain hemorrhage with IA thrombolysis in the carotid territory and a 6.5% risk in the vertebrobasilar territory *(40)*. There is no evidence that the rate of symptomatic brain hemorrhage is lower with IA thrombolysis than with iv thrombolysis, but direct comparisons are difficult. In an uncontrolled series, Gönner et al. *(52)* reported a 4.7% rate of symptomatic brain hemorrhage in 42 patients treated with IA thrombolysis. This series differed from PROACT II in that only 26 out of the 42 patients received heparin; the remainder received aspirin. The higher rate of ICH with neurological deterioration with IA rpro-UK in PROACT II (10.2 %) compared to intravenous t-PA in the National Institute of Neurological Disorders and Stroke (NINDS) (6.4%) *(1)*, the Alteplase ThromboLysis for Acute Noninterventional Therapy in Ischemic Stroke (ATLANTIS) (7.2%) *(53)*, and ECASS II (8.8%) studies *(54)* must be understood within the context of the greater baseline stroke severity, longer time to treatment, and 66% MCA recanalization rate in PROACT II. The median baseline NIHSS score in ATLANTIS and ECASS II was 11, in NINDS 14, and in PROACT II 17. Greater baseline stroke severity was first associated with increased intracranial hemorrhage risk in NINDS and ECASS I. All symptomatic ICH in PROACT II occurred in patients with a baseline NIHSS score of 11 or more, and in NINDS the rate of symptomatic brain hemorrhage in patients with a NIHSS of more than 20 was 18%.

Although brain hemorrhage complicating thrombolysis for acute stroke likely reflects reperfusion of necrotic tissue, several intravenous thrombolysis series have found no direct relationship between recanalization and hemorrhage risk *(55,56)*. Kidwell et al. *(57)* retrospectively reviewed 89 patients treated with IA thrombolysis at their center and found that the leading predictors of any hemorrhage in this population were the baseline NIHSS score, platelet count, glucose level, and a longer time to recanalization. Also, this uncontrolled series from Kidwell et al. showed a strong trend toward a higher rate of hemorrhagic transformation in patients without recanalization vs with recanalization (54% vs 33%, respectively; $p = 0.1$). The amount of ischemic damage is a key factor in the development of brain hemorrhage after thrombolysis induced recanalization. Major early CT changes and severity of the initial neurological deficit, both indicators of the extent of ischemic damage, are some of the best predictors for the risk of hemorrhagic transformation *(56,58)*.

Several other factors have been associated with hemorrhage after thrombolysis for both stroke and myocardial infarction, including thrombolytic dose *(59)*, blood pressure *(56,60,61)*, advanced age, prior head injury *(62)*, and blood glucose greater than 200 mg/dL. Levels of blood matrix metalloproteinase-9 (MMP-9) in patients prior to thrombolytic therapy has been shown to be a risk factor for hemorrhagic transformation *(63)*, although a specific genotypic relationship could not be elucidated *(64)*. Other studies to identify patients at risk have used advanced T2-weighted magnetic resonance imaging (MRI) sequences such as gradient echo planar imaging to identify patients with a history of microbleeds that may predispose to a higher rate of hemorrhagic transformation during thrombolysis *(65)*. Adjunctive antithrombotic therapy may also play a role during IA thrombolysis. Age was the most important risk factor in one of the largest series of thrombolysis-related ICH *(62)*. A relationship between advanced age and hemorrhage was demonstrated in the NINDS *(1)* and ECASS trials *(54,58)*. Although there is no strict age cutoff for administering thrombolytics for stroke, physicians need to take age into account, especially in patients over age 75 when determining the risk of angiography and IA thrombolysis.

INTRAVENOUS VS INTRA-ARTERIAL THROMBOLYSIS

There have been no randomized studies comparing recanalization rates and clinical outcomes between iv thrombolysis and IA thrombolysis. Limited data suggest, however, that intravenous t-PA may be relatively ineffective in patients with ICA or MCA occlusion. Tomsick et al. *(66)* reported that iv t-PA given less than 3 h from stroke onset was ineffective in patients with a baseline NIHSS score of 10 or more and a hyperdense MCA sign (signifying MCA occlusion) on CT.

Endo et al. *(67)* retrospectively reviewed 33 consecutive patients with occlusion of the cervical ICA. The first 12 patients were treated with intravenous t-PA or intravenous UK with posttreatment angiograms or sonograms failing to show recanalization. Nine of these patients died and the remainder had a poor outcome (defined as being incapable of independent living). The remaining 21 patients were treated with IA thrombolysis, of these 8 successfully recanalized, 4 of whom recovered with none or minimal neurological deficits. Of the 13 patients treated with IA thrombolysis who failed to recanalize, all had poor outcomes similar to the intravenous thrombolysis group.

It may be feasible to combine intravenous and IA thrombolysis. The Emergency Management of Stroke (EMS) Bridging trial *(68)* employed a novel design to investigate the safety of combined intravenous and IA t-PA. Patients with an NIHSS 6 or more were randomized within 3 h from symptom onset to receive 0.6 mg/kg intravenous t-PA (n = 17) or placebo (n = 18) over 30 min followed by angiography. If a thrombus was present, patients in both groups then received local IA t-PA, up to a total of 20 mg over 2 h. For patients with M1, M2, or PCA occlusion, there was complete (n = 6) or partial (n = 3) recanalization in all intravenous plus IA cases. For IA-only cases, there were no cases of complete recanalization, four with partial, and two with no recanalization. However, all three cases of major bleeding occurred in the combined intravenous plus IA group. Ernst et al. *(69)* retrospectively reviewed 20 consecutive acute ischemic strokes treated using a modified EMS Bridging trial intravenous and IA t-PA protocol. Ten patients (50%) had minimal or no neurological deficits (modified Rankin score ≤1), whereas another 3 patients (15%) had minor neurological deficits. One patient (5%) had a symptomatic ICH. These favorable outcomes were achieved despite a high-median baseline NIHSS of 21 (range 11–31). The better than expected outcomes in this study may attributed to the relatively short average time to intravenous thrombolysis (2 h and 2 min) and IA thrombolysis (3 h and 30 min).

A suggested treatment algorithm in patients with MCA occlusion is provided in Fig. 4. Patients presenting to the hospital less than 3 h from stroke onset should undergo noninvasive screening to detect for an MCA occlusion. Intravenous t-PA would be given, but if the MCA is still occluded between 3 and 6 h, then the patient would go to angiography for "rescue" IA thrombolysis. Alternatively, the patient could go directly to angiography if IA thrombolysis is available in less than 60 min, or an 0.6 mg/kg loading dose of intravenous t-PA (15% as a bolus over 1 min and the remainder infused over 30 min) could be initiated prior to angiography as in the (EMS) Bridging trial. This would allow outlying community hospitals to start intravenous t-PA and then provide transport of the patient to a regional stroke center for definitive diagnosis and treatment.

LIMITATIONS OF INTRA-ARTERIAL THROMBOLYSIS

A major issue regarding access to IA thrombolysis for treatment of acute ischemic strokes is that it requires the ready availability of a neurointerventionalist and a stroke team. Such expertise is not currently available in most community hospitals across the United States and is limited to large academic centers *(70,71)*. Another limitation of IA thrombolysis is the additional time required to begin treatment compared to iv thrombolysis. In PROACT II, the average time from arrival to the hospital to the initiation of IA r-proUK was 3 h. There are also concerns regarding the invasiveness of the technique and procedural risks not inherent to iv thrombolysis. However, serious procedural complications were uncommon in PROACT I and II, and cerebral angiography in experienced centers is associated with a morbidity of only 1.4%, and a rate of permanent neurological complications and death of 0.1 and 0.02%, respectively.

SPECIAL SETTINGS FOR INTRA-ARTERIAL THROMBOLYSIS

IA thrombolysis may be useful in situations where intravenous thrombolysis carries an excessive bleeding risk. Patients with recent non-ICH, recent surgery or arterial puncture, and patients on systemic anticoagulation were excluded from the NINDS trial because of their perceived increased risk of hemorrhagic complications. IA thrombolysis, by delivering smaller doses of thrombolytics directly into the affected blood vessel, offers the potential to treat such patients with a lesser risk of hemorrhage. Katzan et al. *(72)* used IA thrombolysis to treat six patients who developed acute strokes in the postoperative period after open heart surgery. Although the series was small and only one patient improved

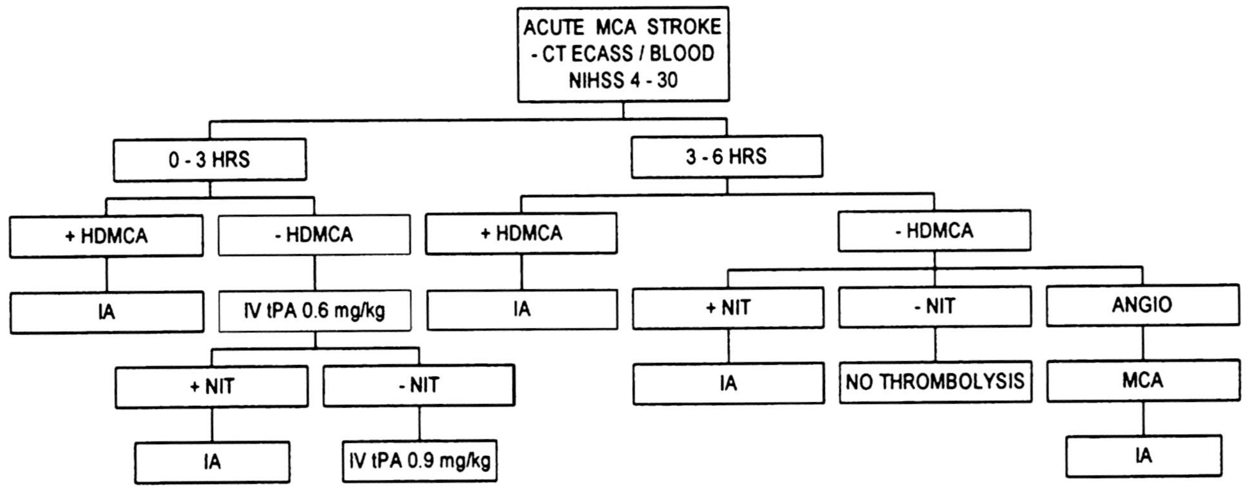

HDMCA = HYPERDENSE MIDDLE CEREBRAL ARTERY
NIT = NON-INVASIVE TESTS
NIHSS = NATIONAL INSTITUTES OF HEALTH STROKE SCALE
IA = INTRA-ARTERIAL THROMBOLYSIS
IV = INTRAVENOUS
tPA = TISSUE PLASMINOGEN ACTIVATOR
ECASS = EUROPEAN COOPERATIVE ACUTE STROKE STUDY

Fig. 4. Potential thrombolysis algorithm for acute MCA occlusion.

dramatically, the authors were able to show the relative safety and feasibility of the procedure as only one minor bleeding complication occurred.

In 1998, Cronqvist et al. *(73)* published their results on local IA fibrinolysis of thromboemboli occurring during endovascular treatment of intracerebral aneurysms. In 19 patients, iatrogenic occlusions occurred in either the MCA, anterior cerebral artery, or basilar artery during the neuro-interventional procedure. Utilizing a combination of UK and mechanical clot fragmentation, they were able to achieve complete recanalization in 10 patients (53%) and partial recanalization in the other 9 patients (47%). Fourteen patients (74%) had a good to excellent recovery and there was good correlation with complete recanalization and improved clinical outcome.

Intravenous thrombolysis has not been studied in retinal ischemia. The series by Weber et al. *(74)* of 17 patients, and the smaller series of 3 patients by Padolecchia et al. *(75)* have shown the safety and efficacy of super selective IA thrombolysis in cases of central retinal artery occlusion. In both groups there were no hemorrhagic complications and there were significant improvements in visual acuity. In the series by Weber et al., 17.6% of patients recovered completely and their patients faired better than historical controls.

MECHANICAL CLOT DISRUPTION AND REMOVAL

Recanalization efficacy of cerebral vessels is limited when thrombolytic agents alone are used. Therefore, neuro-interventionalists are now investigating a variety of mechanical techniques to maximize the speed and completeness of recanalization. Several devices ranging from simple baskets and corkscrews, to more complex lasers and ultrasonic catheters have entered clinical trials *(76)*.

The AngioJet NV150 Rheolytic Thrombectomy System (Possis Medical) is a device which utilizes high velocity saline infusion and the Bernoulli principle of fluid mechanics to extract a clot from a vessel the size of the MCA. The Thrombectomy in Middle Cerebral Embolism (TIME) Trial was the first US Food and Drug Administration (FDA)-approved study combining mechanical thrombectomy with IA thrombolytic agent (t-PA) in patients with MCA occlusion of less than 6 h duration. This phase I safety trial of the NV 150 neurocatheter enrolled 20 patients with a 30% successful recanalization rate. TIME was halted in 2003 by the manufacturer because of the low rate of recanalization.

The EKOS MicroLysUS catheter employs an ultrasonic transducer at the microcatheter tip to loosen the thrombus and promote penetration of the thrombolytic agent into the clot matrix *(77)*. The EKOS catheter is being employed in the ongoing Interventional Mangement of Stroke (IMS) trial of combined iv and IA t-PA.

The Concentric MERCI Retriever (Concentric Medical, Inc.) is a flexible, tapered nickel-titanium wire with a helical shaped distal tip which can be deployed intra-arterially to entrap and retrieve large vessel intracerebral clots. The MERCI trial enrolled 121 patients with an acute MCA, ICA, carotid-T or vertebral basilar (VB) occlusion of less than 6 h duration, some of whom also received IA thrombolytics *(78)*. Entry criteria for MERCI were very similar to PROACT II except occlusions were not restricted to the MCA and there was no randomized control group. The study population had a relatively high stroke severity. The median NIHSS was 19 and 40% of patients had a baseline NIHSS greater than 20. Only 3% of patients had a baseline NIHSS between 6 and 10. One hundred and fourteen patients were treated using the MERCI device; 7 patients were not treated after the guidewire was placed for unspecified reasons. Median time to IA treatment was 6.1 h. Recanalization was achieved in 54% (61 of 114) of patients (ICA 57%; MCA 51%; VB 58%). Device-related serious adverse events occurred in 4 patients (3.5%; dissection in 2 and anterior cerebral artery emboli during MCA retrieval in 2). The symptomatic brain hemorrhage rate was 8% (PROACT II 10%), 5% with the retriever alone but 24% in patients who also received IA thrombolytic agent. The 90-d mortality rate was high at 40% (PROACT II 25%) possibly reflecting the high-baseline stroke severity and distribution of vascular occlusions. Although not a clinical efficacy trial, 37% of patients with MCA occlusion ($n = 65$) achieved a modified Rankin Score (mRS) of 2 or less at 90 d. This compares with the historical control rate of 25% and treated (IA proUK) rate of 40% in PROACT II. Although not a randomized, controlled trial, the results of MERCI are similar to PROACT II. The FDA recently approved the concentric retriever for thrombus removal in acute stroke. Interventionalists will likely use the device first before adding a thrombolytic agent. Clinical efficacy trials are planned (MR RESCUE).

SUMMARY AND FUTURE DIRECTIONS

Intra-arterial thrombolysis is an established treatment option for patients with acute ischemic stroke caused by large vessel cerebrovascular occlusions. In the carotid territory, the efficacy of IA thrombolysis in patients with MCA occlusion of less than 6 h duration has been demonstrated in the PROACT trials. The thrombolytic agent used in the PROACT trials, r-proUK, is not currently FDA approved. Urokinase has been re-introduced to the market by Abbott within the past year. Although there is no evidence that IA UK is superior to IA t-PA, there is more aggregate experience with IA UK. More data are needed on the dosing and safety of IA alteplase and new thrombolytic agents such as desmoteplase, tenecteplase, and reteplase in acute ischemic stroke.

Recanalization and clinical outcome are less predictable with occlusions at the ICA origin, the intracranial carotid T-bifurcation, or in the vertebrobasilar circulation. This may partly reflect the fact that most MCA occlusions are a result of soft clot from cardiac embolism or fresh thrombus from a proximal atherosclerotic plaque. The low TIMI 3 recanalization rate in PROACT II (20%) indicates residual thrombus is frequently present after IA thrombolysis. There is no consensus on how to deal with distal embolization, re-occlusion, or underlying atherostenosis complicating IA stroke thrombolysis. These issues, and the role of clot composition in recanalization efficacy, require further study. Future trials of IA thrombolysis should seek guidance from proposed trial design and reporting standards which have been recently published *(79)*.

Intra-arterial stroke thrombolysis is still evolving and there has been no standardization of patient selection, neuro-interventional techniques, or adjunctive therapy. Mechanical clot removal using devices designed for this purpose, new catheter techniques, and new adjunctive antithrombotic agents should improve the degree, speed and safety of IA recanalization. The number of patients subjected to unnecessary angiography can be reduced by the emergent performance of non-invasive screening, a capability many centers do not currently have. In addition, patient selection and the treatment window may be better defined by using new technologies such as perfusion-diffusion MRI *(80)*. Lastly, IA thrombolysis can be combined not only with intravenous thrombolysis, but also with cytoprotective strategies to improve patient outcomes after acute ischemic stroke in the near future, if these current clinical studies prove safe and efficacious.

REFERENCES

1. The National Institute of Neurological Disorders and Stroke rt-PA Stroke Study Group: Tissue Plasminogen Activator for Acute Ischaemic Stroke. *N Engl J Med* 1995; 333:1581–1587.
2. Wolpert SM, Bruckmann H, Greenlee R, et al. Neuroradiology evaluation of patients with acute stroke treated with recombinant tissue plasminogen activator. *AJNR* 1993; 14:3–13.
3. Tomsick T, Brott T, Barsan W, et al. Thrombus localization with emergency CT. *Am J Neuroradiol* 1992;12:257–263
4. Leary MC, Kidwell CS, Villablanca P, et al. Validation of computed tomography middle cerebral artery "dot" sign. *Stroke* 2003;34:2636–2640.
5. Schellinger PD, Jansen O, Fiebach JB, et al. Monitoring intravenous recombinant tissue plasminogen activator thrombolysis for acute ischemic stroke with diffusion and perfusion MRI. *Stroke* 2000;31:1318–1328.
6. Lev MH, Segal AZ, Farkas J, et al. Utility of perfusion-weighted CT imaging in acute middle cerebral artery stroke treated with intra-arterial thrombolysis. *Stroke* 2001;32:2021–2028.
7. Higashida RT, Halbach VV, Tsai FY, Dowd CF, Hieshima GB. Interventional neurovascular techniques in acute thrombolytic therapy for stroke. In: T Yamagushi, E Mori, K Minematsu, GJ del Zoppo, eds. *Thrombolytic Therapy in Acute Ischemic Stroke III*. Tokyo:Springer-Verlag, 1995, pp.294–300
8. del Zoppo GJ, Higashida RT, Furlan AJ, et al. PROACT: A Phase II Randomized Triof Recombinant Pro-Urokinase by Direct Arterial Delivery in Acute Middle Cerebral Artery Stroke. *Stroke* 1998; 29:4–11.
9. Furlan A, Higashida R, Wechsler L, Gent M et al. PROACT II: Intera-artrerialprourokinase for acute ischemic stroke. A Randomized Controlled Trial. *JAMA* 1999; 282:2003–2011.
10. Liberatore GT, Samson A, Bladin C, et al.Vampire bat salivary plasminogen activator (desmoteplase): a unique fibrinolytic enzyme that does not promote neurodegeneration. *Stroke* 2003 Feb;34(2):537–543.

11. Wallace RC, Furlan AJ, Moliterno DJ, et al. Basilar artery rethrombosis: Successful treatment with platelet glycoprotein Iib/IIIa receptor inhibitor. *Am J Neuroradiol* 1997;18:1257–1260.
12. Eckert B, Koch C, Thomalla G, et al. Acute basilar artery occlusion treated with combined intravenous abciximab and intra-arterial tissue plasminogen activator. *Stroke* 2002;33:1424–1427.
13. Lee DH, Jo KD, Kim HG, et al. Local intra-arterial urokinase thrombolysis of acute ischemic stroke with or without intravenous abciximab: A pilot study. *J Vasc Interv Radiol* 2002;13:769–773.
14. Adams HP, Bogousslavsky J, Barnathan E, et al. Preliminary safety report of a randomized trial of abciximab (ReoPro[R]) in acute ischemic stroke. *Cerebrovasc Dis* 1999;9(suppl 1):127.
15. Pessin M, del Zoppo GJ, Furlan AJ. Thrombolytic treatment in acute stroke: review and update of selective topics. In: Moskowitz MA, Caplan LR , eds. *Cerebrovascular Diseases. Nineteenth Princeton Stroke Conference*. Boston:Butterworth-Heinemann, 1995, pp. 409–418.
16. del Zopo GJ, Sasahara AA. Interventional use of plasminogen activators in central nervous system diseases. *Med Clin N Am* 1998;82(3):545–568.
17. Hoffman AI, Lambiase RE, Haas RA, Rogg JM, Murphy TP. Acute verterbrobasilar occlusion: Treatment with high-dose intraarterial urokinase. *AJR* 1999;172:709–712.
18. Cross DT, Moran CJ, Akins PT, et al. Intraarterial thrombolysis in vertebrobasilar occlusion. *AJNR* 1996;17:255–262.
19. Sussman BJ, Fitch TSP. Thrombolysis with fibrinolysin in cerebral arterial occlusion. *JAMA* 1958;167:1705.
20. Atkin N, Nitzberg S, Dorsey J. Lysis of intracerebral thromboembolism with fibrinolysin. Report of a case. *Angiology* 1964;15:436.
21. Labauge R, Blard JM, Salvaing P, et al. Traitment fibrinolytique et anticoagulant dans 37 cas d'occlusions arterielles, cervicocerebrales d'origin thrombo-embolique. In: *Proceedings of the Fifth International Congress on Thromboembolism*. Bologna, 1978. Pisa, Quaderni della Coagulazione, 1980, pp 362–364.
22. Zeumer H, Hundgen R, Ferbert A, Ringelstein EB. Local intraarterial fibrinolytic therapy in inaccessible internal carotid occlusion. *Neuroradiology* 1984;26:315–317
23. del Zoppo GJ, Ferbert A, Otis S, et al. Local intra-arterial fibrinolytic therapy in acute carotid territory stroke. A pilot study. *Stroke* 1988;19:307–313.
24. Mori E, Tabuchi M, Yoshida T, Yamadori A. Intracarotid urokinase with thromboembolic occlusion of the middle cerebral artery. *Stroke* 1988;19:802–812.
25. Theron J, Courtheoux P, Casasco A, et al. Local intra-arterial fibrinolysis in the carotid territory. *AJNR* 1989;753–765.
26. Zeumer H, Freitag HJ, Zanella F, Thie A, Arning C. Local intra-arterial fibrinolytic therapy in patients with stroke: urokinase versus recombinant tissue plasminogen activator (r-TPA). *Neuroradiology* 1993;35:159–162.
27. Higashida RT, Halbach VV, Barnwell SL, Dowd CF, Hieshima GB.Thrombolytic therapy in acute stroke.. *J Endovasc Surg*.1994;1:4–15.
28. Freitag HJ, Becker V, Thie A, et al. Plasminogen plus rt-PA improves intra-arterial thrombolytic therapy in acute ischemic stroke. In: t Yamugushi, e Mori, K Minematsu, GJ del Zoppo, eds. *Thrombolytic Tehrapy in Acute ischemic Stroke ILL*. Tokyo:Springer-Verlag , 1995, pp 271–278.
29. Matsumoto K, Satoh K. Intra-arterial therapy in acute ischemic stroke. In: Yamagushi T, Mori E, K Minematsu, GJ del Zoppo, eds. *Thrombolytic Tehrapy in Acute Ischemic Stroke III*. Tokyo: Springer-Verlag, 1995, pp279–287.
30. Goto K, Ogata N. A central intra-arterial thrombolysis using a newly developed low friction guidewire/catheter system. In: T Yamagushi, E Mori, K Minematsu, GJ del Zoppo, eds.*Thrombolytic Therapy in Acute Ischemic Stroke III*. Tokyo:Springer-Verlag 1995, pp. 301–306.

31. Sasaki O, Takeuchi S, Koike T, et al. Fibrinolytic therapy for acute embolic stroke: intravenous, intra-carotid and intra-arterial local approaches. *Neurosurgery* 1995;36:246–253.
32. Gönner F, Remonda L, Mattle H, Sturzenegger M, et al. Local intra-arterial thrombolysis in acute ischemic stroke. *Stroke* 1998;29:1894–1900.
33. Lansberg MG, Tong DC, Norbash AM, Yenari MA, Moseley ME. Intra-arterial rtPA treatment of stroke assessed by diffusion- and perfusion-weighted MRI. *Stroke* 1999;30:678–680.
34. Qureshi AI, Suri MFK, Shatla AA, et al. Intra-arterial recombinant tissue plasminogen activator for ischemic stroke: an accelerating dosing regimen. *Neurosurgery* 2000;47:473–479.
35. Qureshi AI, Ali Z, Suri MFK, et al. Intra-arterial third generation recombinant tissue plasminogen activator (reteplase) for acute ischemic stroke. *Neurosurgery* 2001;49:41–50.
36. Hahnel S, Schellinger PD, Gutschalk A, et al. Local intra-arterial fibrinolysis of thromboemboli occurring during neuroendovascular procedures with recombinant tissue plasminogen activator. *Stroke* 2003;34:1723–1729.
37. Eckert B, Kucinski T, Neumaier-Probst E, et al. Local intra-arterial fibrinolysis in acute hemispheric stroke: effect of occlusion type and fibrinolytic agent on recanalization success and neurological outcome. *Cerebrovasc Dis* 2003;15:258–263.
38. Arnold M, Nedeltchev K, Mattle HP, et al. Intra-arterial thrombolysis in 24 consecutive patients with internal carotid T occlusions. *J Neurol Neurosurg Psychiatry* 2003;74:739–742.
39. Furlan AJ. Natural history of atherothromboembolic occlusion of cerebral arteries: carotid versus vertebrobasilar territories. In: Hacke W, del Zoppo GJ, Hirschberg M, eds. *Thrombolytic Therapy in Acute Ischemic Stroke.* New York: Springer-Verlag, 1991, pp.71–76
40. Katzan IL, Furlan AJ. Thrombolytic therapy. In: Fisher M andBogousslavsky J, eds. *Current Review of Cerebrovascular Disease, 3rd Edition.* Boston: Butterworth Heinemann, 1999, pp. 185–193.
41. Hacke W, Zeumer H, Ferbert A, et al. Intra-arterial thrombolytic therapy improves outcome in patients with acute vertebrobasilar occlusive disease. *Stroke* 1988;19:1216–1222.
42. Schumacher m, Siekmann R, Radu W, Wakhloo AK. Local intra-arterial fibrinolytic therapy in vetebrobasilar occlusion. In: BL Bauer, M. Brock, M Klinger. *Advances in Neurosurgery* 1994;22:30–34.
43. Eckert B, Koch C, Thomalla G, Roether J, Zeumer H. Acute basilar artery occlusion treated with combined intravenous abciximab and intra-arterial tissue plasminogen activator. *Stroke* 2002;33:1424–1427.
44. Brandt T, von Kummer R, Muller-Kuppers M, et al. Thrombolytic therapy of acute basilar artery occlusion, variables affecting recanalization and outcome. *Stroke* 1996;27:875–881.
45. Cross DT, Moran CI, Akins P, et al. Relationship between clot location and outcome after basilar artery thrombolysis. *Am J Neuroradiol* 1997; 18:1221–1228.
46. Huemer M, Niederwieser V, Ladurner G. Thrombolytic treatment for acute occlusion of the basilar artery. *J Neurol Neurosurg Psychiatry* 1995;58:227–228.
47. Wijdicks EF, Nichols DA, Thielen KR, et al. Intra-arterial thrombolysis in acute basilar artery thromboembolisms: The initial Mayo Clinic experience. *Mayo Clin Proc* 1997;72:1005–1013.
48. Clark W, Barnwell S, Nesbit G, et al. Efficacy of intra-arterial thrombolysis of basilar artery stroke (abstr). *J Stroke Cerebrovasc Dis* 1997;6:457.
49. Zeumer H, Freitag HJ, Grzyska U, et al. Local intra-arterial fibrinolysis in acute vertebrobasilar occlusion. *Neuroradiology* 1989;31:336–340.
50. Becker KJ, Monsein LH, Ulatowski J, et al. Intraarterial thrombolysis in vertebrobasilar occlusion. *AJNR* 1996;17:255–262.
51. Mitchell PJ, Gerraty RP, Donnan GA, et al. Thrombolysis in the vertebrobasilar circulation: the Australian urokinase stroke trial. *Cerebrovasc Dis* 1997;7:94–99.
52. Gönner F, Remonda L, Mattle H, Sturzenegger M, et al. Local intra-arterial thrombolysis in acute ischemic stroke. *Stroke* 1998;29:1894–1900.

53. Clark WM, Albers GW, for the ATLANTIS Stroke Study Investigators. The ATLANTIS rt-PA (alteplase) acute stroke trial: Final results (abstract). *Stroke* 1999;30:234.
54. Hacke W, Kaste M, Fieschi C, et al. Randomized double-blind placebo-controlled trial of thrombolytic therapy with intravenous alteplase in acute ischemic stroke (ECASS II). *Lancet* 1998;352:1245–1251.
55. von Kummer R, Hacke W. Safety and efficacy of intravenous tissue plasminogen activator and heparin in acute middle cerebral artery stroke. *Stroke* 1992;23:646–652.
56. The NINDS t-PA Stroke Study Group. Intracerebral hemorrhage after intravenous t-PA therapy for ischemic stroke. *Stroke* 1997;28:2109–2118.
57. Kidwell CS, Saver JL, Carneado J, et al. Predictors of hemorrhagic transformation in patients receiving intra-arterial thrombolysis. *Stroke* 2002;33:717–724.
58. Hacke W, Kaste M, Fieschi C, et al. Intravenous thrombolysis with recombinent tissue plasminogen activator for acute hemispheric stroke. The European Cooperative Acute Stroke Study (ECASS). *JAMA* 1995;274:1017–1025.
59. Gore JM, Sloan M, Price TR, et al. Intracerebral hemorrhage, cerebral infarction, and subdural hematoma after acute myocardial infarction and thrombolytic therapy in the thombolysis in myocardial infarction study. Thrombolysis in myocardial infarction, phase II, pilot and clinical trial. *Circulation* 1991;83:448–459.
60. Simoons MI, Maggioni AP, Knatterud G, et al. Individual risk assessment for intracranial hemorrhage durinig thrombolytic therapy. *Lancet* 1993;342:1523–1528.
61. Anderson JL, Karagounis L, Allen A, et al. Older age and elevated blood pressure are risk factors for intracerebral hemorrhage after thrombolysis. *Am J Cardiol* 1991;68:166–170.
62. Gebel M, Sila CA, Sloan MA, et al. Thrombolysis-related intracranial hemorrhage: a radiographic analysis of 244 cases from the GUSTO-1 trial with clinical correlation. *Stroke* 1998;29:563–569.
63. Montaner J, Molina CA, Monasterio J, et al. Matrix metalloproteinase (MMP-9) pretreatment level predicts intracranial hemorrhagic complications after thrombolysis in human stroke. *Circulation* 2003;107:598–603.
64. Montaner J, Fernandez-Cardenas I, Molina CA, et al. Safety profile of tissue plasminogen activator treatment among stroke patients carrying a common polymorphism (C1562T) in the promoter region of matrix metalloproteinase-9 gene. *Stroke* 2003;34:2851–2855.
65. Kidwell CS, Saver JL, Villablanca JP, et al. Magnetic resonance imaging detection of microbleeds before thrombolysis. *Stroke* 2002;33:95–98.
66. Tomsick T, Brott T, Barsan W, et al. Prognostic value of the hyperdense middle cerebral artery sign and stroke scale score before ultraearly thrombolytic therapy. *Am J Neurorad* 1996;17:79–85.
67. Endo S, Kuwayama N, Hirashima Y, Akai T, Nishijima M, Takaku A. Results of urgent thrombolysis in patients with major stroke and atherothrombotic occlusion of the cervical internal carotid artery. *AJNR* 1998;19:1169–1175.
68. Emergency Management of Stroke (EMS) Investigators: Combined intra-arterial and intravenous tPA for stroke (abstract). *Stroke* 1997; 28:273.
69. Ernst R, Pancioli A, Tomsick T, et al. Combined intravenous and intra-arterial recombinant tissue plasminogen activator in acute ischemic stroke. *Stroke* 2000;31:2552–2557.
70. Grotta J. t-PA-The best current option for most patients. *N Engl J Med* 1997;337:1310–1312.
71. Caplan LR, Mohr JP, Kitler JP, et al. Thrombolysis-notr a panacea for ischemic stroke. *N Engl J Med* 1997;337:1309--1310.
72. Katzan IL, Masaryk TJ, Furlan AJ, et al. Intra-arterial thrombolysis for perioperative stroke after open heart surgery. *Neurology* 1999;52:1081–1084.
73. Cronqvist M, Pierot L, Boulin A, et al. Local intraarterial fibrinolysis of thromboemboli occurring during endovascular treatment of intracerebral aneurysm: a comparison of anatomic results and clinical outcome. *AJNR* 1998;19:157–165.

74. Weber J, Remonda L, Mattle HP, et al. Selective intra-arterial fibrinolysis of acute central retinal artery occlusion. i1998;29:2076–2079.
75. Padolecchia R, Puglioli M, Ragone MC, Romani A, Collavoli PL. Superselective intraarterial fibrinolysis in central retinal artery occlusion. *AJNR* 1999;20:565–567.
76. Nesbit GM, Luh G, Tien R, Barnwell SL. New and future endovascular treatment strategies for acute ischemic stroke. *J Vasc Interv Radiol* 2004;15:S103–S110.
77. Mahon BR, Nesbit GM, Barnwell SL, et al. North American clinical experience with the EKOS MicroLysUS infusion catheter for the treatment of embolic stroke. *AJNR* 2003;24:534–538.
78. Starkman S, and MERCI Trial Investigators. Results of the Combined Mechanical Embolus in Cerebral Ischemia (MERCI) I and II Trials. *Abstracts of the 29th International Stroke Conference*, Presented February 6, 2004.
79. Higashida RT, Furlan AJ. Trial design and reporting standards for intra-arterial cerebral thrombolysis for acute ischemic stroke. *Stroke* 2003;34:109–137.
80. Albers GW. Expanding the time window for thrombolytic therapy in acute stroke. The potential role of acute MRI for patient selection. *Stroke* 1999;30:2230–2237.

11 Combinations of Intravenous and Intra-Arterial Thrombolysis

Matthew L. Flaherty, MD
and Joseph Broderick, MD

Contents

INTRODUCTION

The purpose of this chapter is to introduce physicians to the concept of a combined intravenous/intra-arterial (IA) approach to vascular recanalization. Current experience is limited but the concept is attractive and worthy of further study. To understand the potential advantages of a combined approach, it is

From: *Current Clinical Neurology: Thrombolytic Therapy for Acute Stroke, Second Edition*
Edited by: P. D. Lyden © Humana Press Inc., Totowa, NJ

helpful to first examine the known advantages and limitations of intravenous and IA delivery of thrombolytic agents. The basic rationale for IA thrombolysis is presented in Chapter 10. Here we discuss some of the limitations of IA therapy.

INTRAVENOUS RECOMBINANT TISSUE PLASMINOGEN ACTIVATOR FOR ACUTE ISCHEMIC STROKE: EFFICACY AND KNOWN LIMITATIONS

Intravenous recombinant tissue plasminogen activator (rt-PA) administered to appropriately selected patients within 3 h of ischemic stroke onset was shown to reduce morbidity compared to placebo in the National Institute of Neurological Disorders and Stroke (NINDS) rt-PA Stroke Trial (*see* Chapter 7) *(1)*. The time from stroke onset to initiation of thrombolytic therapy has been demonstrated to be the most critical predictor of effectiveness *(2,3)*. In the initial analysis of the NINDS rt-PA Stroke Trial, the odds ratio for a favorable outcome in rt-PA-treated patients compared to placebo did not differ between those enrolled from 0 to 90 min and 91 to 180 min from symptom onset. However, further analysis was subsequently performed to test whether there was a time to treatment effect on 24-h improvement, 3-mo favorable outcome, or the rate of intracerebral hemorrhage (ICH) after adjusting for potential confounders that may have masked a relationship between time-to-treatment and rt-PA effectiveness (*see* Chapter 8) *(2)*. When differences in patient baseline characteristics were considered, patients treated with rt-PA within 0–90 min from stroke onset were more likely to show improvement at 24 h and at 3 mo (compared to placebo-treated patients) than patients who were treated with rt-PA at 90–180 min. No relationship between time-to-treatment and occurrence of ICH was seen, possibly owing to low power *(2)*. A recent pooled analysis of randomized rt-PA trials (NINDS rt-PA Stroke Trial parts I and II, European Cooperative Acute Stroke Study [ECASS] I, ECASS II, Alteplase ThromboLysis for Acute Noninterventional Therapy in Ischemic Stroke parts A and B) enrolling patients within 6 h of stroke onset confirmed that earlier treatment was associated with a higher odds of a favorable recovery, with the greatest benefit noted in patients in whom treatment was begun within 90 min *(3)*. Thus, time to initiation of thrombolytic therapy and restoration of blood flow is critical for clinical benefit, even within the first 3 h from onset.

Intravenous rt-PA has known limitations. For example, intravenous rt-PA administered within 8 h of symptom onset reopens only 30–40% of occluded major intracranial trunk arteries within 1–2 h of treatment as determined by cerebral angiography *(4–6)*. Although patients in the NINDS rt-PA Stroke Trial with a high National Institute of Health Stroke Scale (NIHSS) score (severe stroke) did better when treated with intravenous rt-PA than with placebo, the overall prognosis of these patients was poor *(1,7)*. Only 21% of patients with an

NIHSS score of 10 or more at the start of intravenous rt-PA treatment had an NIHSS score of 0 to 1 at 3 mo. In addition, patients with a high NIHSS score are highly likely to have an occlusion of a major intracranial and/or major extracranial artery *(2)*.

Given that the large majority of patients with a high NIHSS score have an occlusion of a major extracranial or intracranial trunk artery and that intravenous rt-PA alone often fails to open major arterial occlusions despite rapid administration, the overall poor response in patients with high NIHSS scores in the NINDS rt-PA Stroke Trial is not surprising.

INTRA-ARTERIAL THROMBOLYTIC THERAPY: POTENTIAL ADVANTAGES AND KNOWN LIMITATIONS

Intra-arterial therapy by a selective microcatheter has the advantage of delivering a thrombolytic agent or device directly at the site of an occluded intracranial artery (*see* Chapter 10). This is true even if a more proximal artery, such as the internal carotid artery (ICA), is occluded.

Administration of rt-PA or urokinase (UK) via microcatheter at the site of thrombus has been reported to fully or partially recanalize occluded arteries in 50–82% of patients *(9–13)*. The rate of symptomatic ICH in these uncontrolled series of IA thrombolytic therapy has been relatively low (an average rate of approx 10%). Heparin administration has generally been included in IA thrombolytic protocols.

The only published randomized studies of IA thrombolytic therapy are the Pro-Urokinase in Acute Cerebral Thromboembolism (PROACT) I and II studies, which compared pro-urokinase (pro-UK) plus intravenous heparin to IA placebo plus intravenous heparin *(9,10)*. PROACT I demonstrated a recanalization rate of 58% after 2 h of infusion of pro- UK plus heparin in 26 patients compared to 14% after an infusion of a placebo plus heparin in 14 patients *(10)*. The rate of symptomatic hemorrhage in a subgroup treated with 6 mg of pro-UK plus a 100 U/kg bolus of heparin followed by 1000 U of heparin/h for 4 h was 27%. For this reason, the heparin dose was decreased to a 2000 U bolus followed by a 500 U/h infusion for 4 h. The hemorrhage rate in the patients treated with 6 mg of pro-UK and "low-dose" heparin was 7%. Although the recanalization rate in the pro-UK-treated group was significantly greater than in placebo-treated patients, neurological outcome was not significantly different between pro-UK and placebo-treated patients.

The PROACT II Study was published in December 1999 *(9)*. Of 180 patients with angiographically proven M1 or M2 occlusions enrolled within 6 h of symptom onset, 121 patients were randomized to receive 9 mg of pro-UKplus heparin (low-dose) and 59 patients were randomized to receive placebo plus low-dose heparin. Of patients in the pro-UK group, 40% had a modified Rankin score (mRS) of 0–2 at 3 mo compared to 25% of control patients ($p = 0.04$, stratified by NIHSS score at baseline). Whereas Thrombolysis in Myocardial Infarction (TIMI) grade 3 flow (complete opening of the arterial occlusion) was achieved in only 19% of patients who received pro-UK after 2 h of therapy (as compared to 2% of placebo patients), TIMI 2 or 3 flow (complete or partial reopening) was achieved in 66% of patients who received pro-UK. The rate of symptomatic ICH in the pro-UK group was 10%. Even though the absolute difference between groups was moderate in effect, the Food and Drug Administration (FDA) requested an additional study because of the borderline statistical significance of the overall result. In addition, the small number of control patients in the study ($n = 59$, 2 to 1 randomization design) makes it difficult to adjust for differences in baseline variables between the two groups that may affect interpretation of the study results.

Although IA administration of thrombolytic agents appears to produce higher rates of recanalization than intravenous rt-PA, and the rate of ICH is similar to that seen in the NINDS rt-PA Stroke Trial, the IA approach also has limitations. The most important limitation of IA therapy has been the time from symptom onset to initiation of therapy and the time to recanalization once therapy has begun. For example, in the PROACT II study, the median time from symptom onset to initiation of IA treatment was 5.3 h and only one patient had pro-UK started within 3 h *(9)*. In addition, the median time for recanalization in IA studies with reported data is approx 2 h from start of IA therapy. Two published reports of IA thrombolytic therapy from Japan and Switzerland indicate that treatment begun within 3–4 h of symptom onset is associated with higher rates of recanalization and better outcome *(11,13)*.

In summary, intravenous rt-PA administered within 3 h of symptom onset is the only FDA-approved treatment for acute ischemic stroke. The major limitation of this approach is that intravenous rt-PA opens a minority of large intracranial arterial occlusions in a time frame that is likely to improve patient outcome. IA therapy is associated with higher rates of arterial recanalization, but causes a longer delay from symptom onset to treatment. The PROACT II study suggests that IA thrombolytic therapy at longer time windows may be effective in highly selected groups of patients with acute ischemic stroke. Whatever method of arterial recanalization is utilized, the time from symptom onset to recanalization appears to be the key determinant of effectiveness.

COMBINED INTRAVENOUS/INTRA-ARTERIAL RECOMBINANT TISSUE PLASMINOGEN ACTIVATOR: RATIONALE AND PRIOR EXPERIENCE

Combined intravenous and IA delivery of thrombolytic drug has several potential advantages. First, a combined approach allows intravenous thrombolytic therapy as quickly as possible in order to minimize the time from stroke onset to recanalization. The addition of IA therapy following intravenous rt-PA adds the advantage of demonstrating whether or not a clot remains and whether more thrombolytic drug or other methods to recanalize the occluded artery are needed. A potential risk of a combined approach is the need to perform a femoral artery puncture after the recent administration of intravenous rt-PA.

Emergency Management of Stroke Trial

From December 1994 to December 1995, and prior to regulatory approval of intravenous rt-PA for acute ischemic stroke, several investigators from the NINDS rt-PA Stroke Trial initiated a study which attempted to combine the advantages of intravenous and IA rt-PA *(8)*. The Emergency Management of Stroke (EMS) Trial, a randomized controlled study, was designed to test feasibility and provide preliminary data regarding the relative benefits and risks of combined intravenous rt-PA (0.6 mg/kg over 30 min) and IA rt-PA therapy (up to 20 mg delivered over 2 h at the clot), compared to intravenous placebo plus IA rt-PA therapy. Intravenous treatment in the EMS Trial was to be started within 3 h of stroke onset. The inclusion/exclusion criteria for the EMS Pilot Trial were identical to that of the NINDS rt-PA Stroke Trial except that patients with an NIHSS score of 4 or less were excluded, higher baseline systolic blood pressure was allowed (190 systolic as compared to 185 systolic in the NINDS trial), and patients older than 85 yr were excluded (the NINDS trial had no upper age limit). The only computed tomography (CT) exclusion for either trial was the presence of hemorrhage on the baseline CT.

The total number of patients in the EMS study was small (N = 35; combined intravenous/IA rt-PA group n = 17; intravenous placebo plus IA rt-PA group n =18). The pilot study was not powered to examine efficacy differences between the two treatment groups, but rather to demonstrate feasibility and safety of the combined strategy. The combined intravenous/IA rt-PA group had a higher median NIHSS score (16, interquartile range 9–21) than the IA rt-PA-only group (11, interquartile range 9–16). This imbalance in NIHSS scores is important for the interpretation of angiographic results in the EMS Study because the baseline NIHSS score correlated extremely well with the presence or absence of a clot at angiography. For example, 78% of patients with an NIHSS score of at least 10 had a demonstrable IA clot at angiography.

Perhaps because of the imbalance in baseline NIHSS scores between treatment groups, recanalization in the combined intravenous/IA rt-PA treatment group was not significantly greater than recanalization in the IA-only group. For those patients whose angiogram demonstrated a remaining arterial thrombus, recanalization was significantly greater in the combined intravenous/IA group than in the IA-only group (Table 1). The proportion of improved outcomes (prospectively defined as a 7-point improvement of the NIHSS score at 7–10 d) did not differ between groups (both groups = 24%).

Table 1
Post-Treatment Arterial Patency in Emergency Management of Stroke Trial
(Results in Those With Clot on Initial Angiogram)

	Intravenous/Intra-arterial[a] *n = 11 (with clot)*		*Placebo* *n = 10 (with clot)*	
TIMI Score	*n (%)*	*(artery)*	*n (%)*	*(artery)*
0	0 (0%)		2 (20%)	M_2, M_1
1	2 (18%)	2-ICA	3 (30%)	M_1, ICA, M_1+ICA
2	3 (27%)	2-M_1, M_2	4 (40%)	2-M_2,2-M_1, Basilar
3	6 (54%)	3-M_1, 2-M_2, 1-M_1	1 (10%)	ICA

[a] Intravenous/intra-arterial group has better arterial patency by regression analysis at $p = 0.03$ using a central interpretation of the angiograms.

M_1, first part of middle cerebral artery; M_2, second part of middle cerebral artery; ICA, internal carotid artery.

The prospectively determined primary safety measure for the EMS Trial was life-threatening bleeding during the first 24 h after therapy. There were no symptomatic or asymptomatic intracerebral hematomas in the 35 EMS patients. One symptomatic hemorrhagic infarction occurred during the first 24 h among 18 patients treated with placebo/IA rt-PA therapy. One confused patient in the combined intravenous/IA treatment group removed her femoral sheath postprocedure and suffered a retroperitoneal hemorrhage with resulting hypotension requiring blood transfusion. She subsequently developed myocardial ischemia and eventually died. Finally, one patient in the combined group had an unrecognized aortic dissection and developed a hemopericardium following intravenous rt-PA but prior to IA therapy.

Two symptomatic hemorrhagic infarctions occurred in the combined intravenous/IA group 24–72 h after treatment. Asymptomatic hemorrhagic infarction during the first 72 h was also noted more frequently in the intravenous/IA group ($n = 5$) than in the IA-only group ($n = 1$). Mean rt-PA doses administered were 56 mg ± 11 mg in the intravenous/IA group and 11 mg ± 10 mg in the IA-only treatment group. Median time from symptom onset to initiation of intravenous therapy was 2.6 h. Delays in initiating angiography and achieving recanalization are presented in Table 2.

The results of combined intravenous/IA rt-PA in the EMS Trial for patients with an M1 or M2 occlusion were compared with the results of the PROACT II study. The number of patients is small but there was a trend toward better outcomes (Rankin of 0–2 57% EMS, 40% PROACT II, same median NIHSS score at baseline for EMS and PROACT II patients) and better rates of TIMI grade 3 flow (complete recanalization) in the patients treated with combined intravenous/IA rt-PA as shown in Table 3.

Table 2
Time Intervals—Emergency Management of Stroke Trial

	Median number of hours	
	Intravenous/intra-arterial	*Placebo/intra-arterial*
Time from stroke onset to intravenous treatment (n = 35)	2.6	2.7
Time from stroke onset to start of angiogram (n = 35)	3.3	3.0
Time from stroke onset to recanalization for those who had clot at angiogram	6.3	5.7

Table 3
EMS, IMS, and PROACT II Trials: Patients With M1 M2 Clot—TIMI Flow After Therapy

	TIMI grade 3 (%)	*TIMI grade 2 or 3 (%)*
PROACT II		
Placebo (n = 59)	2	18
PROACT II		
Pro-UK (n = 121)	19	66
EMS		
Intravenous/IA rt-PA (n = 9)	67	100
IA rt-PA alone (n = 6)	0	50
Total (n = 15)	40	80
IMS		
Intravenous/IA rt-PA (n =30)	13	67

EMS, Emergency Management of Stroke; IMS, Interventional Management of Stroke; TIMI, Thrombolysis in Myocardial Infarction; IA, intra-arterial; rt-PA, recombinant tissue plasminogen activator; pro-UK, pro-urokinase.

Interventional Management of Stroke Study

The Interventional Management of Stroke (IMS) Study was undertaken to test the feasibility and safety of a combined intravenous/IAapproach to recanalization in a larger group of ischemic stroke patients *(14)*. It was designed as a multicenter, open-label, single-arm study comparing eligible patients treated with an intravenous/IA rt-PA protocol to historical subjects of similar age and baseline NIHSS score from the NINDS rt-PA Stroke Trial. Entry criteria were similar to the NINDS trial except for exclusion of (1) patients older than 80 yr old, (2) patients with a baseline NIHSS of 9, and (3) patients with large regions

(33% middle cerebral artery territory) of hypodensity on baseline CT. Maximal allowable blood pressure was 190 systolic and 110 diastolic. Patients enrolled in the IMS Study were treated with low-dose intravenous rt-PA (0.6 mg/kg, 15% as a bolus over 1 min followed by the remainder over 30 min) and up to 22 mg of IA rt-PA if clot was identified at angiography. Intravenous and IA rt-PA was to begin within 3 and 5 h of stroke onset, respectively. A 2000 U bolus of heparin was administered before IA rt-PA therapy and a low-dose infusion (40 U/h) was continued until the catheter was removed. The primary safety endpoint of the trial was life-threatening bleeding within 36 h of rt-PA infusion (symptomatic intracerebral hematoma/hemorrhagic infarction or systemic bleeding requiring transfusion of at least 3 U of blood or major surgical intervention). Although the study was not powered for efficacy, the primary outcome endpoint was an mRS of 0–1 at 3 mo. Secondary outcome measures included rates of TIMI grade II or III flow at the completion of angiography, an mRS of 0–2 at 3 mo, and other 3-mo-endpoints from the NINDS rt-PA Stroke Trial. Additional secondary endpoints were also identified based on a prospective analysis of the most sensitive endpoints from the NINDS rt-PA Stroke Trial *(14,15)*.

Of 1477 subjects screened over 9 mo, 80 patients were enrolled. Only 1 patient was lost to follow-up. Median time from symptom onset to intravenous rt-PA administration was 140 min, whereas median time to start of IA rt-PA was 212 min, compared to a median 90 min for the intravenous rt-PA in the NINDS rt-PA trial *(1)*. Both mean and median NIHSS scores for IMS patients were 18.

Combined intravenous/IA therapy proved comparatively safe in the selected patients. Whereas the mortality rate and rate of symptomatic ICH were similar between IMS subjects and rt-PA-treated subjects in the NINDS rt-PA Stroke Trial, the rate of asymptomatic ICH during the first 36 h was higher in the IMS study (43% vs 6%). However, only 6 (7.5%) subjects had PH2 type hematomas that have been associated with neurological deterioration and poor outcome *(16)*. In addition, the overall rate of ICH in the IMS study was similar to that in the PROACT II study (54%) *(9)*. IMS subjects with occlusions of the ICA, with or without distal occlusions, were particularly likely to have hemorrhagic change (20 of 28 [71%]). By comparison, only 15 of the 36 (42%) subjects with occlusions in the MCA or vertebral artery system had hemorrhagic change. Symptomatic ICH was more common in IMS and NINDS rt-PA patients than NINDS placebo patients (IMS patients 6.3%, NINDS rt-PA patients 6.6%, NINDS placebo patients 1.0%, Table 4).

Outcome was better in IMS subjects than matched NINDS placebo-treated subjects, with 30 and 18% of respective patients achieving an mRS of 0–1 at 3 mo (odds ratio 2.26, 95% confidence interval 1.15–4.47). IMS subjects had similar 3-mo primary and secondary outcomes as rt-PA-treated NINDS patients, although odds ratios trended in favor of IMS subjects (Table 5).

Table 4
Safety Results: IMS and NINDS rt-PA Trial Cohorts (Ages 18–80 and Baseline NIHSS ≥10)

	IMS Study (n = 80)	*NINDS Placebo (n = 211)*	*p-Value*[a]	*NINDS rt-PA (n = 182)*	*p-Value*[b]
Mortality at 3 mo	13/80 (16%)	50/211 (24%)	0.17	39/182 (21%)	0.33
Symptomatic ICH ≤36 h	5/80 (6.3%)	2/211 (1.0%)	0.018	12/182 (6.6%)	0.91
PH2 ICH ≤36 h	6/80 (7.5%)	1/211 (0.5%)	0.002	6/182 (3.4%)	0.20
Asymptomatic ICH[c] ≤36 h	34/80 (43%)	12/211 (5.7%)	<0.0001	11/182 (6.0%)	<0.0001
Serious systemic bleeding events ≤36 h	3%	0.5%	0.18	1%	0.58

[a]*p*-value from c^2 test comparing IMS to NINDS-placebo.
[b]*p*-value from c^2test comparing IMS to NINDS-rtPA.
[c]Includes subjects categorized as hyperdense infarcts in the NINDS rt-PA Stroke Trial that are categorized as hemorrhagic infarction (HI) in IMS Study.
IMS, Interventional Management of Stroke; NINDS, National Institute of Neurological Disorders and Stroke; rt-PA, recombinant tissue plasminogen activator; NIHSS, National Institute of Health Stroke Scale; ICH, intracerebral hemorrhage.

For subjects receiving IA rt-PA in addition to intravenous rt-PA, rates of TIMI 3 and TIMI 2 or 3 recanalization were 11% (7 of 62) and 56% (35 of 62). Among these patients, achievement of TIMI 2 or 3 flow was associated with a better outcome (mRS 0–1 at 3 mo) than TIMI 0 or 1 flow ($p = 0.013$). Rates of recanalization for subjects with M1 or M2 clot without ICA occlusion are compared to the PROACT II and EMS trials in Table 3. Initiation of IA rt-PA within 3 h of stroke onset was associated with a trend toward better outcome compared to initiation after 3 hours ($p = 0.095$).

Two patients in the IMS study did not have an angiogram owing to breakdown of angiographic equipment (one) and symptomatic ICH from IV rt-PA prior to angiography (one). A third patient who had an MRA that showed no clot in the visualized arteries and concomitant resolution of his neurological deficit did not undergo angiography. At the time of baseline angiography, an additional 13 patients treated with intravenous rt-PA had no major clot in any major arterial trunk, with only stenoses of major arteries (nine patients) or distal sluggish or absent flow in M4 branches (four patients) (Table 6). It is likely that

Table 5
3-Mo Outcome: IMS and NINDS rt-PA Trial Cohorts
(Ages 18–80 and Baseline NIHSS ≥10)

	IMS Study (80)	*NINDS Placebo (211)*	*Odds Ratio[a] (95% CL)*	*NINDS rt-PA (182)*	*Odds Ratio[b] (95% CL)*
mRS (0–1) at 90 d	24/80 (30%)	38/211 (18%)	2.26 (1.15, 4.47)	59/182 (32%)	1.00 (0.51–1.96)
NIHSS score ≤1 at 90 d	22/80 (28%)	31/211 (15%)	2.51 (1.21, 5.18)	45/182 (25%)	1.45 (0.73, 2.90)
Barthel (95–100) at 90 d	37/80 (46%)	63/211 (30%)	2.17 (1.20, 3.91)	76/182 (42%)	1.39 0.76, 2.54)
Glasgow (91) at 90 d	27/80 (34%)	47/211 (22%)	1.91 (1.01, 3.60)	63/182 (35%)	1.12 (0.59, 2.14)
Global Test			2.36[c] (1.35, 4.14)		1.35[d] (0.78, 2.37)
mRS (0–2) at 90 d	34/80 (43%)	59/211 (28%)	2.18 (1.20, 3.99)	71/182 (39%)	1.28 (0.70, 2.33)
NIHSS score ≤2 at 90 d	25/80 (31%)	42/211 (20%)	2.11 (1.08, 4.13)	60/182 (33%)	1.08 (0.57, 2.06)
NIHSS score ≤2 at 24 h	11/80 (14%)	7/211 (3%)	5.39 (1.80, 16.19)	26/182 (14%)	1.77 (0.71, 4.39)

[a]From logistic regression model for favorable outcome adjusted by baseline NIHSS score, age, and time-to-treatment (continuous) comparing IMS to NINDS-placebo.

[b]From logistic regression model for favorable outcome adjusted by baseline NIHSS score, age, and time-to-treatment (continuous) comparing IMS to NINDS-rt-PA cohort.

[c]From global test adjusted for baseline NIHSS score, age, gender, and time-to-treatment (continuous) comparing IMS to NINDS-placebo.

[d]From global test adjusted for baseline NIHSS score, age, gender, and time-to-treatment (continuous) comparing IMS to NINDS-rt-PA cohort.

IMS, Interventional Management of Stroke; NINDS, National Institute of Neurological Disorders and Stroke; rt-PA, recombinant tissue plasminogen activator; NIHSS, National Institute of Health Stroke Scale; mRS, modified Rankin score.

some of these patients would have had major arterial occlusions at angiography had intravenous rt-PA not been administered prior to angiography. Thus, the reported overall recanalization rate of the combined approach in the IMS study is likely an underestimate.

The EMS and IMS studies suggest that combined intravenous/IA therapy is feasible and potentially superior to intravenous therapy alone, particularly for patients with large strokes. Figure 1 illustrates the logistics of intravenous/IA use

Table 6
Locations of Arterial Occlusive Lesions at Baseline Angiogram

	n	*Recanalization # TIMI 2–3, 3 (n = 64)*	*Rankin (%) (n = 79)* 0–1	0–2	*Death (%)*
ICA occlusion[a] + distal embolus	5	1,0	1 (20)	1 (20)	2 (40)
ICA stenosis[b] + distal embolus	15	8, 2 (Two perforations – No IA diagnosis)	3 (20)	3 (20)	3 (20)
C5,6,7 (T)	7	4,1	0	1 (14)	2 (28)
C5 + M2	1	0	0	0	0
M1	16	13,2	4 (25)	6 (38)	3 (19)
M2	12	6,2	4 (33)	9 (75)	1 (8)
M3,4	3	1,0	1(33)	1(33)	0
M1 + A1/A2	2	1,0	1 (50)	1 (50)	0
Vertebrobasilar	3	1,0	2 (66)	3 (100)	0
No AOL	3	No IA Rx	3 (100)	3 (100)	0
ICA stenosis [b]	3	No IA Rx	1 (33)	2 (66)	0
ICA stenosis <20%	1	No IA Rx	1 (100)	1(100)	0
MCA distal/stenosis	4	No IA Rx	1 (25)	1(25)	0
VB stenosis	2	No IA Rx	1 (50)	1 (50)	1 (50)
MRA Only	1	No IA Rx	1 (100)	1 (100)	0
No angiogram	2	No IA Rx	0	0	1 (50)
Total	80	35, 7	24 (30%)	34 (43%)	13 (16%)

[a]Two ICA dissections.
[b]ICA stenosis ≥70%.
TIMI, Thrombolysis in Myocardial Infarction; ICA, internal carotid artery; IA, intra-arterial; AOL, arterial occlusive lesion; MCA, middle cerebral artery; VB, vertebrobasilar; MRA, magnetic resonance angiogram; Rx, treatment.

in the case a patient treated at the University of Cincinnati with combined therapy. Intravenous rt-PA was begun within 95 min of onset at a local community hospital by a stroke-team physician. The patient was then transferred to University Hospital where a cerebral angiogram was performed immediately. At angiography (and after 30 mg of intravenous rt-PA) she had an occlusion of the left ICA terminus and MCA (Fig. 1A). An additional 12 mg of rt-PA at the site of the clot plus mechanical manipulation via the guidewire and catheter completely restored blood flow in the occluded arteries at 3 h and 20 min from the onset of symptoms (Fig. 1B). The patient's baseline NIHSS score was 24. After res-

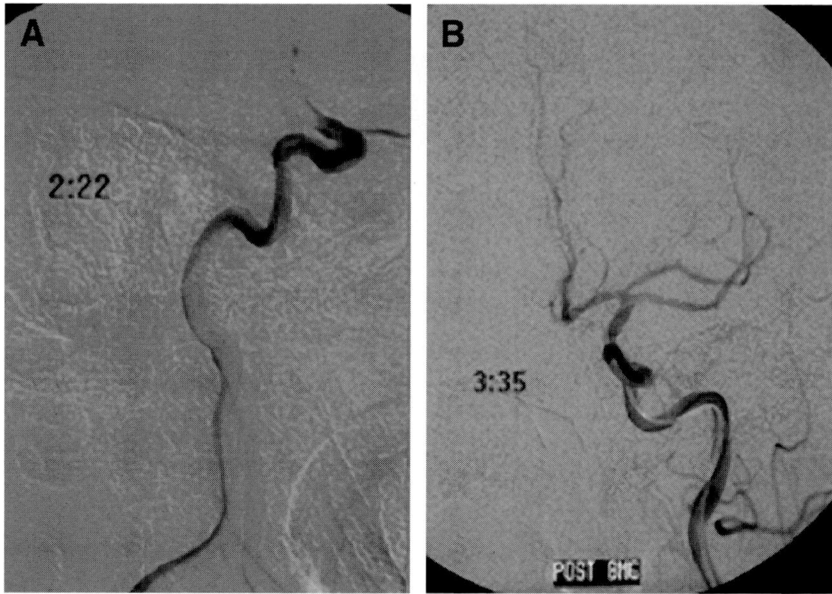

Fig. 1. (A) Intraluminal clot in ICA terminus 60 min after iv t-PA began and 2 h and 20 min after onset of stroke symptoms. **(B)** Complete recanalization after additional IA t-PA 3 h and 30 min after onset of stroke symptoms.

toration of blood flow she immediately improved (turning to a physician and asking "What happened?") and at 24 h after stroke onset had an NIHSS score of 1 with a normal CT scan (Fig. 2).

The following data illustrate that a combined approach can help to minimize the time to treatment and recanalization, can be used to help titrate the amount of thrombolytic drug delivered, and can be associated with excellent outcome.

- 12:00 PM: Patient witnessed to have a sudden onset of aphasia and right-sided weakness.
- 12:08 PM: 911 called.
- 12:15 PM: Ambulance at patient's home.
- 12:28 PM: Patient arrives at the emergency department (ED) of a community hospital.
- 12:40 PM: Stroke Pager called, CT scan ordered.
- 12:48 PM: CT scan completed: hyperdense left MCA, no hemorrhage.
- 13:00 PM: Stroke-team physician arrives. NIHSS score 24.
- 13:18 PM: Intravenous rt-PA bolus given. Infusion begun.
- 13:33 PM: Leaves outside emergency room in ambulance for University of Cincinnati.

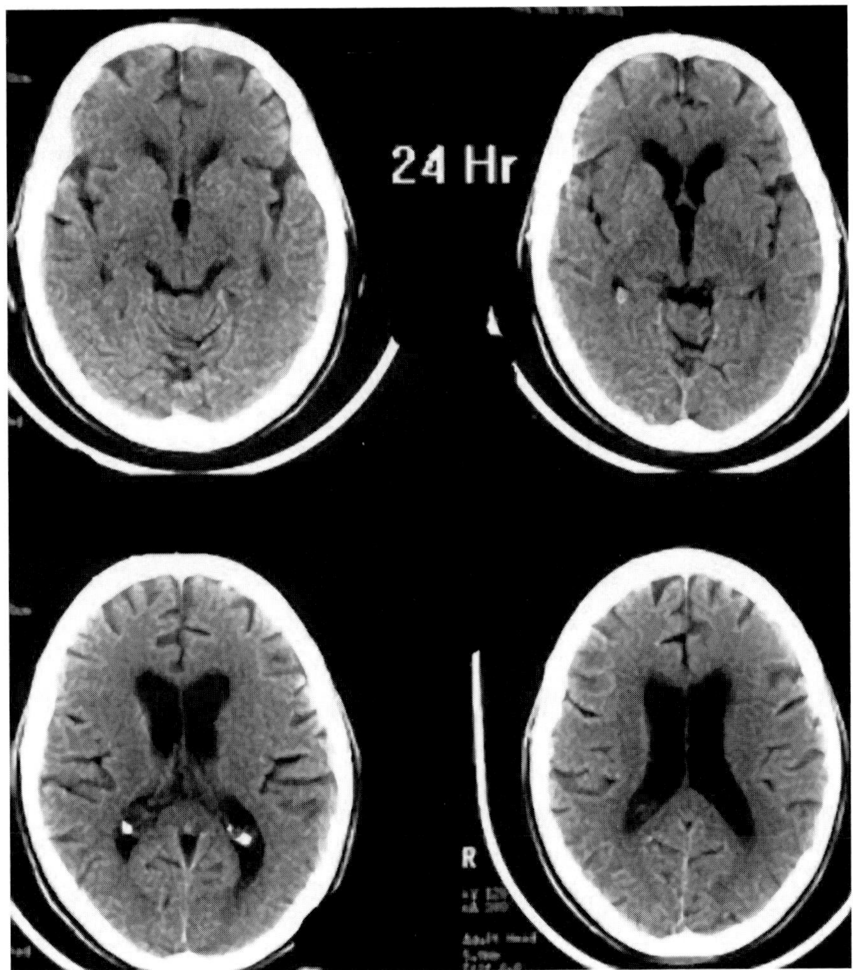

Fig. 2. 24-h CT of patient treated with combined iv/IA t-PA.

- 13:49 PM: Arrives at University of Cincinnati.
- 14:03 PM: Angiography begun.
- 14:20 PM: At clot. ICA terminus clot with extension into MCA. Patient receives 4 mg rt-PA bolus within clot. Infusion at 10 mg/h of rt-PA begun IA.
- 15:15 PM: Trickle of flow seen in the MCA. NIHSS score 23.
- 15:20 PM: Complete opening of the ICA and MCA. NIHSS score 7.
- 15:50 PM: Arrives in ICU. NIHSS score 3.
- 12:00 PM: 24-h NIHSS score 1.
- Discharged home 6 d later with NIHSS score 0.

COMBINED INTRAVENOUS/INTRA-ARTERIAL APPROACH: CARDIOLOGY EXPERIENCE

Many investigators in cardiology have already embraced the concept of a combined intravenous/IA approach in patients with acute myocardial infarction. This combined intravenous/IA approach is illustrated by the Plasminogen Activator-Angioplasty Compatibility Trial (PACT) *(17)*. This double-blind, randomized trial addressed: angiographic patency following lower dose rt-PA (50 mg) or placebo, and the need for rescue angioplasty. Time-to-treatment was 2.7 h in the 606 randomized patients. TIMI-3 flow (full perfusion) at the first angiogram (median 50 min after treatment) was achieved in 33% of the low-dose rt-PA patients compared to 15% of the placebo patients. There were no clinically significant differences in safety endpoints including groin hematoma (a peripheral bleeding complication rate of 8% in both groups). These patency results for lower dose rt-PA in the PACT study are almost identical to the 60 min patency results reported in the Reteplase vs Alteplase in Acute Myocardial Infarction (RAPID) trial for full-dose rt-PA *(18)*. In the RAPID trial, 100 mg of alteplase was administered over 3 h to patients with acute myocardial infarction as part of a randomized comparison study of rt-PA with reteplase. TIMI-3 patency was achieved in 33% of the 101 patients randomized to rt-PA. In summary, twice as many patients treated with intravenous t-PA compared to placebo-treated patients had restored blood flow by the time of angiography, obviating the need for angioplasty.

The results support the concept of a combined intravenous/IA approach as opposed to an IA-alone approach and provide evidence for comparable clot-lysis capability of lower dose intravenous rt-PA as compared to full-dose intravenous rt-PA. These studies also support data in ischemic stroke patients that intravenous rt-PA alone recanalizes only one-third of occluded intracranial arteries.

WHICH IS SUPERIOR: COMBINED INTRAVENOUS/INTRA-ARTERIAL THERAPY OR THE CURRENTLY APPROVED DOSE OF INTRAVENOUS RECOMBINANT TISSUE PLASMINOGEN ACTIVATOR?

There are no randomized trials that compare combined intravenous/IA rt-PA to the currently approved dose of intravenous rt-PA or placebo. Thus, the efficacy of a lower dose of intravenous rt-PA followed by IA rt-PA has yet to be demonstrated. Whether the higher rates of recanalization demonstrated in the EMS and IMS studies are associated with improved efficacy compared to full-dose intravenous rt-PA can only be answered by a randomized study. The patient selection for such a trial will be critical. It is likely that patients with low NIHSS scores and a smaller area of affected brain would benefit most with intravenous rt-PA because they are much less likely to have occlusions of major intracranial arteries. The IMS study limited intravenous/IA treatment to patients with a NIHSS score of at least10 to increase the likelihood of selecting patients with a major IA occlusion. The IMS study also addressed logistical issues that must be surmounted, such as more rapid initiation of intravenous and IA rt-PA.

At best, the combined intravenous/IA approach may offer a modest improvement over the currently approved dose of intravenous rt-PA. Other innovative means of arterial recanalization will assume greater importance in the coming years. These include mechanical devices to remove or fragment clots via the catheter *(19)* and the addition of other agents such as platelet glycoprotein IIb/IIIa receptor antagonists *(1,20–22)* or substrates for rt-PA such as plasminogen *(23)*. Whatever combination of agents or methods is tested, the primary goal will be shortening the time from symptom onset to recanalization of the occluded artery. We will likely follow the steps of cardiologists who have used a multipronged approach that reopens occluded coronary arteries with drugs and mechanical devices, and that depends on the availability of technology and expertise at a given hospital.

REFERENCES

1. NINDS rt-PA Stroke Study Group. Tissue plasminogen activator for acute ischemic stroke. *NEJM* 1995;333:1581–1587.
2. Marler JR, Tilley B, Lu M, et al. Earlier treatment associated with better outcome: The NINDS rt-PA Stroke Study. *Neurology* 2000;55:1649–1655.
3. ATLANTIS, ECASS, and NINDS rt-PA Study Group Investigators. Association of outcome with early stroke treatment: pooled analysis of the ATLANTIS, ECASS, and NINDS stroke trials. *Lancet* 2004;363:768–774.
4. Wolpert S, Bruckmann H, Greenlee R, Wechsler L, Pessin M, del Zoppo G, and the rt-PA Acute Stroke Study Group. Neuroradiologic evaluation of patients with acute stroke treated with recombinant tissue plasminogen activator. *AJNR* 1993;14:3–13.
5. Yamaguchi T, Hayakawa T, Kiuchi H, for the Japanese Thrombolysis Study Group. Intravenous tissue plasminogen activator ameliorates the outcome of hyperacute embolic stroke. *Cerebrovascular Dis* 1993;3:269–272.
6. Mori E, Yoneda Y, Tabuchi M, et al. Intravenous recombinant tissue plasminogen activator in acute carotid artery territory stroke. *Neurology* 1992;42:976–982.
7. NINDS t-PA Stroke Study Group. Generalized efficacy of t-PA for acute stroke: Subgroup analysis of the NINDS t-PA Stroke Trial. *Stroke* 1997;28:2119–2125.
8. Lewandowski CA, Frankel M, Tomsick TA, et al. Combined intravenous and intra-arterial rt-PA versus intra-arterial therapy of acute ischemic stroke: Emergency Management of Stroke (EMS) Bridging Trial. *Stroke* 1999;30:2598–2605.
9. Furlan A, Higashida R, Wechsler L, et al. Intra-arterial prourokinase for acute ischemic stroke. The PROACT II Study: A randomized controlled trial. Prolyse in acute cerebral thromboembolism. *JAMA* 1999;282:2003–2011.
10. del Zoppo G, Higashida R, Furlan A, Pessin M, Rowley H, Gent M, and the PROACT Investigators. PROACT: A phase II randomized trial of recombinant pro-urokinase by direct arterial delivery in acute middle cerebral artery stroke. *Stroke* 1998;29:4–11.
11. Gonner F, Remonda L, Mattle H, et al. Local intra-arterial thrombolysis in acute ischemic stroke. *Stroke* 1998;29:1894–1900.

12. Zeumer H, Freitz HJ, Zanella F, Thie A, Arning C. Local intra-arterial fibrinolytic therapy in patients with stroke: Urokinase versus recombinant tissue plasminogen activator (rt-PA). *Neuroradiology* 1993;35:159–162.
13. Endo S, Kuwayama N, Hirashima Y, Akai T, Nishijima M, Takaku A. Results of urgent thrombolysis in patients with major stroke and atherothrombotic occlusion of the cervical internal carotid artery. *Am J Neuroradiol.*1998;19:1169–1175.
14. IMS Study Investigators. Combined intravenous and intra-arterial recanalization for acute ischemic stroke: The Interventional Management of Stroke (IMS) Study. *Stroke* 2004; 35:904–912.
15. Broderick JP, Lu M, Kothari R, et al. Finding the most powerful measures of the effectiveness of tissue plasminogen activator in the NINDS t-PA Stroke Trial. *Stroke* 2000;31:2335–2341.
16. Berger C, Fiorelli M, Steiner T, et al. Hemorrhagic transformation of ischemic brain tissue: Asymptomatic or symptomatic? *Stroke* 2001;32:1330–1335.
17. Ross AM, Coyne KS, Reiner JS, et al. A randomized trial comparing primary angioplasty with a strategy of short-acting thrombolysis and immediate planned rescue angioplasty in acute myocardial infarction: The PACT Trial. *J Am Coll Cardiol* 1999;34:1963–1965.
18. Smalling RW, Bode C, Kalbfleisch J, et al, and the RAPID Investigators. More rapid, complete, and stable coronary thrombolysis with bolus administration of reteplase compared with alteplase infusion in acute myocardial infarction. *Circulation* 1995;91:2725–2732.
19. Leary MC, Saver JL, Gobin YP, et al. Beyond tissue plasminogen activator: Mechanical intervention in acute stroke. *Ann Emerg Med* 2003;41:838–846.
20. Wallace RC, Furlan AJ, Molterno DJ, Stevens GH, Masaryk TJ, Perl JN. Basilar artery rethrombosis: Successful treatment with platelet glycoprotein IIb/IIIa receptor inhibitor. *Am J Neuroradiol* 1998;18:125–160.
21. EPILOG Investigators. Effect of the platelet glycoprotein IIb/IIIa receptor inhibitor abciximab with lower heparin doses in ischemic complications of percutaneous coronary revascularization. *NEJM* 1997;336:1689–1696.
22. Straub S, Junghans U, Jovanovic V, Wittsack HJ, Seitz RJ, Siebler M. Systemic thrombolysis with recombinant tissue plasminogen activator and tirofiban in acute middle cerebral artery occlusion. *Stroke* 2004;35:705–709.
23. Freitag HJ, Becker V, Thie A, et al. Lys-plasminogen as an adjunct to local intra-arterial fibrinolysis for carotid territory stroke. *Neuroradiology* 1996;38:181–185.

III

Using Thrombolysis for Acute Stroke

12 Thrombolysis in Vertebrobasilar Occlusive Disease

Louis R. Caplan, MD

Contents

INTRODUCTION

Most experience with thrombolysis involves patients with cerebral hemisphere ischemia related to thromboembolic disease within the anterior (carotid arterial) territory (*see* Chapters 2 and 7). Although less experience has been gained in patients with posterior circulation (vertebrobasilar [VB] arterial) thromboembolism, most such data has concerned patients whose arterial lesions were documented before and after thrombolysis.

INTRA-ARTERIAL THROMBOLYSIS

The first published study of intra-arterial (IA) treatment of patients with VB territory thromboembolism was from investigators in Aachen,Germany *(1)*. Hacke and colleagues treated 65 patients with recent occlusions of the intracranial vertebral arteries (ICVAs) or basilar artery (BA). Two-thirds were treated within 24 h. One group of 43 patients was given IA thrombolytics (either urokinase [UK]-plasminogen activator or streptokinase). Another 22 patients were treated with anti-thrombotics. Among those given thrombolytics, survival occurred only in those that recanalized after treatment. None of the patients treated with

From: *Current Clinical Neurology: Thrombolytic Therapy for Acute Stroke, Second Edition*
Edited by: P. D. Lyden © Humana Press Inc., Totowa, NJ

Table 1
Intra-Arterial Thrombolysis Outcomes

	Antithrombotic diagnosis	*Thrombolytic therapy-recanalyzed*	*Thrombolytic therapy (not recanalized)*
n	22	19	24
Survived	3	13	0
Favorable	3	10	0

Adapted from ref. *1*.

thrombolytics that did not recanalize survived. Three of the patients treated with anti-thombotics survived, all in favorable condition *(1)*. Table 1 summarizes the results of this study and the arterial lesions are shown in Fig. 1.

Table 2 shows the results of other relatively large studies ($N \geq 9$) of IA thrombolysis in patients in whom angiography confirmed intracranial posterior circulation occlusion before IA thrombolysis *(1–8)*. The location of the arterial occlusions in those series that contained this detailed data *(1–5,7)* are shown in Fig. 1.

In most studies, thrombolytic drugs were given more than 8 h after stroke onset. Despite this late treatment, 56% of arteries recanalized. The outcomes were rather poor, with only about one-quarter of patients judged as "good" after treatment. These studies did yield hope that VB intracranial occlusions could be opened even after the first 6–8 h in some patients, even those with severe neurological deficits. Time to treat, on average, was longer in patients who survived than in those who succumbed.

Brandt et al. analyzed the variables among their 51 patients to determine what factors predicted good outcome *(3)*. A summary of their data is tabulated in Table 3. Embolic occlusions that were mostly proximal in the BA and were short in patients who had developed good collaterals were predictors of good outcome and recanalization. Patients who were comatose or tetraplegic, as well as patients with leukoariosis (perhaps because small artery disease limited available collaterals), tended to have poor outcomes *(3)*.

A variety of different drugs at different doses had been used in the studies listed in Table 2. Eckert and colleagues analyzed the data from their 83 posterior circulation IA thrombolytic cases to compare the results among the various regimes used (*see* Table 4) *(8)*. More patients recanalized using tissue plasminogen activator (t-PA) than with UK although the outcomes were not substantially different. A t-PA dose of 30–80 mg did not produce better outcomes or more recanalization than a dose of 10–20 mg but did result in more brain hemorrhages. Giving recombinant tissue plasminogen activator (rt-PA) with plasminogen led to better recanalization, better outcomes, and no higher frequency of

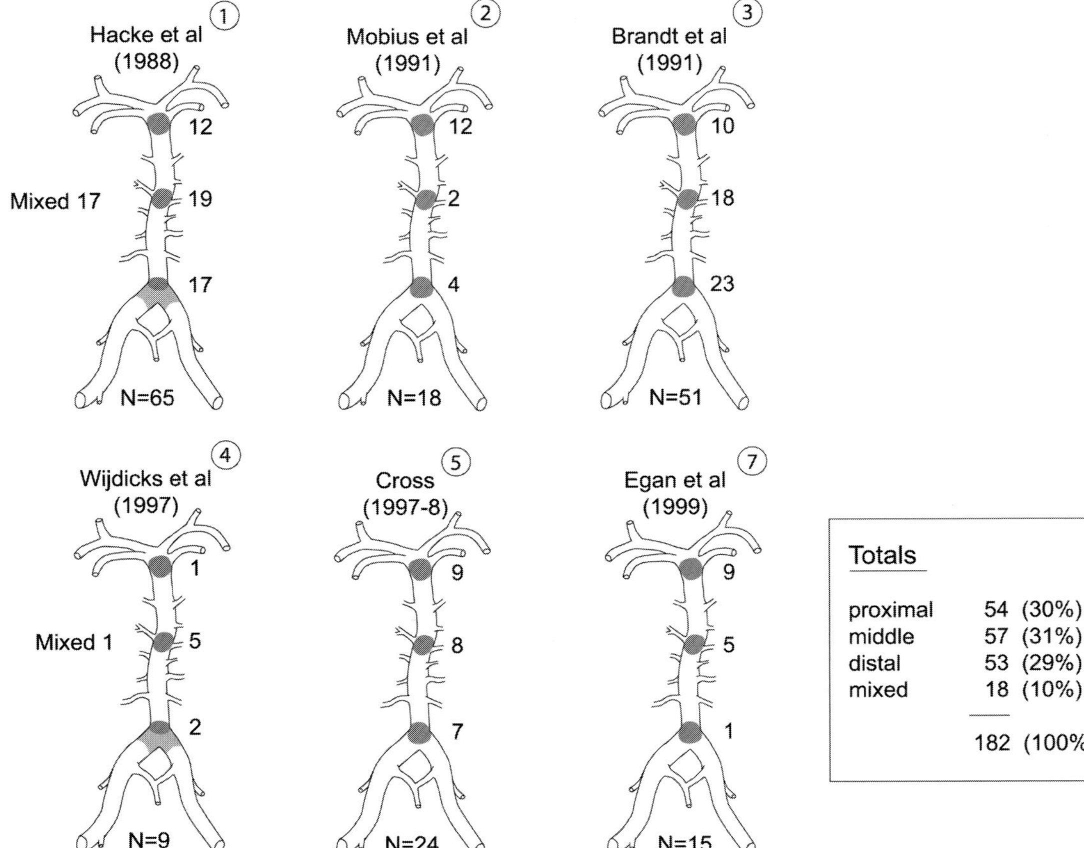

Fig. 1. Arterial occlusive lesions found in reports of intra-arterial thrombolysis in patients with basilar artery occlusive disease.

Table 2
Intra-Arterial Thrombolysis—Basilar Artery Occlusions

Study (yr)	*n*	*Time to treat (h)*	*Recanalize*	*Outcome* good	*Outcome* bad	*Outcome* dead
Hacke (1988) *(1)*	43	29 <24h	13 (30%)	10	3	30
Mobius (1991) *(2)*	18	Not stated	14 (78%)	6	6	4
Brandt (1996) *(3)*	51	8.8	26 (51%)	10	6	35
Wijdicks (1997) *(4)*	9	6.1 (2–13)	8 (89%)	5	2	2
Cross (1997) *(5)*	24	20.5 (1–82)	13 (65%)	6	3	15
Mitchell (1997) *(6)*	16	15 (5–31)	13 (82%)	9	2	5
Egan (1999) *(7)*	15	12.3 (4–48)	12 (80%)	4	6	5
Eckert (2002) *(8)*	83	8 (3–18)	54 (60%)	19	14	50
Totals	259		153 (56%)	27%	16%	57%

Table 3
Variables and Outcomes in the Series of Brandt et al. *(3)*

Variable	*Survived (n = 16)*	*Dead (n = 35)*
Age*	44.4 yr	59.6 yr
Rapid course	3 (19%)	16 (46%)
Tetraplegia*	1 (6%)	15 (43%)
Coma	6 (38%)	20 (58%)
Leukoariosis*	0	9 (26%)
Mechanism*		
thrombosis	1 (6%)	15 (43%)
embolism	15 (94%)	20 (58%)
Occlusion length*		
short	16 (100%)	19 (55%)
long	0	16 (46%)
Occlusion site*		
caudal	3 (19%)	20 (58%)
Middle	8 (50%)	10 (29%)
distal	5 (31%)	5 (14%)
Collaterals*		
good	14 (88%)	18 (51%)
poor	2 (12%)	17 (49%)
Recanalize*		
yes	14 (88%)	12 (34%)
no	2 (12%)	23 (66%)
Time to treat (min)	597 ± 359	496 ± 384

Table 4
Thrombolytic Drug Comparisons in the Eckert et al. Study *(8)*

Drug	*n = 83*	*Recanalize*	*Outcome*			*Hemorrhage*
			Good	*Bad*	*Died*	
Urokinase						
750,000–1.5 million	23	39%	17%	26%	57%	4%
rt-PA 10—20 mg	17	71%	18%	6%	76%	6%
rt-PA 30–80 mg	24	67%	17%	20%	63%	17%
rt-PA + plasminogen	19	89%	42%	11%	47%	5%

rt-PA, recombinant tissue plasminogen activator.

hemorrhages *(8)*. In this study, 8 of the 83 patients were first given IA thrombolysis but if recanalization was incomplete and the BA showed significant residual stenosis, angioplasty was performed successfully in all 8 patients, 4 of whom survived with "favorable" outcomes. The outcomes in these patients who had angioplasty was better than in comparable patients who did not reperfuse and did not have angioplasty *(8)*.

Cross and his Mayo Clinic colleagues commented on the relationship of time to treat with outcomes among their 24 thrombolysed patients *(5)*. Treatment of patients with BA occlusions was often effective many hours after symptom onset. Good outcome did not correlate with time to treat. Early treatment did not guarantee good outcome. None of the seven patients treated within 10 h had a good outcome. All patients with good outcomes had symptom durations of more than10 h (4 of 13) *(5)*. Patients treated at 36 and 82 h had good outcomes (modified Rankin score [mRS] = 1) and patients treated at 72 and 79 h had fair outcomes (mRS = 2).

Outcomes in the single study of IA thrombolysis in patients with bilateral vertebral artery disease were very poor *(9)*. Two of the patients had bilateral occlusions in the neck, whereas nine had bilateral ICVA occlusions. At the time of treatment with UK (average 22.5 h), three of the patients were comatose and tetraplegic and eight were alert, four with hemiparesis. Only one patient was considered to have an embolic occlusion, the remainder had *in situ* thrombosis. Eight patients recanalized but two of these rethrombosed. Only two of the patients survived; the other nine died. Two patients had bleeding—one subdural and one both intracerebral and intraventricular—and both died *(9)*.

INTRAVENOUS THROMBOLYSIS

There have been three reports of intravenous thrombolysis in patients with VB disease *(10–12)*. von Kummer et al. reported the only study in which angiography was performed before and after intravenous thrombolysis *(10)*. They treated five patients, four with BA and one with bilateral ICVA occlusions, with intravenous rt-PA within 6 h of symptom onset *(10)*. Minor partial reperfusion developed in two patients at 6 h and complete reperfusion in one patient by transcranial Doppler (TCD) at 24 h. Three patients died and one remained "locked-in."

In the other two studies, angiography was not performed. Grond et al. treated 12 patients who had "typical progressive brainstem symptoms" with intravenous t-PA within 3 h *(11)*. At the time of treatment, 2 patients were comatose and tetraplegic and 3 others had impaired alertness with tetraparesis in 2; all other patients had cranial nerve and/or motor signs. Five patients had BA stenosis determined by magnetic resonance angiography (MRA) and/or TCD, one shown by TCD before treatment. Stroke mechanisms were atherothrombotic in 6, embolic in 2, and vertebral artery dissection in 1. Of the 12 patients, 10 had favorable outcomes: 7 excellent, 3 good, 1 poor, and 1 dead *(11)*.

Montavont and colleagues in Lyon treated 18 patients with VB disease with t-PA within 7 h *(12)*. Computed tomography preceded treatment but MRA was often done after treatment. Of the 18 MRAs, 12 showed eight ICVA or BA occlusions and 3 posterior cerebral artery occlusions. Three months after treatment, 5 of the 8 patients with ICVA/BA occlusions had good outcomes and 10 of the 18 patients were independent; 2 had died and 6 were in poor condition.

CONCLUSIONS

Much is to be learned especially about intravenous thrombolysis in patients with lesions determined before treatment. No information is available concerning treatment of patients with extracranial and ICVA occlusions, the two most common arterial occlusive lesions within the posterior circulation *(13)*. The time window is longer in posterior circulation disease than in the anterior circulation and hemorrhagic complications are fewer. The effectiveness and safety of intravenous vs IA treatment in patients with known arterial lesions and mechanisms needs to be compared. It has to be determined when to use other adjuvant methods such as angioplasty/stenting, mechanical clot removal, or ultrasound energy with or instead of thrombolysis. Finally, anti-thrombotic strategies (glycoprotein IIb/IIIa inhibitors, heparins, ximelagratran, antiplatelets) to use before, during, and after thrombolysis need to be explored.

REFERENCES

1. Hacke W, Zeumer H, Ferbert A, Bruckmann H, del Zoppo G. Intra-arterial thrombolytic therapy improves outcome in patients with acute vertebrobasilar occlusive disease. *Stroke* 1988;19:1216–1222.
2. Mobius E, Berg-Dammer E, Kuhne D, Nahser HC. Experience with 18 patients in Thrombolytic therapy in acute ischemic stroke. In: *Local Thrombolytic Therapy in Acute Basilar*

Artery Occlusion, Hacke W, del Zoppo GJ, Hirschberg M, eds. Heidelberg:Springer-Verlag, 1991, pp. 213–215.

3. Brandt T, von Kummer R, Muller-Kuppers M, Hacke W. Thrombolytic therapy of acute basilar artery occlusion. Variables affecting recanalization and outcome. *Stroke* 1996:27:875–881.
4. Wijdicks EFM, Nichols DA, Thielen KR et al. Intra-arterial thrombolysis in acute basilar artery thromboembolism: the initial Mayo Clinic experience. *Mayo Clin Proc* 1997;72:1005–1013.
5. Cross DT, DT, Moran CJ, Akins PT, Angtuaco E, Diringer MN. Relationship between clot location and outcome after basilar artery thrombosis. *AJNR* 1997;18:1221–1228.
6. Mitchell PJ, Gerraty RP, Donnan GA et al. Thrombolysis in the vertebrobasilar circulation: the Australian Urokinase Stroke Trial. *Cerebrovasc Dis* 1997;7:94–99.
7. Egan R, Clark W, Lutsep H, Nesbit G, Barnwell S, Kellogg J. Efficacy of intraarterial thrombolysis of basilar artery stroke. J *Stroke Cerebrovasc Dis* 1999;8:22–27.
8. Eckert B, Kucinski T, Pfeiffer G, Groden C, Zeumer H. Endovascular therapy of acute vertebrobasilar occlusion: early treatment onset as the most important factor. *Cerebrovasc Dis* 2002;14:42–50.
9. Becker KJ, Monsein LH, Ulatowski J, Mirski M, Williams M, Hanley DF. Intraarterial thrombolysis in Vertebrobasilar occlusion. *AJNR* 1996;17:255–262.
10. von Kummer R, Forsting M, Sartor K, Hacke W. Intravenous recombinant tissue plasminogen activator in acute stroke. In: *Thrombolytic Therapy in Acute Ischemic Stroke,* Hacke W, del Zoppo GJ, Hirschberg M, eds. Berlin:Springer-Verlag, 1991, pp. 161–167.
11. Grond M, Rudolf J, Schmulling S, Stenzel C, Neveling M, Heiss-W-D. Early intravenous thrombolysis with recombinant tissue-type plasminogen activator in vertebrobasilar ischemic stroke. *Arch Neurol* 1998;55:466–469.
12. Montavont A, Nighoghossian N, Derex L, et al. Intravenous r-tPA in vertebrobasilar acute infarcts. *Neurology* 2004;62:1854–1856.
13. Caplan LR, Wityk RJ, Glass TA, et al. New England medical center Posterior Circulation registry. *Ann Neurol* 2004;56:389–398.

13 Thrombolytic Therapy in Stroke Patients

Patrick D. Lyden, MD

CONTENTS

INTRODUCTION

The use of tissue plasminogen activators (t-PA) for acute stroke was proven safe and effective in the National Institutes of Neurologic Disorders and Stroke (NINDS) study of t-PA for acute stroke, published in 1995 *(1)*. The therapy was approved by the US Food and Drug Administration (FDA) in 1996, and endorsed by the American Heart Association, American Academy of Neurology, and National Stroke Association in 1997 *(2–4)*. Nevertheless, some authorities argued that thrombolytic therapy with t-PA for stroke was still not ready for general use, leaving the practitioner in an awkward position *(5)*. Since the original approval, there have been several reports that bear on some of the questions raised by skeptics. What have we learned since the original study to answer

From: *Current Clinical Neurology: Thrombolytic Therapy for Acute Stroke, Second Edition*
Edited by: P. D. Lyden

remaining concerns about thrombolytic stroke therapy? Are data available now, that were not available previously, to reassure neurologists that it is now time to expand their use of thrombolytic therapy for stroke patients? The extension of thrombolytic therapy into the community—that is outside of specialized academic medical centers—is presented in Chapter 9. In the previous edition of this book, the case for limiting the use of thrombolytic therapy was eloquently made by Dr. Lou Caplan; for this edition, in Chapter 14, Dr. Caplan continues to point out the limitations of our understanding of thrombolysis, while making a case in favor of limiting thrombolytic use to specialized centers. Here, we will present the case in favor of thrombolytic therapy under the current guidelines.

The available data support six basic contentions: (1) t-PA for stroke therapy is cost effective, despite the high cost of the drug itself and the stroke teams to give it; (2) community-based practicing neurologists can use t-PA for acute stroke and obtain the same good results seen in the original research study; (3) additional support for the first study conclusions comes from long-term follow up of the original patients and from analysis of the computed tomography (CT) scan data; (4) angiograms are probably not necessary prior to administering t-PA; (5) There are no particular subgroups from whom t-PA should be withheld, such as those with very large strokes; and (6) other groups, using other drugs such as pro-urokinase (pro-UK), have found beneficial effects of thrombolytic therapy for stroke. On the other hand, there still remains considerable room for improvement, and we are far from having the ideal thrombolytic agent. Let us consider these contentions in turn.

t-PA IS COST EFFECTIVE

Since the initial publication of the NINDS Recombinant Tissue Plasminigen Activator Stroke Trial results, NINDS investigators have published additional data and analyses, which is presented in Chapter 8. It is critical to understand that rigorous methodology was used in that analysis to estimate the likelihood that the cost estimates were correct *(6)*. Certain assumptions about stroke costs and outcomes were based on data from the literature and from the original study. Then, to account for possible errors in those assumptions, a simulation method was used to vary the values of those assumptions. For example, the authors estimated that the cost of in-patient rehabilitation might be $21,233, but in the simulation, this assumption was varied from $10,000 to $40,000. For a cohort of 1000 t-PA-treated patients, the net cost savings in the first year were estimated to be $4 million; the sensitivity analysis from the simulations indicated a probability of 93% that the estimate is correct. Thus, thrombolytic stroke therapy joins a very small number of therapies that not only save disability, but also save dollars. To put these results in perspective, it is important to remember how few other therapies result in net cost savings to the health care system; two traditional examples are prenatal care and early childhood vaccinations *(7–11)*. These therapies cost money to administer, but overall there is a net cost reduction owing to lower disease incidence.

In recent years, further studies have confirmed that thrombolytic therapy is, overall, revenue saving to the health care system, even after factoring in the costs of the stroke teams, the evaluations on "mimic" patients, and the hemorrhages that result in some cases *(12,13)*. It is clear from these analyses, however, that the protocol must be followed rigorously; a greater number of protocol deviations can turn the equation around, and end up costing the system considerably.

THROMBOLYTIC THERAPY CAN BE GIVEN OUTSIDE OF ACADEMIC MEDICAL CENTERS

It has been stated that the NINDS investigators were a select group of neurologists with special expertise, and that the study hospitals were unusual places where t-PA could be used safely *(14,15)*. It was hypothesized that in wider clinical practice the risk of the drug, a hemorrhage rate of 6.4%, would be higher, fewer patients would benefit, and practicing neurologists would not meet the strict requirement for prompt evaluation and treatment *(5)*. In support of this, the Cleveland Area Stroke Team surveyed local hospitals about their experience with thrombolytic therapy *(16)*. A total of 3948 patients were admitted with a primary diagnosis of stroke (using the International Classification of Diseases, Ninth Revision, code 434 or 436). Of these patients, the authors could find records and study the use of t-PA in 70 patients (1.8%). Of these, in 50% there were protocol variations, and in 11 (15.7%) there were symptomatic hemorrhages. These data suggest that perhaps the benefit of the thrombolytic stroke therapy may not accrue in a community application. In many respects, however, the study was flawed. Most importantly, the charts were located and reviewed retrospectively, so there is a high likelihood of selection bias: bad cases are more likely to be found than good cases. The study does illustrate nicely, however, that few patients are receiving t-PA for their stroke. Similarly, in Rio de Janiero, only 5 of 56 evaluated patients could be treated, primarily as a result of lack of symptom recognition, transfer delay, or late CT scan *(17)*. In a distressing eight patients, the CT scan could not be performed in a timely manner.

Whereas it is true that all investigators in the original study were trained to follow the study protocol properly, including video certification using the National Institutes of Health Stroke Scale (NIHSS) *(18,19)*, it is also true that a majority of patients were enrolled at community hospitals, not academic medical centers. In the original trial, over two-thirds of the patients were enrolled at non-academic medical centers. The investigators involved, however, were trained by the investigative team, and could have enjoyed some special advantage that would not be available in wider clinical use. To determine whether the study results could be replicated in practice, several groups have studied thrombolytic therapy in large numbers of stroke patients, known as post-marketing or phase IV studies. The results of these studies are summarized in Chapter 9. Note especially Table 1 in that chapter: the outcome response rate varies from about one-third to more than 50%. Overall, it is now clear that community-based neurologists can deliver the drug with statistics that mirror the original study *(20)*.

In Alberta, Canada, the stroke center examined 68 consecutive patients treated by general neurologists (non-stroke specialists) in an academic medical center *(21)*. A favorable outcome, as defined by the NIHSS, was noted in 38% by 3 mo after treatment. Using the modified Rankin scale (mRS), a favorable outcome occurred in 57% by 3 mo. Symptomatic hemorrhages occurred more often in patients in whom the protocol was violated (27%) than in those in whom the protocol was followed (5%). Similar results were obtained in communities around the world, as summarized in Chapter 9.

The largest phase IV study of thrombolytic therapy was organized by the maker of t-PA, Genentech *(22)*. This prospective, multicenter study was conducted at 57 US medical centers, of which 24 were academic and 33 were community. In this series, the hemorrhage rate was 3.3%, and as expected, one-half of these patients died. After 30 d, 35% of the patients had very favorable outcomes; 43% were functionally independent. Protocol violations were noted in 32.6%. A similar registry is underway in Europe to track thrombolytic effectiveness after approval in 2003 by the European authorities.

Most notable of all, in Cleveland, a community training program was instituted in the very medical centers where so many protocol violations were detected in the Cleveland area study mentioned earlier. A re-survey was done, and a significant improvement in protocol violations and a reduction in complication rates were detected *(23)*. It would appear that community use of thrombolytics is safe and effective, as long as the protocol is followed.

These reports of community experiences are limited by the unavoidable fact that they cannot be blinded or placebo-controlled. At this time, however, it is fair to conclude that if the NINDS protocol is followed scrupulously, then outcome results similar to the original study can be obtained in community hospitals. It remains speculative, but a reasonable presumption, that violating the protocol necessarily results in higher rates of complications. The notion that somehow the investigators in the original trial treated patients differently than practicing clinicians has been put to rest. No matter what the background, training, or experience of the physician, if the protocol is followed, the same benefits will accrue.

THE ORIGINAL RESULTS ARE CONFIRMED ON LONG-TERM FOLLOW-UP

There is always a question as to whether good results seen early after therapy can still be detected some time after the therapy. In the initial report, the effect of thrombolysis was confirmed 3 mo after stroke. Next, the beneficial effects of thrombolytic stroke therapy were confirmed by following the patients in the original study for up to 1 yr *(24)*. These data are presented in more detail in Chapter 8. Only 22 patients (out of 624) were lost to follow-up, 14 in the t-PA group and 8 in the placebo group. In order to avoid biasing the results toward benefit in the t-PA group, each of these missing patients was assigned the most unfavorable outcome; that is, the analysis was biased slightly in favor of the placebo group. When the patients were assessed 6 and 12 mo after thrombolytic stroke therapy, the results were nearly exactly the same as in the original publication. Using a global test to simultaneously describe the results of three outcome measures, the odds ratio (OR) of a near complete recovery after t-PA was 1.7 (OR 95% confidence interval [CI] 1.3 to 2.3), compared to placebo (p = 0.0013). Looking at the individual measures of outcome, patients are 30 to 50% more likely than placebo-treated patients to have minimal or no disability 1 yr after thrombolytic stroke therapy. In addition to the long-term functional data, the volume of infarction seen on CT scans 3 mo after thrombolytic therapy was analyzed; there was a significant effect: median stroke volume was 25.5 cm^3 in placebo-treated, vs 15.5 cm^3 in t-PA-treated, patients (p = 0.039) *(25)*.

VASCULAR IMAGING IS UNNECESSARY PRIOR TO THROMBOLYTIC THERAPY

The need for vascular imaging prior to stroke thrombolysis remains controversial, at least for some (*see* Chapter 14). The argument may be summarized by the contention that thrombolytic therapy could be given needlessly to some patients unless an image of the occluded artery is first obtained. That is, if the patient has no documented vascular occlusion, then thrombolytic therapy should not be used *(5)*. In rebuttal, consider two important points. First, using the NINDS thrombolysis protocol, very few patients were treated "needlessly". In the placebo group, only 2% of patients exhibited no neurological deficit (NIHSS score = 0) when examined 24 h after stroke *(1)*. These 2% of patients included patients with transient ischemic attacks (TIA) and perhaps other non-stroke etiologies. No hemorrhages or other thrombolytic side effects occurred in these patients. At 3 mo after their strokes, all of these patients were independent in activities of daily living; none suffered hemorrhage *(26)*. Thus, it seems unlikely that vascular imaging prior to thrombolytic stroke therapy would add any benefit, because the protocol allows the proper selection of suitable patients. That is, if the protocol is followed correctly, there is only a 2% chance of treating a non-stroke etiology with thrombolysis. No harm occurred to any of the TIA patients who received t-PA.

The second rebuttal point is that the press of time requires prompt intervention, and vascular imaging requires precious time. An angiography team requires at least 60 min to mobilize and obtain the first images, even in the most dedicated centers *(27)*. During those 60 min, brain-cell death continues and the chances for a good outcome decline. Alternatives to invasive angiography await further development. Transcranial ultrasound techniques are improving, but do not visualize the intracerebral circulation in a majority of acute stroke patients. Novel techniques, such as spiral CT angiography and xenon enhanced CT may hold promise, but will require carefully designed, properly controlled trials to assure reliability. In the meantime, vascular imaging seems to be neither required, nor desirable, prior to thrombolytic stroke therapy. On the other hand, magnetic resonance imaging (MRI) techniques continue to improve (*see* Chapter 17). As magnetic scanners become as ubiquitous as CT, and as perfusion and angiographic methods improve, MRI may become the imaging procedure of choice for acute stroke. It remains problematic, however, to assure that hemorrhage detection proceeds accurately. There are two risks, under-call and over-call. The MRI sequences used to detect blood are extremely sensitive; more sensitive than CT; we do not know if "blood on the MRI scan" is as obvious a contraindication to thrombolytic therapy as "blood on the CT scan." In particular, the risk of thrombolysis in the setting of large ischemic stroke that contains a small amount of MRI-detectable petechial hemorrhage is unknown. On the other hand, in some centers thrombolysis is withheld unless MRI perfusion shows a deficit larger than the diffusion-weighted lesion (so-called mismatch). This practice is not yet validated, and will lead to under utilization of treatment in patients who could benefit (*see* Chapter 17).

The advantage of intravenous thrombolytic therapy is that active treatment is delivered to patients within a reasonable time frame. Is it harmful to administer t-PA to patients in whom no blockage can be documented on angiogram? The evidence is to the contrary: in the subgroup analysis of the NINDS t-PA study the group of patients who were thought to have lacunes responded to therapy as well as or better than other subgroups *(28)*. It is well appreciated that for patients with lacunar-syndrome presentations, angiography is inadequate to document the level of arterial occlusion. Because these patients responded to thrombolytic therapy, it can be inferred that thrombosis occurs in lacunar syndromes and that angiography will not document this thrombus. Furthermore, the safety of thrombolytic therapy in this subgroup of "angio-negative" strokes is proven.

On the other hand, one important advantage of angiography is that intra-arterial (IA) therapy could be delivered directly into the clot *(29)*. Trials of IA urokinase showed benefit: 180 patients were treated within 6 h of stroke onset with intravenous low-dose heparin and IA pro-UK *(30)*. IA pro-UK significantly improved the proportion of good outcomes from 25 to 40% ($p < 0.05$). Hemorrhages were seen in 10%, consistent with other thrombolytic trials. This study demonstrated that thrombolysis with IA pro-UK is safe and effective up to 6 h after stroke. More recently, mechanical devices used to retrieve the clot showed promise in pilot trials.

SUBGROUP SELECTION IS STILL NOT JUSTIFIED

It is widely argued that because the full range of potentially salvageable stroke patients is not known, we should treat no one until we know precisely which patient subgroups do respond to thrombolytic therapy. This argument can be supported by examining the response rate in the original report and in subsequent analyses: a minority (30 to 50%) of t-PA-treated patients enjoys a full recovery. Furthermore, every clinician desires to find the best possible candidate for therapy, and to attempt to "target" treatment at the subgroup of patients that is most likely to respond. On the other hand, a majority of patients enjoy some benefit from t-PA, albeit not a complete cure *(28)*. This discrepancy derives from the statistical method that was used in the original report; the primary outcomes were reported in terms of complete or nearly complete recoveries, without mentioning the benefits accrued in those patients who had less than a complete recovery. For example, patients who have a severe deficit on admission (pretreatment) and are over the age of 75, appear to improve significantly compared to placebo-treated patients in the same subgroup (*see* Fig. 4 in Chapter 8). These patients do not achieve the criteria for a complete recovery with either placebo or t-PA treatment, but there are more patients with a mild deficit, and fewer patients with a moderate or severe deficit, in the t-PA-treated group. That is, patients in this subgroup are too ill to recover completely, but t-PA treatment may improve their outcome from severe to mild. Similar analyses can be presented for other types of patients as well. The NINDS investigators examined the original data for *any* subgroup of patients in whom t-PA was unlikely to benefit, and therefore could be withheld. A similar analysis was conducted to try to identify subgroups of patients who were more likely than others to suffer hemorrhagic complications *(31)*. The analysis included multiple sequential statistical analyses, and various combinations of baseline data were analyzed. From the analyses of baseline variables, such as age, stroke deficit, presence of diabetes, presence of prior stroke, and other important factors, no subgroup could be identified for whom thrombolytic stroke therapy can be particularly recommended or prohibited. At present, therefore, the wisest course for the active clinician is to prescribe t-PA to patients who fulfill the criteria as outlined in the original protocol. Withholding therapy in some subgroup of patients hoping to target treatment to a more-likely-to-respond group is unwise.

THE POSITIVE RESULTS HAVE BEEN CONFIRMED USING OTHER PROTOCOLS AND OTHER DRUGS

Since the original report of the NINDS Stroke Trial, additional confirmations of the value of thrombolytic therapy for stroke, including the pro-UK trial that was discussed above, have now been published. In the first report of the European

Cooperative Acute Stroke Study (ECASS), there was no statistically significant benefit for t-PA. Upon re-analysis, however, using the data methods developed for the NINDS study, a clear benefit was seen: the global odds ratio for favorable outcome was 1.5 (95% CI 1.1 to 2.0, $p = 0.008$) *(32)*. Furthermore, in ECASS, most patients were enrolled within 6 h of stroke onset, but 87 patients were enrolled within the 3-h time limit used in the NINDS study *(33)*. The global odds ratio for favorable outcome was 2.3 (95% CI 0.9–5.3, $p = 0.07$), which is not statistically significant due to the small sample size. To examine these potentially positive findings further, a confirmatory study was conducted (ECASS II) *(34)*. The primary endpoint of this study, the global odds ratio for a favorable outcome (score of 0 or 1) on the mRS, was negative. However, there were significantly more patients who scored well on the Rankin (mRS = 0, 1, or 2) in the t-PA-treated (54.3%) vs placebo-treated (46%) patients, ($p = 0.024$). In this trial, there were quite conservative inclusion criteria, resulting in an excess of mild patients in the study. For this reason, the beneficial effect of t-PA could have been diluted, resulting in lower statistical power.

Using a completely different type of drug, the defibrinogenating agent ancrod, a group of investigators also found benefit for patients treated within 3 h. Ancrod causes a reduction in fibrinogen, prolongation of the prothrombin time, reduced serum viscosity, and perhaps a thrombolytic effect *(35,36)*. In this trial, patients were treated within 3 h of stroke onset with a 72-h infusion of ancrod; the dose was adjusted to lower the fibrinogen to a target level. Preliminary data indicated a treatment benefit: there was a favorable outcome (mRS = 0 or 1) in 41.1% of patients, compared to 35.3% in placebo treated patients ($p < 0.05$). Unfortunately, if the fibrinogen were lowered excessively, there were more symptomatic intracranial hemorrhages (ICHs).

CONCLUSIONS

The data collected and analyzed during the first years of the stroke thrombolytic era suggest that this new therapy withstands the test of time. The benefits persist over the long term, and are realized by clinically active neurologists practicing in typical community settings. Several groups have confirmed the value of thrombolytic stroke therapy when given within 3 h of stroke onset; pooled analysis shows that treatment between 3 and 6 h after stroke is of some benefit, and lacks significantly increased risk compared to under 3-h treatment *(37)*. No specific subgroup can be found at particularly increased risk or benefit, suggesting that the original guidelines for selecting patients must be followed. Yet, the success of thrombolytic therapy, even at a distance of a few years, still raises a number of questions. Did we test the right dose and timing of drug administration? Might other thrombolytic drugs, or other dosing schedules, prove more beneficial? How can we increase the success rate to something greater than

50%? Will neuroprotectants add benefit or reduce risk, when combined with thrombolytic therapy? How do we extend the 3-h limit, without increasing the numbers of pointless treatments? Most importantly, what can be done to educate more patients and potential stroke-witnesses about the signs of stroke and the need for immediate medical attention?

Thrombolytic stroke therapy represents something of a novel situation for clinically active neurologists. Heretofore, the general strategy in neurology has been to minimize disability while doing no harm. It is a rare situation when the active neurologist must choose a therapy that has side effects but also has a net benefit: the first therapy for stroke is also the first therapy for which neurologists must urgently present difficult choices to patients and families for an immediate decision. Without question, this is an uncomfortable situation for all. However, now that the results of the NINDS t-PA study have been well digested, criticized, confirmed, supplemented with additional data, and diffused widely, it is time to take this bull by the horns. It is no longer appropriate to wait for further developments in this field: more than 11 patients per hour have a disabling stroke in America. Although more and more stroke patients receive thrombolytic therapy, it is still true that a majority of eligible patients do not receive it. The dictum *primum no nocere* still applies: we must do no harm, either by actively committing an act or by withholding a proven therapy through inaction.

REFERENCES

1. NINDS rt-PA Stroke Study Group. Tissue plasminogen activator for acute ischemic stroke. *N Engl J Med* 1995; 333(24):1581–1587.
2. Report of the Quality Standards Subcommittee of the American Academy of Neurology. Thrombolytic therapy for acute ischemic stroke—Summary Statement. *Neurology* 1996; 47:835–839.
3. Adams HP, Jr., Brott TG, Furlan AJ, et al. Guidelines for thrombolytic therapy for acute stroke: A supplement to the guidelines for the management of patients with acute ischemic stroke. *Circulation* 1996; 94:1167–1174.
4. Lyden PD, Grotta JC, Levine SR, et al. Intravenous thrombolysis for acute stroke. *Neurology* 1997; 49:14–29.
5. Caplan L, Mohr JP, Kistler JP, Koroshetz W. Should thrombolytic therapy be the first-line treatment for acute ischemic stroke? Thrombolysis—not a panacea for ischemic stroke. *New Engl J Med* 1997; 337:1309–1310.
6. Fagan SC, Morgenstern LB, Petitta A, et al. Cost-effectiveness of tissue plasminogen activator for acute ischemic stroke. *Neurology* 1998; 50:883–890.
7. Schoenbaum SC, Hyde JN, Baroshesky L, Crampton K. Benefit-cost analysis of rubella vaccination policy. *N Engl J Med* 1976; 294:306–310.
8. Koplan JP, Schoenbaum SC, Weinstein MC, Fraser DW. Pertussis vaccine—an analysis of benefits, risks and costs. *N Engl J Med* 1979; 301:906–911.
9. Koplan JP, Preblud SR. A benefit-cost analysis of mumps vaccine. *Am J Dis Child* 1982; 136:362–364.
10. Cutting WA. Cost-benefit evaluations of vaccination programmes. *Lancet* 1980; 8195 pt 1:634–635.

11. Avruch S, Cackley AP. Savings achieved by giving WIC benefits to women prenatally. *Public Health Rep* 1995; 110:27–34.
12. Sandercock P, Berge E, Dennis M, et al. Cost-effectiveness of thrombolysis with recombinant tissue plasminogen activator for acute ischemic stroke assessed by a model based on UK NHS costs. *Stroke* 2004; 35(6):1490–1497.
13. Wein TH, Hickenbottom SL, Alexandrov AV. Thrombolysis, stroke units and other strategies for reducing acute stroke costs. *Pharmacoeconomics* 1998; 14(6):603–611.
14. Furlan A, Kanoti G. When Is thrombolysis justified in patients with acute ischemic stroke? a bioethical perspective. *Stroke* 1997;(28):214–218.
15. del Zoppo G. Acute stroke: on the threshold of a therapy? *New Engl J Med* 1995; 333:1632–1633.
16. Katzan I, Furlan AJ, Lloyd L, et al. Use of tissue-type plasminogen activator for acute ischemic stroke: The Cleveland area experience. *JAMA* 2000; 283(9):1151–1158.
17. Andre C, Moraes-Neto J, Novis S. Experience with t-PA treatment in a large south american city. *J Stroke Cerebrovasc Dis* 1998; 7(4):255–258.
18. Lyden P, Brott T, Tilley B, et al. Improved reliability of the NIH stroke scale using video training. *Stroke* 1994; 25:2220–2226.
19. Albanese MA, Clarke WR, Adams HP Jr., Woolson RF. Ensuring reliability of outcome measures on multicenter clinical trials of treatments for acute ischemic stroke: the program developed for the trial of ORG 10172 in acute stroke treatment (TOAST). *Stroke* 1994; 25:1746–1751.
20. Graham GD. Tissue plasminogen activator for acute ischemic stroke in clinical practice: a meta-analysis of safety data. *Stroke* 2003; 34(12):2847–2850.
21. Buchan A, Barber P, Newcommon N, et al. Effectiveness ot t-PA in acute ischemic stroke. *Neurology* 2000; 54:679–684.
22. Albers GW, Bates V, Clark W, et al. Intravenous tissue-type plasminogen activator for treatment of acute stroke: the standard treatment with alteplase to reverse stroke (STARS) study (STARS). *JAMA* 2000; 283:1145–1150.
23. Katzan I, Hammer M, Furlan A. Quality improvement and tissue-type plasminogen activator for acute ischemic stroke. a Cleveland update. *Stroke* 2003; 34:799–800.
24. Kwiatkowski TG, Libman R, Frankel M, et al. Effects of tissue plasminogen activator for acute ischemic stroke at one year. *N Engl J Med* 1999; 340:1781–1787.
25. NINDS rt-PA Stroke Study Group. Effect of intravenous recombinant tissue plasminogen activator on ischemic stroke lesion size measured by computed tomography. NINDS; The National Institute of Neurological Disorders and Stroke (NINDS) rt-PA Stroke Study Group. *Stroke* 2000; 31:2912–2919.
26. Lyden P, Lu M, Kwiatkowski TG, et al. Thrombolysis in patients with transient neurologic deficits. *Neurology* 2001; 57:2125–2128.
27. del Zoppo G.J., Higashida RT, Furlan A, et al. PROACT: A phase II randomized trial of recombinant pro-urokinase by direct arterial delivery in acute middle cerebral artery stroke. *Stroke* 1998; 29:4–11.
28. The NINDS t-PA Stroke Study Group. Generalized Efficacy of t-PA for Acute Stroke. subgroup analysis of the NINDS t-PA stroke trial. *Stroke* 1997; 28:2119–2125.
29. Hacke W, Zeumer H, Ferbert A, Bruckmann H, del Zoppo G. Intra-arterial thrombolytic therapy improves outcome in patients with acute vertebrobasilar occlusive disease. *Stroke* 1988; 19:1216–1222.
30. Furlan A, Higashida RT, Wechsler L,et al. Intra-arterial Prourokinase for Acute Ischemic Stroke. *JAMA* 1999; 282(21):2003–2008.
31. The NINDS t-PA Stroke Study Group. Intracerbral hemorrhage after intravenous t-PA therapy for ischemic stroke. *Stroke* 1997; 28(11):2109–2118.

32. Hacke W, Bluhmki E, Steiner T, et al. Dichotomized efficacy end points and global end-point analysis applied to the ECASS intention-to-treat data set. *Stroke* 1998; 29:2073–2075.
33. Steiner T, Bluhmki E, Kaste M, et al. The ECASS 3-hour cohort. *Cerebrovasc Dis* 1998; 8:198–203.
34. Hacke W, Kaste M, Fieschi C, et al. Randomised double-blind placebo-controlled trial of thrombolytic therapy with intravenous alteplase in acute ischaemic stroke (ECASS II). *Lancet* 1998; 352:1245–1251.
35. The Ancrod Stroke Study Investigators. Ancrod for the treatment of acute ischemic brain infarction. *Stroke* 1994; 25:1755–1759.
36. Sherman DG, Atkinson RP, Chippendale T, et al. Intravenous ancrod for treatment for acute ischemic stroke. *JAMA* 2000; 283(18):2395–2403.
37. Hacke W, Donnan G, Fieschi C, et al. Association of outcome with early stroke treatment: pooled analysis of ATLANTIS, ECASS, and NINDS rt-PA stroke trials. *Lancet* 2004; 363(9411):768–774.

14 Stroke Thrombolysis

The Present Guidelines and Policies for Clinical Use Should Be Changed

Louis R. Caplan, MD

Contents

INTRODUCTION

Although 8 yr have passed since the Food and Drug Administration (FDA) released tissue plasminogen activator (t-PA) for use in the United States to treat patients with acute ischemic stroke, thrombolysis is still very controversial. Clearly, thrombolysis is a step forward but there remain problems with its use, and with the guidelines and policies that direct its application.

Although we finally have a drug that is generally acknowledged to be effective in stroke patients, problems still abound. Doctors and medical centers have been slow to deliver thrombolytics. Only about 1–2% of acute stroke patients are given thrombolytics. About 5% of patients who arrive at medical centers and are eligible to be given thrombolytic agents under present guidelines actually receive it. Many hospitals, doctors, ambulance services, and emergency room units are still not adequately prepared to handle acute stroke patients. There are not enough doctors available who are sufficiently trained and experienced in

From: *Current Clinical Neurology: Thrombolytic Therapy for Acute Stroke, Second Edition*
Edited by: P. D. Lyden © Humana Press Inc., Totowa, NJ

managing acute stroke patients. Emergency physician organizations have not supported thrombolysis, setting doctors against doctors. Doctors are being sued for allegedly inappropriately giving or not giving thrombolytic drugs to patients. In the author's opinion, the guidelines and policies need to be updated.

THE PRESENT GUIDELINES AND THEIR SHORTCOMINGS

The present recommendations for thrombolytic use were reported by American Heart Association *(1)* and American Academy of Neurology *(2)* committees. These recommendations were based on the National Institutes of Neurologic Disorders and Stroke (NINDS) *(3)* protocol, essentially only repeat the inclusions and exclusions used in that trial, and are substantially the same. Conducting trials is very different from caring for sick patients *(4–8)*. The same specified treatments are given in trials to all eligible patients depending only on randomization. But doctors take care of individual patients and must weigh the risks and benefits of all possible treatments in complex situations that may not have been studied or analyzed in trials. Information from trials must be weighed according to the context of specific treatment decisions in individual patients. Although there may be general evidence that thrombolysis is effective using NINDS guidelines, there may be no evidence that it is effective or ineffective for a given vascular lesion unless it has been specifically tested for that lesion. Even when it has been tested for that lesion, coexisting factors in that particular patient often complicate the decision. Therapeutic decisions are often difficult and complex. They require experienced physicians. Evidence from trials, past experience, and knowledge of the patient, the disease, and the wishes of all concerned are required to make difficult therapeutic decisions. Rarely have the inclusions and exclusions of a trial been used as the guidelines for treating individual patients.

There are also ethical considerations in translating randomized trials into clinical practice. Can a physician, in good conscience, give a patient a potentially hazardous medication when that patient might not have the disorder that the medicine treats?

Suppose it was well documented that thrombolytic drugs were effective in treating 85 patients among a large group of 100 patients who had acute brain ischemia. If among those 100 patients there were 5 who might not have the disorder the drug treats effectively, then treatment exposes 5 patients to harm needlessly. Would it be appropriate to give all 100 the drug, possibly sacrificing the 5 "innocent" individuals?

Using an analogy, suppose that radiation therapy was 85% effective in patients with undefined lumps that appeared as mass lesions on brain imaging scans, but 5% of the patients did not have tumors and would be harmed by the radiation. Would we radiate all 100 or instead insist on a definitive diagnosis of cancer before radiation? Even though a treatment is effective in most patients, the

Table 1
Analysis From Six Randomized Trials of the Odds Ratio of Good Outcome According to Timing of Intravenous Thrombolysis

Time epoch	*Odds ratios*
1–1.5 h	2.8 $p < 0.0001$
1.5–3 h	1.5 $p < 0.01$
3–4.5 h	1.4 $p < 0.02$
4.5–6 h	1.2 $p < 0.26$

doctor and the patient need to decide if the benefit is more than the risk in a particular situation.

Most authorities agree that thrombolysis can be effective if given within 3 h following present guidelines, but are the present guidelines optimal? Could thrombolytic treatment be improved? Are there patients now excluded that could respond to treatment? Are there some patients now treated under the guidelines who should not be treated because of little likelihood of success and high risk of hemorrhage or edema?

The major criticisms of the present guidelines include:

1. The rigid time limit for treatment is 3 h.
   Patients do not change from queens to pumpkins as the clock strikes 3. Some patients have sizable infarcts at 1 and 2 h after symptom onset that pose a risk for hemorrhage and edema if thrombolytics are given. Some patients respond well after the 3-h limit. Analysis of pooled data from six t-PA trials shows that the earlier patients are treated the higher the likelihood of a favorable outcome (*see* Chapter 7). Treatment after 3 h, especially between 3 and 4.5 h, was also effective, but not as effective as earlier treatment (Table 1). Results from both intravenous and intra-arterial (IA) trials that included angiography before and after treatment showed that recanalization and good outcomes often developed in patients treated 6 and 8 hs after onset *(5,7,8)*. Some patients treated with IA thrombolytics have done well even when treated after 12 h.
2. Exclusion of patients who awaken with deficits or in whom time of onset is uncertain.
   Studies have shown that most ischemic strokes occur during the morning after awakening *(9)*. Contrary to previous teaching, ischemic strokes are not very common during sleep. It is often difficult for patients to know if they awakened with the deficit or developed it after awakening. When there are no accurate reliable observers with the patient, it is often difficult to judge when the symptoms and signs began. This is especially true in patients with right cerebral hemisphere strokes who are anosognosic for their deficits. In a 3-yr analysis at

a hospital in Calgary of why stroke patients were excluded from treatment, Barber et al. found that 24.2% of 1168 acute stroke patients were excluded because of an uncertain time of onset *(10)*. In these patients and those who may have awakened with a deficit *(11)*, modern brain and vascular imaging can define the presence, location, and size of infarction, and the presence and location of a vascular occlusive lesion*(12–18)*. This information along with the clinical findings can be used to guide treatment decisions.

3. Exclusion of patients with minor or significantly improving deficits.
   In the Calgary study, among 314 acute ischemic stroke patients admitted within the 3-h time limit, 13.1% were excluded because of mild stroke and 18.2% were excluded because of improvement after onset *(10)*. The presence of slight deficits and improvement were understandably used as exclusions in the NINDS trial because most patients in those categories do well. These patients would not have represented good targets for statistically significant treatment effects because the outlook is so good without treatment. But all experienced stroke clinicians have seen many patients who are not badly off on admission or who show improvement who subsequently worsen and even suddenly crash and develop severe neurological deficits. A third of patients in the Calgary study considered to have mild or improving deficits during the initial evaluation were either dependent or dead at the time of hospital discharge *(10)*. Staroselskaya et al. have shown that patients with persistent vascular occlusions who have a major perfusion–diffusion mismatch on magnetic resonance image (MRI) worsen during hospitalization if the occlusive lesion does not open *(16)*. Although appropriate for use in trials, these exclusions are not appropriate for general use, but are situations in which brain and vascular imaging are very important.
   Another problem with slight deficits is that the volume of brain infarction as determined by MRI does not correlate well with the National Institutes of Health (NIH) stroke scale in patients with right hemisphere and posterior circulation ischemia *(11,19)*. Patients with cognitive and behavioral abnormalities related to right cerebral hemisphere infarcts may have low NIH stroke scale scores yet be quite disabled and have relatively large infarcts *(11)*. Posterior circulation patients with hemianopia, diplopia, or ataxia may have low NIH stroke scale scores and yet have disabling brainstem, cerebellar, and posterior hemisphere strokes *(19)*.
4. Exclusion of patients with seizures at or near onset.
   Seizures are now a contraindication for thrombolysis. However some stroke patients, especially those with embolism, do have seizures soon after embolism. As far as is known, a convulsion does not increase the risk of thrombolysis per se. The reason for this exclusion in the NINDS trial is understood. Most seizures are not caused by acute strokes and using the history and computed tomography (CT) alone it would be very difficult for an inexperienced physician to diagnose an acute stroke in a patient who presents post-ictally or who has a seizure under observation. However, acute brain ischemia can be recognized using modern brain and vascular imaging in patients with seizures *(20)*. Furthermore, patients

with brainstem ischemia often have convulsive-like movements that are difficult to differentiate from seizures by inexperienced doctors *(21,22)*. Seizures are another situation in which imaging can be very helpful in diagnosis and selecting treatment.

5. No guides as to who should treat and in what setting.
   Whenever possible, thrombolytic drugs should be given only by physicians experienced in treating stroke patients. Optimally, the patient should be studied at an expert stroke center that has a team of physicians, including neurologists and neurosurgeons, trained and experienced in stroke care. The expert stroke center should have modern brain and vascular imaging technology and have protocols for rapid examinations and imaging. The present guidelines, however, do not designate personnel or location for treatment. The European equivalent of the US FDA does designate physicians trained and experienced in stroke care as the treating physicians. Dedicated stroke centers are also more common in Europe than in the United States, and there are policies in many European cities that facilitate delivery of acute stroke patients to the hospitals that have stroke centers. Unfortunately, many hospitals in the United States are not adequately prepared. They have insufficient technology and personnel. Most emergency physicians are not adequately trained in neurology. Using only clinical history and examination and CT scan during a very short period of time, they understandably do not feel qualified or comfortable in using thrombolytic drugs, agents that have significant risks. Mostly for this reason (in the author's opinion) the emergency physician societies have not supported the present thrombolytic guidelines.
   Hospitals and medical facilities designate privileges according to training and experience. The privilege to perform surgery and various diagnostic procedures depends on demonstration of training, experience, and competence in those procedures. Should the privilege and responsibility of giving thrombolytic drugs to acute stroke patients be different?
6. No mention of vascular imaging studies.
   Ischemic stroke is a vascular disease. Acute and chronic treatment of patients with brain ischemia is aimed at the nature, location, and severity of the causative cervico-cranial, vascular, cardiac, and hematological abnormalities that caused the stroke. The present guidelines do not recommend, or even mention, the potential utility of vascular imaging. Technology advances have led to the availability of three noninvasive techniques that can safely and quickly yield reliable data about the presence of occlusive lesions within the arteries of the neck and head since the NINDS trial was planned. In addition, studies of patients who have had intravenous and IA thrombolysis who have had arterial occlusive lesions shown before and after thrombolysis yields important data about what lesions are likely to respond to treatment at what time and using what route of administration *(5,7,8)* (Tables 2 and 3). Because brain imaging is required before thrombolysis, magnetic resonance angiography (MRA) or computed tomography angiography (CTA) can be performed at the same time as brain

Table 2
What Has Been Learned About IA Thrombolysis in Patients Studied Angiographically

1. Mechanical clot disruption is important.
2. Embolic occlusions recanalize better than *in situ* thrombi.
3. Angioplasty/stenting is often needed to keep the recanalized artery open.
4. Mainstem MCA and basilar artery occlusions seem to respond best. Branch MCA occlusions do not respond as well.
5. Clinical improvement highly correlates with recanalization.
6. Although time matters there is no linear relation between time of treatment and recanalization or outcome in patients with basilar artery occlusion.
7. Hemorrhages occur in about 10–20% of treated patients.

IA, intra-arterial; MCA, middle cerebral artery.

Table 3
What Has Been Learned About Intravenous Thrombolysis in Patients Studied Angiographically

1. In aggregate, considering all patients, treatment is effective.
2. The earlier the treatment the more likely it will be effective.
3. Recanalization correlates with outcome.
4. Thrombolysis is likely to be mostly ineffective in recanalizing some arterial lesions— ICA T-portion, basilar artery—although more research is needed
5. Branch arterial occlusions respond better than large artery neck lesions. MCA occlusions respond much better than ICA occlusions that have embolized intracranially.
6. Hemorrhage is an important risk.
7. Patients with severe clinical deficits and those with substantial infarcts shown by brain imaging at the time of thrombolysis have a higher rate of brain hemorrhage than those with minor deficits and no or little infarction.

ICA, intracranial artery; MCA, middle cerebral artery.

MRI and CT imaging without appreciable loss of time in many medical centers. Extracranial and transcranial ultrasound can also be performed quickly and safely and is very reliable in showing occlusions of large arteries—the targets of thrombolytic treatment. The updated guidelines should include an option for vascular studies if felt useful by the treating physicians.

Some vascular lesions that cause brain ischemia are not likely to be treated effectively by thrombolytic drugs including the following:

- Pre-occlusive atherostenosis.
- Vasoconstriction without superimposed thrombosis (e.g., related to migraine).

- Embolism of substances other than red erythrocyte-fibrin clots (such as cholesterol crystals, atheromatous plaques, bacteria, myxoma material, fat, air, calcium fragments from plaques and valves, and white platelet-fibrin thrombi). Other vascular lesions are likely not to be benefited by thrombolysis but need further research including: emboli that have passed, and penetrating artery disease related ischemia.

7. Adherence to the present guidelines will stop important research in patients arriving within 3 h.

   There is much that we do not know about thrombolysis (Table 4). If the present guidelines are followed, in relation to the 3-h time window, we will never know which thrombolytic drug should be given to which patients with what vascular occlusive lesions and what extent of brain ischemia. t-PA works but is treatment optimal? We now have the noninvasive technology and manpower to try to answer these questions but advancement in knowledge will not occur as quickly as it might if the present guidelines are rigidly adhered to.

POLICIES ALSO NEED TO BE CHANGED

Shortly after approval of t-PA by the FDA for use in acute ischemic stroke, a meeting was sponsored in 1996 by NINDS to attempt to encourage all hospitals to become able to deliver thrombolytic agents for acute stroke patients according to the guidelines and the results of the NINDS trial. The general policy followed since that time has been to encourage all hospitals to become able to give t-PA. Medico-legal suits have been brought against doctors and hospitals when patients have not been given t-PA.

This author believes that this policy was ill conceived and has failed. Only a very small fraction of eligible patients are treated with thrombolysis. Many hospitals simply cannot become capable of giving thrombolytics in an acceptable manner. There are not enough trained stroke clinicians, and many hospitals do not have the personnel, experience, and technology to handle acute stroke patients in a satisfactory manner. Economic constraints also limit these hospitals. They cannot do everything for all patients.

Stroke and neurology are complex. The health care system recognized the need for specialized centers handling complex disorders when they encouraged a system for management of patients with severe trauma. Trauma centers were designated and systems set in motion to deliver patients to those centers whenever possible. Is acute stroke that different? It is suggested that a system be set in motion to designate highly capable expert stroke centers and primary stroke centers. There should be objective criteria that consider personnel, experience, technology, throughput, and systems in these centers. Centers with adequate personnel and systems but not meeting criteria for expert centers could be designated as primary stroke centers by published criteria and review. Every effort should be then made to get patients to the highest-level stroke center. If that is not possible in a rural area, hospitals not meeting criteria could connect by telemedicine with higher centers for advise in individual patients. Hospitals in urban and suburban areas could choose not to accept acute stroke patients when a qualified center is available nearby and patients can and should be diverted to those centers.

WHAT WE HAVE LEARNED ABOUT THROMBOLYSIS

In early studies performed since the 1980s, acute stroke patients were screened clinically and by CT, then angiography was performed. If an intracranial arterial occlusion was shown, thrombolytic drugs were administered into the clots either by IA or iv. Follow-up angiography was performed after treatment to assess recanalization. Both anterior and posterior circulation thromboembolism were treated. These studies were observational only since controls were seldom used and patients were not randomized but successive patients meeting protocol requirements were treated *(5,7,8)*. Unfortunately, the results of these early studies were not included in the publications of the results of the NINDS and European Cooperative Acute Stroke Study randomized trials. The randomized Prolyse in Acute Cerebral Thromboembolism trials of IA prourokinase also added to the knowledge base *(23,24)*. Conclusions from IA studies are shown in Table 2 and conclusions from intravenous studies are shown in Table 3.

Some vascular occlusive lesions are not likely to respond well to intravenous therapy but might respond better to IA therapy including the following:

1. Internal carotid artery (ICA) occlusions in the neck with embolism to the intracranial ICA or middle cerebral arteries.
2. Intracranial ICA occlusions.
3. Mainstem middle cerebral artery occlusions near the origin.
4. Basilar artery occlusions.
5. Occlusion of the bilateral vertebral arteries.
6. Extracranial vertebral artery occlusions with intracranial IA embolism.

There is no credible data concerning patients who have acute ischemia who do not have arterial occlusions. These patients likely have emboli that have passed, occlusion of superficial arteries beyond vascular imaging capability, occlusion of penetrating arteries, or reversible vasoconstriction, or nonvascular causes, such as mitochondrial encephalomyopathy, lactic acidosis, and stroke (MELAS).

We have learned that intravenous thrombolysis can be practiced effectively in the community by experienced clinicians at many selected hospitals.

WHAT WE DO NOT KNOW ABOUT THROMBOLYSIS

Concerning thrombolysis, more is not known than known. Table 4 lists major areas that require further study. This is a short list that could be extended. Clearly, much more research is needed at all potential time levels.

Table 4
What Is Known About Thrombolysis

1. The role of hematological, coagulation, and rheological factors, such as the amount of plasminogen, plasminogen inhibitor, platelet count, etc.
2. The optimal drug to use.
3. Dosage
4. What agents are useful and safe to use with and after thrombolysis and when.
5. What vascular lesions respond best to intravenous vs IA treatment. These routes have not been compared directly in trials.
6. The role of modern brain and vascular imaging in selecting patients for treatment
7. Comparison of thrombolysis with mechanical vascular opening techniques, such as angioplasty/stenting
8. Thrombolysis vs GP IIb/IIIa agents.
9. Thrombolysis combined with neuroprotective strategies

IA, intra-arterial; GP, glycoprotein.

IMAGING ADVANCES SINCE 1990

When the European Cooperative Acute Stroke Study and NINDS trials were planned, available technology was limited. The 1990s witnessed a dramatic up-grade in MRI, CT, and ultrasound technology. Diffusion-weighted (DWI) MRI can predict with reasonable accuracy the location and amount of irreversible ischemic damage soon after symptom onset. T2* weighted (susceptibility) images were able to show acute brain and subarachnoid hemorrhages. MRA was able to show occlusions of neck and large intracranial arteries. Perfusion-weighted MRI showed underperfused brain regions. When DWI, perfusion-weighted, and MRA were combined, clinicians were finally able to determine, quickly and safely, the presence and location of arterial occlusions, the amount of brain likely already infarcted, and the amount of brain threatened by underperfusion.

CT capability also developed. Helical CT scanners became more widely available. They provided films more quickly and accurately than older scanners. Dye injection led to vascular opacification and generation of vascular data. Software allowed rapid reformatting showing a CTA, and late films showed perfusion data because underperfused areas had less dye density.

Clinicians gained experience with Duplex ultrasound scans of the neck arteries. In Germany and elsewhere clinicians became adept at using Doppler ultrasound at the bedside and in the emergency room. Neck and transcranial Doppler was able to accurately show complete occlusions of large arteries in the neck and head. Ultrasound testing was cheap and portable.

In the years since NINDS was reported, doctors have developed the ability to safely and quickly determine the data needed to logically choose acute and subsequent therapy for their acute stroke patients, contingent on availability and the ability to use modern technology, as well as the ability to interpret the results. Since brain imaging was mandated, the addition of CTA to CT and either MRA or DWI to standard MRI takes only a few minutes. The technology greatly aids experienced stroke clinicians. It does not replace the clinical encounter; it merely refines and quantifies the anatomy, pathology, and pathophysiology of the stroke.

SUGGESTIONS (5)

Physicians at medical centers that intend to treat acute stroke patients should develop systems and protocols for rapid delivery, efficient evaluation, and rapid throughput of patients with suspected acute strokes and transient ischemic attacks. Physicians managing the patients should be experienced in stroke care and the technology available must be adequate.

What should be done if a community medical center is not adequately staffed with physicians who are experienced in stroke care and modern technology? There are three viable options.

1. Choose not to accept patients suspected of having acute stroke and divert them to a nearby stroke center if such is available.
2. Upgrade the facility to meet standards and then accept patients. Upgrading requires improving available technology and adding experienced stroke clinicians, and facilitating throughput.
3. If it is not feasible to divert to a nearby facility consider connecting with such a facility by telemedicine or consultative arrangements to facilitate care.

What if a medical center has experienced stroke clinicians and modern technology? How should patients be managed?

1. If the patient is seen within 3 h, the cause is clinically clear (e.g., atrial fibrillation), and CT does not show a large region of hypodensity, it is reasonable to give t-PA using present guidelines without further study.
2. If the cause is not obvious and/or the patient does not meet guidelines (presentation after 3 h, stroke on awakening, >3 h of symptoms, minor or improving deficit, or usual exclusion) then further brain and vascular imaging are recommended This could be MRI with T2*, DWI, MRA, CT with CTA, or CT or MRI with neck and transcranial Doppler.
3. Key to these decisions are knowledge of the presence, location, and nature of arterial occlusion; time since symptom onset, if known; presence and amount of infarction and threatened brain; availability of other potentially effective treatments; and the wishes of patients informed about the risks and benefits of your recommendations.

REFERENCES

1. Adams HP, Brott TG, Furlan AJ, et al. Use of thrombolytic drugs. A supplement to the guidelines for the management of patients with acute ischemic stroke. A statement for Health Care Professionals from a special writing group of the Stroke Council American Heart Association. *Stroke* 1996; 27:1711–1718.
2. Quality Standards Subcommittee of the American Academy of Neurology, Practice advisory: Thrombolytic therapy for acute ischemic stroke- summary statement. *Neurology* 1996;47:835–839.
3. The National Institute of Neurological Disorders and Stroke rt-PA Study Group. Tissue plasminogen activator for acute ischemic stroke. *N Engl J Med* 1995;333:1581–1587.
4. Caplan LR, Mohr JP, Kistler JP, Koroshetz W. Thrombolysis: not a panacea for ischemic stroke. *N Eng J Med* 1997;337:1309–1310, 1313.
5. Caplan LR. Thrombolysis 2004: the good, the bad, and the ugly. Reviews in *Neurological Diseases* 2004;1:16–26.
6. Caplan LR. Evidence-based medicine: concerns of a clinical neurologist. *J Neurology Neurosurg Psychiatry* 2001;71:569–576.
7. Caplan LR. Caplan's Stroke, a clinical approach. Boston:Butterworth-Heinemann, 2000, pp. 119–169.
8. Caplan LR. The case against the present guidelines for stroke thrombolysis. In: *Thrombolytic Therapy for Stroke, 1st Ed.,* Lyden PD ed. Totowa, NJ:Humana Press, 2001, pp.223–235.
9. Marler JR, Price TR, Clark GL, et al. Morning increase in onset of ischemic stroke. *Stroke* 1989;20:473–476.
10. Barber PA, Zhang J, Demchuk AM, Hill MD, Buchan AM. Why are stroke patients excluded from tPA therapy? *Neurology* 2001;56:1015–1020.
11. Fink JN, Kumar S, Horkan C, et al. The stroke patient who woke up. Clinical and radiological features including diffusion and perfusion MRI. *Stroke* 2002;33:988–993.
12. Warach S. New imaging strategies for patients selection for thrombolytic and neuroprotective strategies. *Neurology* 2001; 57(Suppl 2):S48–S52.
13. von Kummer R, Weber J. Brain and vascular imaging in acute ischemic stroke: the potential of computed tomography. *Neurology* 1997;49(Suppl 4):S52–S55.
14. Lee KH, Cho S-J, Byun HS, et al. Triphasic perfusion computed tomography in acute middle cerebral artery stroke. A correlation with angiographic findings. *Arch Neurol* 2000;57:990–999.
15. Fisher M, Prichard JW, Warach S. New magnetic resonance techniques for acute ischemic stroke. *JAMA* 1995;274:908–911.
16. Staroselskaya I, Chaves C, Silver B, et al. Relationship between magnetic resonance arterial patency and perfusion-diffusion mismatch in acute ischemic stroke and its potential clinical use. *Arch Neurol* 2001;58:1069–1074.
17. Wintermark M, Reichhart M, Thiran J-P, et al. Prognostic accuracy of cerebral blood flow measurement by perfusion computed tomography, at the time of emergency room admission, in acute stroke patients. *Ann Neurol* 2002;51:417–432.
18. Nabavi DG, Kloska SP, Nam E-M, et al. MOSAIC: multimodal stroke assessment using computed tomography. Novel diagnostic approach for the prediction of infarction size and clinical outcome. *Stroke* 2002;33:2819–2826.
19. Linfante I, Llinas R, Schlaug G, Chaves C, Warach S, Caplan LR. Diffusion-weighted imaging and NIH Stroke Scale in the acute phase of posterior circulation stroke. *Arch Neurol* 2001;58:621–628.
20. Selim MH, Kumar S, Fink Jn, Schlaug G, Caplan LR, Linfante I. Seizures at stroke onset: should it be an absolute contraindication to thrombolysis. *Cerebrovasc Dis* 2002;14:54–57.
21. Ropper AH. "Convulsions" in basilar artery occlusion. *Neurology* 1988;38:1500–1501.

22. Saposnik G, Caplan LR. Convulsive-like movements in brainstem stroke. *Arch Neurol* 2000;58:654–657.
23. del Zoppo GJ, Higashida RT, Furlan AJ, et al. PROACT: a phase II randomized trial of recombinant pro-urokinase by direct arterial delivery in acute middle cerebral artery stroke. PROACT Investigators. Prolyse in Acute Cerebral Thromboembolism. *Stroke* 1998;29:4–11.
24. Furlan AJ, Higashida RT, Wechsler L, et al. A randomized trial of intra-arterial pro-urokinase for acute ischemic stroke of less than 6 hours duration due to middle cerebral artery occlusion. PROACT Investigators. Prolyse in Acute Cerebral Thromboembolism. *JAMA* 1999;282: 2003–2011.

15 How to Run a Code Stroke

Askiel Bruno, MD

CONTENTS

INTRODUCTION

The demonstration that early thrombolytic therapy for acute cerebral infarction improves outcomes and the Food and Drug Administration (FDA) approval of intravenous recombinant tissue plasminogen activator (rt-PA) for acute cerebral infarction (*see* Chapter 7) stimulated establishment of rapid response stroke teams and certified stroke centers in the United States. The positive results from thrombolytic acute stroke clinical trials were exciting and not surprising given the known pathophysiology of acute cerebral infarction, the similarity of acute stroke to acute myocardial infarction (MI), and the demonstrated benefits of early myocardial reperfusion in acute MI. The need for rapid response teams in acute stroke is based on the evidence that thrombolysis with intravenous rt-PA is effective only within 3 h after stroke onset *(1,2)*. The main risk in thrombolytic therapy for acute stroke is cerebral hemorrhage transformation of an infarct. Fortunately, the benefits of thrombolytic therapy in acute cerebral infarction overshadow the risks and the bleeding can be minimized by careful patient selection according to guidelines (*see* Chapter 18).

From: *Current Clinical Neurology: Thrombolytic Therapy for Acute Stroke, Second Edition*
Edited by: P. D. Lyden

Benefits to acute stroke victims from early hospital arrival extend beyond thrombolytic therapy. Some complications, such as aspiration pneumonia, deep venous thrombosis (DVT), cardiac arrhythmias, and metabolic or hemodynamic derangements can be prevented and treated. Additional complications specific to primary intracranial hemorrhage can also be prevented and treated most effectively when patients present to the hospital early. Thus, *the urgency to bring acute stroke victims to stroke centers is based on the time-sensitive effectiveness of thrombolytic therapy and other therapies to prevent complications*. The reasoning behind the development of certified stroke centers can be compared to the benefits seen in the management of trauma victims through the establishment of certified Level 1 trauma centers. Because approx 700,000 people suffer a stroke in the United States each year, even small improvements in outcomes will affect a large number of patients.

THE STROKE TEAM

The stroke team is the driving force behind an effective code stroke system. Although every medical center has its own unique problems, and every stroke team will be different, there are some common elements that are in important in any setting (Table 1). The team should consist of individuals eager to and capable of improving stroke outcomes. There are considerable advantages to the stroke team including diverse individuals who are visible, readily available, and dedicated to improving acute stroke outcomes. Team availability may be enhanced by a system of pagers linked to a single and stable number so that a single call will activate the stroke team with certainty; changing numbers with every call-schedule change causes confusion and missed opportunities. Communication and teamwork may be enhanced by regular team meetings. Leadership by one individual to oversee, coordinate, and assume responsibility for all the functions of a stroke team is essential, but this individual does not necessarily need to be a neurologist or neurosurgeon; the key criterion is a dedication to optimizing stroke team operations.

Also essential for the existence of an effective stroke team is support from medical center administration. Administrative support may include funding for stroke nurses, computed tomography (CT) technologist 24/7 coverage, and stroke center certification and marketing. Certification as a primary stroke center has recently become available through the Joint Commission on Accreditation of Healthcare Organizations. The requirements for certification are based on the Brain Attack Coalition recommendations that include written care protocols, on-site neuroimaging available at all times, a stroke unit, and outcomes documentation, among others. More information about primary stroke center certification is available at www.jcaho.org.

Table 1
Key Elements of an Effective Stroke Team and Their Advantages

Key elements	*Advantages*
Composition: at least one member from various departments—EMS, emergency medicine, neurology, radiology, surgery, nursing	Diversity in knowledge and talent and broader involvement across medical center
High visibility and availability 24/7 to evaluate acute stroke victims	Stroke awareness and confidence throughout medical center and opportunity to conduct acute stroke clinical trials
Familiarity with all clinical aspects of acute stroke and guidelines for rt-PA therapy	Expert health care delivery
Agreement on the process of acute stroke evaluation and management	Unified approach to consistently high quality acute stroke care
Teamwork: concerted urgent data collection by multiple members	Coordinated and efficient approach to optimal therapy
Eagerness to continually educate community residents and health care providers	Sustained increase in stroke awareness
Acute stroke data collection and computerized storage	Awareness of opportunities for improvement and tracking of trends
Identified leader: to contribute an additional effort to promote the usefulness and maintain the existence of the team and with all other groups for maximal effectiveness	Enhanced communications within team
Stroke center certification	Recognition by community and peers

EMS, emergency medical services; rt-PA, recombinant tissue plasminogen activator.

ON THE SCENE

Community Awareness

First, the patient or a witness must recognize that a probable stroke has occurred. Inability to recognize the symptoms of acute stroke or denial of the symptoms and delayed calling for help is a common reason for delayed presentation and consequent ineligibility for treatment with rt-PA. Various adult community education strategies have shown small improvements in the ability of the general public to recognize stroke symptoms. Better general awareness is likely to increase the proportion of stroke patients presenting within 2 h after symptom onset. Patients presenting beyond 2 h after stroke onset often cannot be fully evaluated for possible thrombolytic therapy within 3 h.

Emergency Medical Services

Ideally, emergency medical services (EMS) should be the system first contacted after stroke symptom onset. It is vital for EMS personnel to be aware of acute stroke symptoms and mechanisms and to have a low index of suspicion for stroke in the appropriate setting. Suspicion of acute stroke should be followed by urgent dispatch of an ambulance equipped at least for basic life support. Once on the scene, EMS personnel follow a set of guidelines that include hemodynamic and respiratory assessments. If the hemodynamic and respiratory parameters are stable and the history is consistent with stroke, a focused neurological assessment can be done to further evaluate for stroke. The Cincinnati Prehospital Stroke Scale *(3)* considers facial drooping, arm drifting from horizontal, and speech disturbance, and is useful in distinguishing stroke from other disorders on the scene. Once acute stroke is determined to be the likely diagnosis, transport to the nearest appropriate emergency department (ED) should proceed without delay.

During transit, other important steps taken by EMS include inserting an intravenous line, measuring capillary blood glucose level, notifying the destination ED that a likely acute stroke victim is on the way, and an initial attempt at establishing the exact time of stroke onset. Neurological deficits in the patient—including neglect or aphasia—may require that a witness be found to estimate the time of stroke onset; if possible the witness should accompany the victim to the hospital or be available for questioning by the stroke team by telephone. Intravenous infusion in the field may include isotonic solutions, such as normal saline, but should not include hypotonic solutions, such as 5% dextrose, as they may predispose to cerebral edema. Notification of the ED that a likely acute stroke victim is on the way should be followed by activation of the stroke team and the CT scanner technologist to expedite assessment once the victim arrives at the ED.

IN THE EMERGENCY DEPARTMENT

Rapid Assessment: Time Is Brain

In many centers, the stroke team functions best if activated before the patient arrives in the ED allowing at least some of the team members to be present when the patient arrives. On arrival at the ED, potential stroke victims should be reassessed without delay. Vital signs and ventilation need to be documented and monitored frequently. Blood should be drawn for laboratory testing. At least one well functioning intravenous line should be available, and although two lines are often recommended, there should be no delay in testing, such as CT brain scanning. Once hemodynamic stability is established, a focused and brief history and physical examination should be done to confirm the likelihood of stroke and to generate a preliminary differential diagnosis. Acute stroke is the likely diagnosis if a focal neurological deficit develops abruptly in the absence of trauma or obvious seizure. If acute stroke is suspected, head CT without contrast should be obtained with minimal delay to rule out conditions other than cerebral infarction—especially hemorrhage—and to look for large ischemic hypodensity. Frank hypodensity that is visible on the initial CT and is greater than one-third of the middle cerebral artery (MCA) territory, has been shown to be a risk for serious hemorrhagic transformation of the infarct (*see* Chapter 16) *(4)* and is currently considered a contraindication to rt-PA therapy. Some stroke centers have protocols for MRI rather than a CT as the initial or only neuroimaging test for acute stroke (*see* Chapter 17).

Focused History

A crucial aspect of acute stroke diagnosis is to establish that lateralized neurological deficits occurred suddenly. It is important to determine if similar symptoms have occurred with a previous stroke, which would suggest that a toxic or metabolic derangement may be causing exacerbation of previous stroke symptoms. Next in urgency is estimation of the time of stroke onset. Patients with acute stroke may inaccurately estimate the time of stroke onset, so ideally a witness should be questioned as well. For patients who wake up with stroke deficits, the time of onset is taken as the last time that they were completely free of the deficits. For most such patients this is usually when they fell asleep the night before, but some patients report awakening in the middle of the night without deficits. A useful technique is the so-called "time-anchor"; some events occur at a specific times that can be linked to the onset of symptoms. For example, if the family was watching television, stroke timing can be related to the beginning or ending of a specific program. The case scenarios at the end of this book include several examples of stroke onset estimation.

Focused Neurological Examination

The initial physical examination should be focused so that only the essential elements needed to make a confident diagnosis of stroke are obtained expeditiously. The neurological deficits may include various combinations depending on lesion location. The mental status is observed as the examiner meets the patient and can be challenging to interpret. The first observation assesses the level of consciousness. If the patient is fully alert, mental deficits, such as aphasia and amnesia, can be interpreted with confidence. However, if the patient is lethargic or stuporous, mental deficits can result from decreased consciousness rather than a focal brain lesion.

Presence of aphasia is usually recognized during an unsuccessful attempt at obtaining the medical history from the patient. There may be decreased comprehension, decreased ability to express oneself fluently, or both. Patients with aphasia usually cannot respond correctly when asked about the current date or place and they often realize their communication deficit and are frustrated by it. Aphasia implies left fronto-temporal brain dysfunction and is often associated with right hemiparesis.

In the presence of decreased consciousness, mental status assessment is more challenging; the severity of mental deficits needs to be judged in relation to the extent of decreased consciousness. Decreased consciousness could result from a stroke, a metabolic or toxic derangement, or may represent a post-ictal state.

The National Institutes of Health Stroke Scale (NIHSS) is useful for quantifying the neurological deficits: the higher the score the greater the deficit. A score of 4 or less usually indicates a mild stroke, but severe aphasia receives a score of only 3, and severe hemianopsia, a 2. Moderate strokes usually score between 5 and15 and severe strokes 20 or higher. Patients with low NIHSS scores (<5) generally do well and patients with high scores (>22) do poorly regardless of treatment. The NIHSS should complement the clinical impression regarding stroke severity when deciding about rt-PA candidacy but should not dictate treatment without physician judgment; the appended cases offer several useful examples of mild strokes (low NIHSS scores) that should be treated.

Differential Diagnosis of Stroke

The most common conditions mimicking acute stroke are post-ictal paralysis, migraine with prolonged aura, and unmasking of old stroke symptoms by toxic or metabolic effects. Patients with history of seizures or any underlying brain lesion can present with post-ictal paralysis. Also, the acute stroke can occasionally cause an early seizure. Toxic or metabolic derangements mimicking acute stroke include a wide spectrum of infections and metabolic abnormalities and this presentation is more likely in the elderly, especially the nursing home resident. Brain tumors, subdural and epidural hematomas, and psychogenic disorders are less likely to mimic acute stroke. With an accurate history, physical examination, and head CT, a confident diagnosis is usually possible by an experienced stroke team.

Acute cerebral infarction is a dynamic process and sometimes patients improve considerably in the ED during preparation for possible rt-PA therapy. This fluctuation usually suggests that rt-PA does not need to be given. However, complete resolution of symptoms within 24 h and absence of stroke on subsequent neuroimaging (suggesting transient ischemic attack) is rare in patients presenting with deficits lasting more than 60 min *(5)*. Most fluctuating patients end up with considerable deficits if not treated aggressively and thrombolytic therapy is often given to patients with an oscillating deficit, even if the deficit is quite mild at the time the decision is made.

Thrombolytic Decision

Often the history and physical examination are completed soon after the head CT is done and the laboratory test results become available. At that time, the decision can be made whether the patient qualifies for intravenous rt-PA therapy. An acute stroke rt-PA assessment sheet (Table 2) may be used during code stroke to provide a visible evolving record of the data for a more rapid and confident treatment decision. The various data items in this sheet could be added as they become available so that it can be clearly and promptly documented that either all criteria for rt-PA treatment are met or that an excluding criterion is present. Weighing the patient or estimating the weight is important because the rt-PA dose is based on weight.

Two other acute stroke treatments showed positive results but are not FDA-approved at this time (*see* Chapter 6). Ancrod, a defibrinogenating drug derived from snake venom, was shown to be effective if administered within 3 h after stroke onset *(6)*. Ancrod was given intravenously over 72 h and boluses were given at 96 and 120 h after stroke onset. The dose was adjusted to keep plasma fibrinogen in a low target range 59–67 mg/dL. The other treatment shown to be effective is intra-arterial pro-urokinase (a urokinase precursor) for patients with middle cerebral artery occlusion treated within 6 h after stroke onset *(7)*. Patients who do not qualify for intravenous rt-PA therapy usually receive standard therapies. Some centers have protocols for using intra-arterial thrombolytics (usually rt-PA), but this is not approved by the FDA.

Other treatment options currently in use but not proven effective and not FDA approved for acute stroke include anticoagulation with heparin or fractionated heparin and antiplatelet drugs. Although long-term anticoagulation with warfarin is effective in preventing thromboembolic events in some patients, anticoagulation during acute stroke has not been established as beneficial in any patient subgroup. Similarly, antiplatelet therapy has been shown to reduce the rate of thromboembolic events following stroke or transient ischemic attack, but it does not need to start on the first day of stroke.

Blood Pressure Management

Fluctuations in blood pressure can have significant effects on cerebral perfusion and stroke outcomes. In one acute cerebral infarction clinical trial, higher doses of intravenous nimodipine were associated with lower blood pressures and worse clinical outcomes *(8)*. There are many anecdotal reports of neurological worsening during acute stroke associated with over-aggressive blood pressure reduction. During acute cerebral ischemia, local autoregulation is impaired and a lower blood pressure can translate into decreased cerebral perfusion and result in increased brain injury. Thus, it is not recommended to lower the blood pressure during acute cerebral infarction unless the systolic reading is more than 220 mmHg and the diastolic reading is more than 120 mmHg, a definite medical

Table 2
Acute Stroke rt-PA Assessment Sheet

Patient Name: ____________________ MR#: ____________________
Date of birth: ____________________ Age (yr): ________ Sex: M ___ F ___
Weight ______________ kg

			Comments
Date and time of stroke onset (last time without neurological deficit)	____________		____________
Time arrived in ED	____________		____________
Time at 3 h after stroke onset	____________		____________
Seizure at stroke onset	Yes	No	____________
Serious head trauma or another stroke in the past 3 mo	Yes	No	____________
Major surgery in the past 14 d	Yes	No	____________
Gastrointestinal or urinary bleeding in the past 21 d	Yes	No	____________
Any past intracranial hemorrhage	Yes	No	____________
Currently taking oral anticoagulant	Yes	No	____________
PT > 15 or INR > 1.7	Yes	No	____________
Platelets < 100,000/mm^3	Yes	No	____________
50 < glucose > 400 mg/dL	Yes	No	____________
Serial BP measurements (must remain <185/110 mmHg)			
Intracranial hemorrhage, other mass lesion or ischemic hypodensity > one-third MCA territory	Yes	No	____________
Additional concerns	Yes	No	____________

Rt-PA given: Yes No If No, why not? ____________________
Minutes from stroke onset to:

CT completion ______ MRI completion ______ Starting intravenous rt-PA: _____

Any complications during hospitalization?: Yes No

____
____
____

rt-PA, recombinant tissue plasminogen activator; ED, emergency department; MR, medical record; PT, prothrombic time; INR, international normalized ratio; BP, blood pressure; MCA, middle cerebral artery; CT, computed tomography; MRI, magnetic resonance imaging.

indication is present, or rt-PA has been given *(9)*. The recommended target decrease in blood pressure is 10–15% if necessary. Table 3 summarizes the recommendations for blood pressure management during acute cerebral infarction.

For patients who may be candidates for rt-PA therapy, gentle blood pressure lowering with nitropaste, or low doses of labetalol (up to 40 mg), is indicated if the blood pressure is somewhat higher than the maximum allowed (185/110 mmHg) (Table 3). If this gentle approach does not bring the blood pressure below 185/110 mmHg, rt-PA should not be given because of increased risk for hemorrhagic transformation of the infarct. Once rt-PA is given, aggressive blood pressure control until the reading is below 180/105 mmHg is recommended. Higher doses of labetalol are recommended (up to 300 mg) and, if insufficient, intravenous nicardipine or nitroprusside can be used. There is no single ideal pressure for all patients. The higher the premorbid blood pressure the riskier it might be to lower it during the acute period (first 48 h). Because wide fluctuations in blood pressure during acute stroke can significantly impact the outcome and because blood pressure can be controlled, it is important to admit acute stroke victims to hospital units able to monitor the blood pressure frequently and use continuous monitoring when needed.

Glucose Level Management

Common symptoms of hypoglycemia are systemic and include adrenergic (diaphoresis, tachycardia, anxiety) and neurological manifestations (tremulousness, dizziness, blurred vision, psychomotor slowing, seizure). However, some of these manifestations may be focal, mimicking a stroke. Thus, capillary glucose should be checked as soon as possible during acute stroke and if below 50 mg/dL, intravenous concentrated dextrose should be given and rt-PA therapy withheld. Patients being treated with glucose lowering drugs are at risk for hypoglycemia.

At the other end of the glucose spectrum is hyperglycemia. Current evidence suggests that hyperglycemia during acute cerebral infarction may augment the brain injury. Secondary observational analyses in clinical trials show a linear relationship between increasing admission glucose level and worse outcomes *(10,11)*. This effect appears to be greater with reperfusion than without it *(12)*, perhaps because hyperglycemia contributes to reperfusion injury. Tight control of hyperglycemia during acute myocardial infarction *(13)* and in critically ill, ventilated, postsurgical patients *(14)* has been shown to improve clinical outcomes compared to usual care with higher glucose levels. Clinical trials for tight glycemic control during acute cerebral infarction are currently in progress.

In addition to exacerbating ischemic brain injury, admission hyperglycemia is associated with symptomatic hemorrhagic conversion of infarcts in patients treated with thrombolytics *(11,15)*. Although tight glycemic control with intra-

Table 3
American Stroke Association Panel Recommendations for Blood Pressure Management During Acute Cerebral Infarction

Blood pressure	*Recommendation*
	Not rt-PA candidate
Systolic ≤220 and diastolic ≤120	Monitor without therapy unless medically necessary, e.g., aortic dissection, acute MI; treat other metabolic derangements, complications, and pain
Systolic >220 or diastolic 121–140	Intravenous Labetalol[a] or Nicardipine[b]; aim for 10–15% BP reduction
Diastolic >140	Intravenous Nitroprusside IV[c]; continuous BP monitoring; aim for 10–15% BP reduction
	rt-PA candidate—pretreatment
Systolic >185 or diastolic >110	Intravenous Labetalol up to 40 mg or Nitropaste 1–2 in; If BP remains >185/110, do not treat with rt-PA
	rt-PA treated—first 24–48 h
Monitor BP at least every 15 min for 2 h, then every 30 min for 6 h, then every 60 min for 16 h	
Systolic 180–230 or diastolic 105–120	Intravenouse Labetalol[a]
Systolic >230 or diastolic 121–140	Intravenous Labetalol[a] or Nicardipine[b]
Diastolic >140	Intravenous Nitroprusside[c]; continuous BP monitoring

[a]10–20 mg intravenous bolus over 1–2 min and may repeat or double every 10 min up to 300 mg or start drip at 2–8 mg/min after first bolus.

[b]Start with 5 mg/h and increase by 2.5 mg/h every 5 min to desired BP (maximum 15 mg/h).

[c]Start with 0.5 μg/kg/min and titrate to desired BP.

rt-PA, recombinant tissue plasminogen activator; MI, myocardial infarction; BP, blood pressure.

venous insulin requires additional effort and cost and is not standard of care, it might be best at this time to monitor elevated glucose levels closely during acute stroke, such as every 4 h, and administer a subcutaneous insulin sliding scale whenever the glucose is more than 200 mg/dL. This seems feasible and safe.

Body Temperature Management

Hypothermia is well known to slow the decay of biological tissues. It makes winter hibernation and successful resuscitation of ice water drowning victims possible. Animal studies consistently show that brain hypothermia slows and decreases the extent of ischemic brain injury *(16)*, but external hypothermia therapy is challenging to apply to human stroke, partly because of a larger head size. Application of hypothermia therapy usually requires admission to an intensive care unit and special labor-intensive procedures. Serious complications related to hypothermia therapy include infections and cardiac arrhythmias.

In two randomized trials, mild hypothermia therapy (core temperature 33°C) with external cooling improved neurological outcomes after cardiac arrest *(17,18)*. In acute stroke, meta-analysis shows that elevated body temperature is associated with worse clinical outcomes than normothermia *(19)*. Pilot studies of the feasibility of therapeutic hypothermia in acute stroke have been done and efficacy trials are anticipated.

The relationship between body temperature and brain injury appears linear within certain parameters. Thus, elevated body temperature during acute stroke likely increases the extent of brain injury compared to normothermia. Although hypothermia therapy in acute stroke is not standard at this time, it might be prudent to carefully monitor body shell temperature (axillary or sublingually) and treat hyperthermia (>98.6°F or >37.0°C) rapidly. Acetaminophen, cool ambient temperature, and cooling blankets or ice packs are relatively simple and safe options to reduce body temperature toward normal.

Stroke Unit Admission

Clinical trials show that admission of acute stroke victims to specialized stroke units results in improved outcomes compared to general hospital wards. One study randomized acute stroke patients to stroke unit (n = 152), general wards (n = 152), or care at home (n = 153) *(20)*. Stroke unit care was associated with significantly lower mortality and disability compared to the other two groups during a 1-yr follow-up. Further analysis of this cohort showed that the improved outcomes are limited to patients with large-vessel disease *(21)*.

Another study randomized 110 acute stroke patients to stroke unit care and 110 to general ward care *(22)*. After a 1-yr follow-up, stroke unit care was associated with a significantly better functional status than general ward care. After 5 yr, stroke unit care was associated with significantly reduced mortality, increased chance of living at home, and better quality of life *(23,24)*. In a meta-analysis of five randomized trials, admission of 551 acute stroke patients to a stroke unit was associated with a 28% reduction in mortality at 3 mo and 22% at 12 mo as compared to 627 admissions to a general ward *(25)*.

Ideally, acute stroke victims should be admitted to a unit, such as an intermediate care unit, where more than minimal monitoring is feasible. Guidelines for monitoring and possible intervention following rt-PA therapy necessitate admission to at least an intermediate care unit. The nurses and other support staff on a dedicated stroke unit could be valuable members of the stroke team.

Data Collection and Storage

Data collection and storage improves stroke team's ability to know the statistics at their stroke center, to look for opportunities to improve care, and to look at important trends. Useful data to collect might include the number of acute stroke victims presenting within a defined time after stroke onset, number treated with intravenous rt-PA, time from ED arrival to CT, time from ED arrival to start of rt-PA, and reasons for exclusion from rt-PA therapy. Such information should optimize efforts to increase the fraction of acute stroke victims treated with rt-PA in that community. Also, this information will be needed by accreditation agencies and might be of interest to the community. To be useful, such data should be stored in appropriate computerized databases and could be de-identified for privacy. Hospital administration can make a significant contribution towards data collection and storage by providing personnel and appropriate equipment for this task.

REFERENCES

1. The NINDS rt-PA Stroke Study Group. Tissue plasminogen activator for acute ischemic stroke. *N Engl J Med* 1995;333:1581–1587.
2. Clark WM, Wissman S, Albers GW, Jhamandas JH, Madden KP, Hamilton S. Recombinant tissue-type plasminogen activator (Alteplase) for ischemic stroke 3 to 5 hours after symptom onset. The ATLANTIS Study: a randomized controlled trial. *JAMA* 1999;282:2019–2026.
3. Kothari RU, Pancioli A, Liu T, Brott T, Broderick J. Cincinnati Prehospital Stroke Scale: reproducibility and validity. *Ann Emerg Med* 1999;33:373–378.
4. The NINDS t-PA Stroke Study Group. Intracerebral hemorrhage after intravenous t-PA therapy for ischemic stroke. The NINDS t-PA Stroke Study Group. *Stroke* 1997;28:2109-2118.
5. Levy DE. How transient are transient ischemic attacks? Neurology 1988;38:674–677.
6. Sherman DG, Atkinson RP, Chippendale T, et al. Intravenous ancrod for treatment of acute ischemic stroke: the STAT study: a randomized controlled trial. Stroke Treatment with Ancrod Trial. *JAMA* 2000;283:2395–2403.
7. Furlan A, Higashida R, Wechsler L, et al. Intra-arterial prourokinase for acute ischemic stroke. The PROACT II study: a randomized controlled trial. Prolyse in Acute Cerebral Thromboembolism. *JAMA* 1999;282:2003–2011.
8. Ahmed N, Nasman P, Wahlgren NG. Effect of intravenous nimodipine on blood pressure and outcome after acute stroke. *Stroke* 2000;31:1250–1255.
9. Adams HP, Jr., Adams RJ, Brott T, et al. Guidelines for the early management of patients with ischemic stroke: a scientific statement from the Stroke Council of the American Stroke Association. *Stroke* 2003;34:1056–1083.
10. Bruno A, Biller J, Adams HP Jr, et al. Acute blood glucose level and outcome from ischemic stroke. Trial of ORG 10172 in Acute Stroke Treatment (TOAST) Investigators. *Neurology* 1999;52:280–284.
11. Bruno A, Levine SR, Frankel MR, et al. Admission glucose level and clinical outcomes in the NINDS rt-PA Stroke Trial. *Neurology* 2002;59:669–674.
12. Alvarez-Sabin J, Molina CA, Montaner J, et al. Effects of admission hyperglycemia on stroke outcome in reperfused tissue plasminogen activator-treated patients *editorial comment. *Stroke* 2003;34:1235–1241.

13. Malmberg K, Ryden L, Efendic S, et al. Randomized trial of insulin-glucose infusion followed by subcutaneous insulin treatment in diabetic patients with acute myocardial infarction (DIGAMI study): effects on mortality at 1 year. *J Am Coll Cardiol* 1995;26:57–65.
14. van den Berghe G, Wouters P, Weekers F, et al. Intensive insulin therapy in the critically ill patients. *N Engl J Med* 2001;345:1359–1367.
15. Kase CS, Furlan AJ, Wechsler LR, et al. Cerebral hemorrhage after intra-arterial thrombolysis for ischemic stroke: the PROACT II trial. *Neurology* 2001;57:1603–1610.
16. Ginsberg MD, Busto R. Combating hyperthermia in acute stroke: a significant clinical concern. *Stroke* 1998;29:529–534.
17. Group THACAS. Mild therapeutic hypothermia to improve the neurologic outcome after cardiac arrest. *N Engl J Med* 2002;346:549–556.
18. Bernard SA, Gray TW, Buist MD, et al. Treatment of comatose survivors of out-of-hospital cardiac arrest with induced hypothermia. *N Engl J Med* 2002;346:557–563.
19. Hajat C, Hajat S, Sharma P: Effects of poststroke pyrexia on stroke outcome: a meta-analysis of studies in patients. *Stroke* 2000;31:410–414.
20. Kalra L, Evans A, Perez I, Knapp M, Donaldson N, Swift CG. Alternative strategies for stroke care: a prospective randomised controlled trial. *Lancet* 2000;356:894–899.
21. Evans A, Harraf F, Donaldson N, Kalra L. Randomized controlled study of stroke unit care versus stroke team care in different stroke subtypes. *Stroke* 2002;33:449–455.
22. Indredavik B, Bakke F, Solberg R, Rokseth R, Haaheim LL, Holme I. Benefit of a stroke unit: a randomized controlled trial. *Stroke* 1991;22:1026–1031.
23. Indredavik B, Slordahl SA, Bakke F, Rokseth R, Haheim LL. Stroke unit treatment. Long-term effects. *Stroke* 1997;28:1861–1866.
24. Indredavik B, Bakke F, Slordahl SA, Rokseth R, Haheim LL. Stroke unit treatment improves long-term quality of life: a randomized controlled trial. *Stroke* 1998;29:895–899.
25. Langhorne P, Williams BO, Gilchrist W, Howie K. Do stroke units save lives? *Lancet* 1993;342:395–398.

16 The Impact of Computed Tomography on Acute Stroke Treatment

Rüdiger von Kummer

CONTENTS

INTRODUCTION

Imaging in Acute Stroke Patients

Computed tomography (CT) was the first modality to image the brain and its pathology in vivo. Before the invention of CT in the early 1970s, brain diseases were categorized according to their clinical phenotype. The term "stroke" originates from these old days of medicine, when brain hemorrhages could not be differentiated from ischemic brain diseases. It is unfortunate that we still use the term "stroke" for different diseases like subarachnoid hemorrhage (SAH), cerebral venous thrombosis, spontaneous intracerebral hemorrhages (ICH), and focal brain ischemia, which should be distinguished even though each may present as "brain attack."

From: *Current Clinical Neurology: Thrombolytic Therapy for Acute Stroke, Second Edition*
Edited by: P. D. Lyden © Humana Press Inc., Totowa, NJ

CT and magnetic resonance imaging (MRI) are today regarded as safe methods to quickly image the skull and its content. They confirm the definite diagnosis of ischemic stroke and detect the pathology of the ischemic brain in individual patients. Compared to MRI, brain imaging with CT is less expensive, quicker, more practical for severely ill patients, and in general easier to interpret. CT is consequently widely used and considered as the method of first choice for differentiating among the stroke syndromes. Moreover, CT imaging of acute stroke pathology allows the early assessment of irreversible ischemic injury *(1)*. In this chapter, we discuss whether this information has an impact on reperfusion strategies.

A CT image of the brain in acute stroke patients is not difficult to read; it is, however, not self-evident. Reading of CT needs training and instruction on how to recognize anatomy and pathology, combined with knowledge about the physical conditions of image contrast *(2)*.

CT BASICS

The image provided by CT consists of a limited number of volume units (voxels). A typical matrix has 256 × 256 voxels or 512 × 512 voxels. The matrix and the slice thickness determine spatial resolution. The X-ray attenuation of each voxel is electronically detected, grouped in relative attenuation values, named Hounsfield Units (HU), between –1023 and +3072 calibrated by the attenuation of water (HU = 0) and air (HU = –1000), and translated into 20 levels of a gray scale, which can be distinguished by the human eye. To enhance contrast resolution, the entire gray scale is used to represent the attenuation of the brain, which normally varies between 0 and 50 HU (Table 1). Another section ("window") of the entire HU scale is used if structures with different attenuation (e.g., the temporal bone) are examined. A typical CT window for the brain has a width of 80 HU. The mean value of such CT windows is called "level" and is responsible for the brightness of the image. X-ray attenuation below the range of the CT window appears as black on the image, above this range as white. A broader window diminishes the contrast between gray and white matter and impairs the detection of subtle changes in X-ray attenuation. If a CT window width of 80 HU is used, each gray level represents 4 HU. The contrast resolution is thus limited to 4 HU and could be enhanced by a reduction of the window width. A smaller window will, however, reduce the signal to noise ratio (Fig. 1).

The electron densities of the substrate under study attenuate X-rays *(3)*. In biological tissue, X-ray attenuation is directly correlated with the tissue-specific gravity *(4)*. The different electron densities of gray and white matter, brain vessels, cerebrospinal fluid (CSF), and skull allow to differentiate these structures on CT and to recognize pathological alterations.

Table 1
X-Ray Attenuation in Cranial Computed Tomography

	X-ray attenuation (HU)
Gray matter	35–45
White matter	20–30
Cerebrospinal-fluid	4–8
Skull	100–1000
Large vessels	40–50
Tissue calcification	80–150
Hematoma	70–90
Fat	–60–70
Air	–1000

HU, Hounsfield Units

TECHNICAL NOTE: HOW TO PERFORM CT IN ACUTE STROKE

If the imaging facility is informed in advance, the scanner can be kept free for the patient with acute stroke. Emergent life support should be continued during the patient's imaging test if necessary. Although a detailed neurological examination is not needed before the brain imaging is done, localizing the stroke to the posterior fossa or the cerebral hemisphere will assist in optimizing the imaging techniques selected.

CT should be performed without contrast with a rapid scan time to reduce motion artifact. A correct head position is crucial to avoid obliquity of the sections. If necessary because of motion artifact, specific section cuts can be repeated. The high density of bone often causes an artifact, which may impair visualization of the lower part of the brain stem in the posterior fossa. Small (<5 mm) transaxial sections from the posterior fossa and the base of the cerebral hemispheres and a broader CT window can minimize this artifact. The rest of the brain is best examined with 8-mm sections. Image windows should be adjusted so that gray and white matter can be easily distinguished and subtle hypodensities are detected. A window width of 70–80 HU at a center of 35–40 HU is recommended. A close communication between the stroke physician and the radiologists or technician performing the scan will enhance the information gained from CT. The image should be optimized for spatial and contrast resolution in the region of interest. Additional bone window views can be performed if head trauma is a possibility, in order to search for skull fractures, subdural air or blood, or effusions in nasal sinuses and middle ear. A contrast-enhanced scan

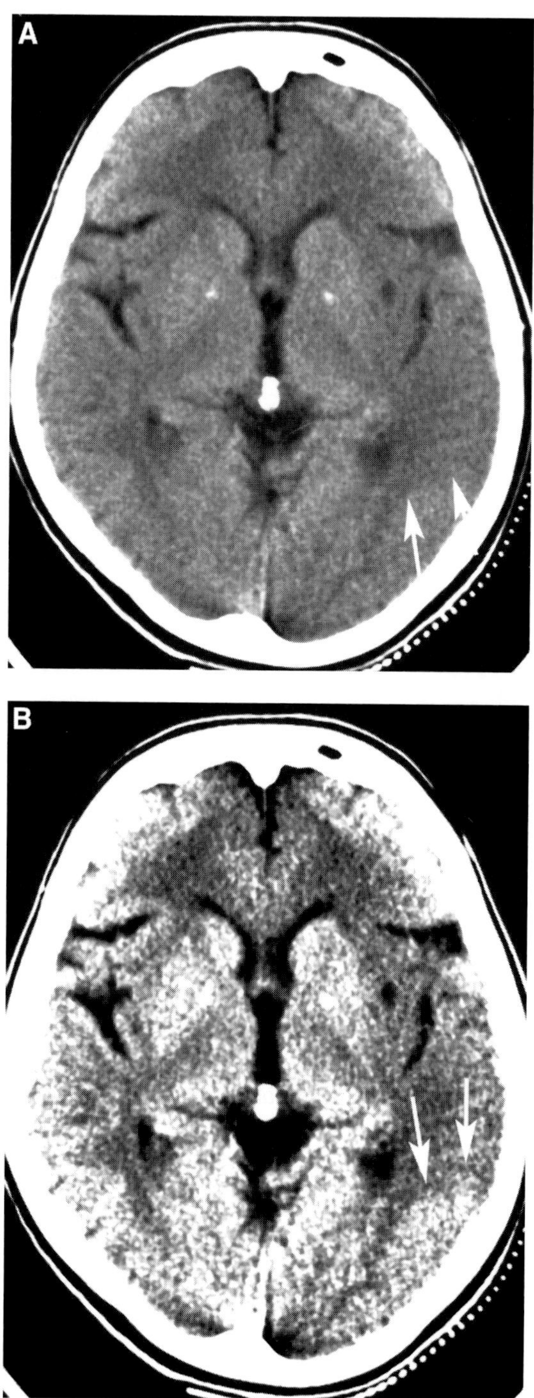
A
B

should be obtained after, if there is suspicion for neoplasm or localized infection and no MRI available. Advanced CT technology provides the opportunity of CT angiography (CTA) and CT perfusion imaging *(5,6)*. A CTA is performed after bolus injection of 130 mL nonionic contrast (injection rate: 4–5 mL/s) with a spiral scan of the brain base and three-dimensional reconstruction of the Circle of Willis on a workstation. Perfusion imaging with CT requires repeated imaging of one or more sections to measure the contrast uptake and clearance curve in each voxel. Parameter images are then calculated for cerebral blood volume (CBV), mean transit times, cerebral blood flow (CBF), or time intervals to the peaks of contrast enhancement—time to peak (Fig. 2) *(7)*.

INTERPRETATION OF CT FINDINGS

Pathological findings on CT in acute stroke patients may be thrombo-embolic occlusion of large vessels, focal brain tissue swelling caused by vasodilatation, ischemic edema, intracranial hemorrhage, focal brain tissue inflammation, or tumor like lesions. CT identifies these findings by detecting changes in X-ray attenuation of normal brain structures, a shift or replacement of brain structures by pathological substrates, or pathological contrast enhancement. A pathological increase in X-ray attenuation is called "hyperdensity," a pathological decrease "hypodensity." These terms are somewhat confusing because they do not define a fixed degree of X-ray attenuation. They are commonly used to characterize the attenuation of a structure in comparison to other tissue (e.g., in saying that a parenchymal hematoma is identified by its hyperdensity if compared with gray matter). These terms are best used, however, to characterize a change in X-ray attenuation by comparing the "density" of an affected structure to its normal "density." The symmetry of the brain structures in transaxial planes facilitates this comparison (e.g., the putamen is best evaluated by comparing its attenuation to that of the contralateral putamen and to that of the head of the caudate nucleus, because the caudate nucleus and the putamen are portions of the same anatomical structure—the striatum) (Fig. 3). It is obvious, that low-technical quality of the scan (motion artifacts, wrong window width or wrong level) and in particular any obliquity of the scan impair the recognition of real changes in X-ray attenuation (Fig. 4).

Fig. 1. (*opposite page*) Two representations of the identical section of a computed tomography (CT) in a patient with acute stroke. Both sections are displayed with the same level, but with a different window width. With a window width of 80 Hounsfield Unit (HU) (**A**), the contrast between normal cortical density and cortical hypodensity is less obvious than with a window width of 31 HU (**B**). The area of hypodensity covers part of the temporal lobe, the entire insular cortex, and the lateral rim of the putamen and is better outlined with the narrrow CT window *(arrows)*. Note the increase of noise in **B**.

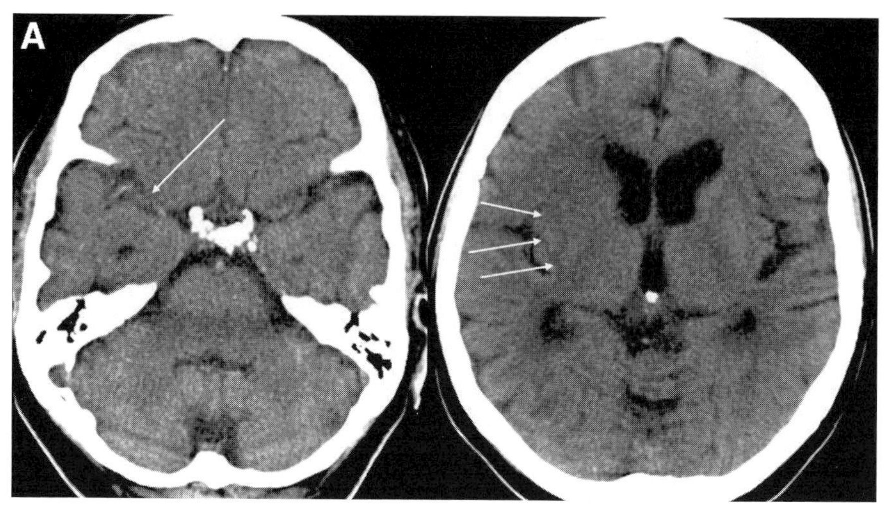
A

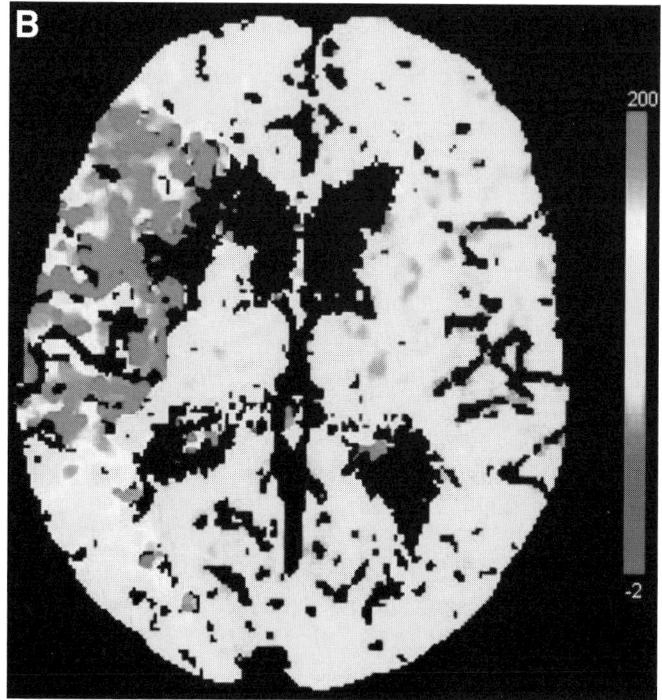
B
200
-2

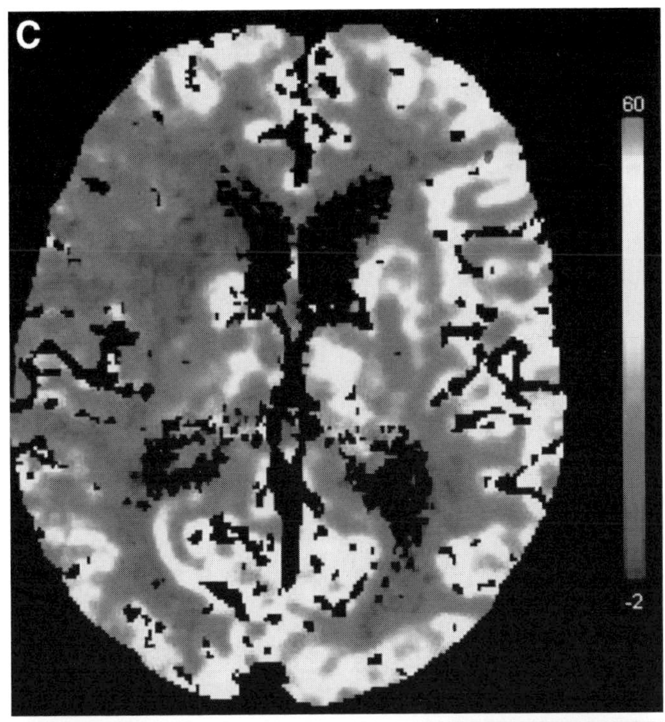
C
60
-2

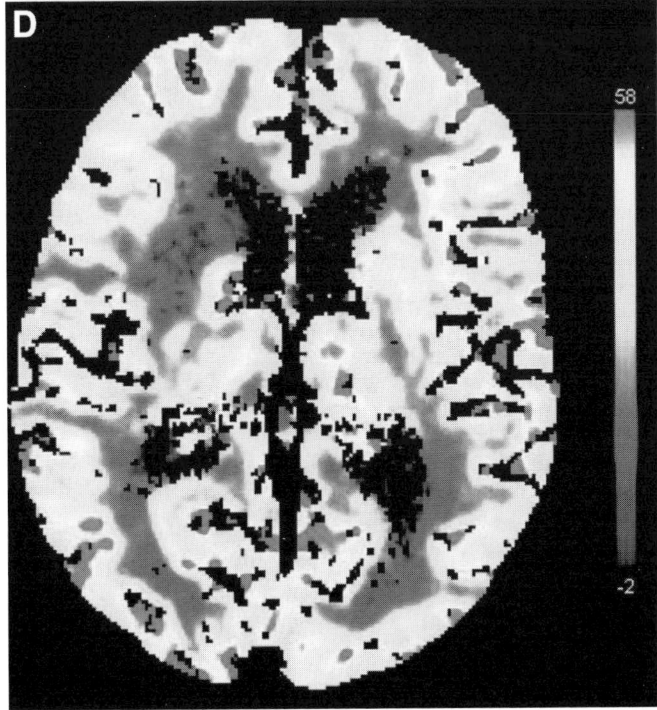
D
58
-2

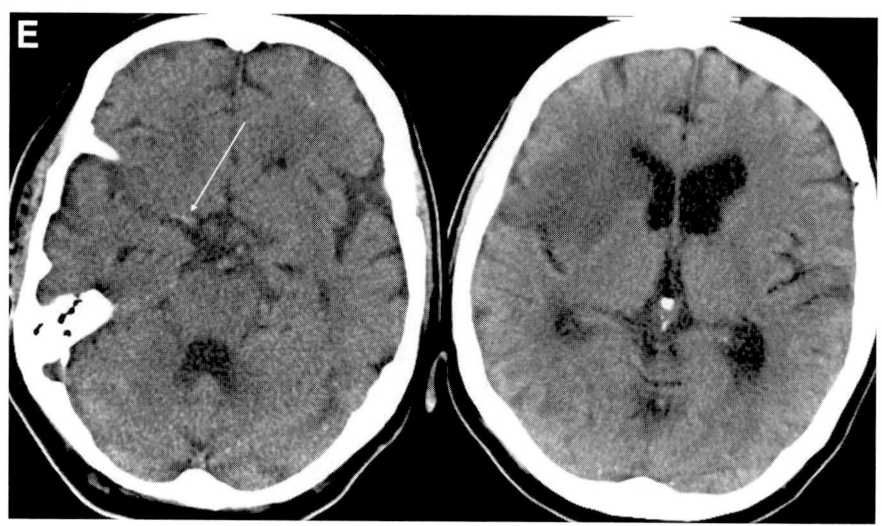

Fig. 2. Computed tomography (CT) and perfusion CT in an 82-yr-old woman 2 h after the onset of a left-sided hemiparesis. The right middle cerebral artery (MCA) trunk is occluded (**A**, *long arrow*) and the putamen and the frontal insular cortex are hypodense (**A**, *short arrows*). The time-to-peak (TTP) map, (**B**) shows an area of delayed contrast inflow exceeding the hypoattenuating volume of brain tissue. No contrast peak could be identified within the right striatum owing to very low blood flow. *See* color insert following p.110. The cerebral blood flow (CBF), (**C**) map shows diminished flow of the area indicated by the TTP map, pronounced in the right striatum and insular cortex. Cerebral blood volume (CBV) (**D**) is diminished only within the right striatum and insular cortex. *See* color insert following p.110. Despite thrombolysis, the right MCA remained occluded (**E**, *long arrow*) as shown on the follow-up CT 1 d later. The infarct covers exactly the tissue volume that was hypodense on the baseline CT and identified by low CBV. The TTP and CBF maps showed a volume of brain tissue with disturbed perfusion that did not convert into infarct until 1 d after stroke onset.

THE DETECTION OF STROKE PATHOLOGY BY CT

Thrombo-embolic occlusion of large brain arteries may result in a segmental hyperdensity of the artery (Fig. 2A,E). This finding is called "hyperdense artery sign" and is highly specific for the obstruction of this artery, if "hyperdensity" is defined as an increased X-ray attenuation of one arterial segment with various length in comparison to other portions of the same artery or its contralateral counterpart *(8)*. A hyperdense middle cerebral artery (MCA) trunk was observed in 48% of patients with angiographically proven MCA trunk occlusion *(9)*. It was recently suggested that the hematocrit of thrombi affects X-ray attenuation and thus the CT detection sensitivity *(10)*: a red thrombus—relatively higher red blood cell content—would be detected more often than a white thrombus—fewer

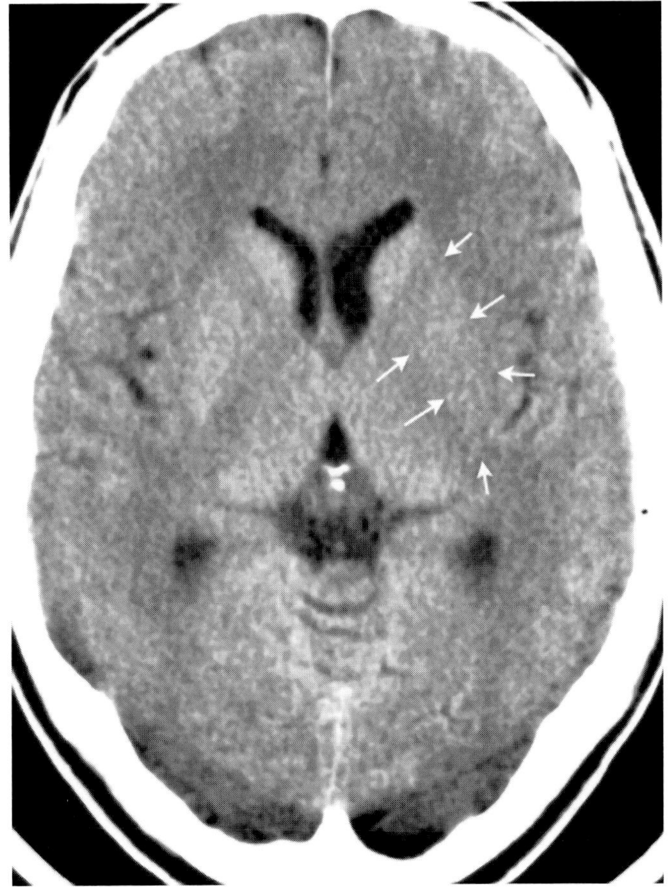

Fig. 3. Hypodensity of the left lentiform nucleus (*arrows*). X-ray attenuation is less in comparison to the right lentiform nucleus, and attenuation of the left putamen is less than the attenuation of the left head of caudate nucleus. With further decline in attenuation, the lentiform nucleus cannot be distinguished from the internal and external capsule; it will be obscured.

red blood cells–on CT. A hyperdense artery is not an "infarct sign," because arteries can occlude without a subsequent or immediate brain infarct as a result of relatively perserved collateral blood supply. A hyperdense MCA trunk in association with normal tissue density may indicate a large tissue volume at risk from hypoperfusion, but no irreversible damage. Nevertheless, a hyperdense MCA trunk is often associated with a severe stroke and large infarct *(11)*. It is, therefore, prudent to carefully examine the territory of a hyperdense artery for parenchymal hypodensity.

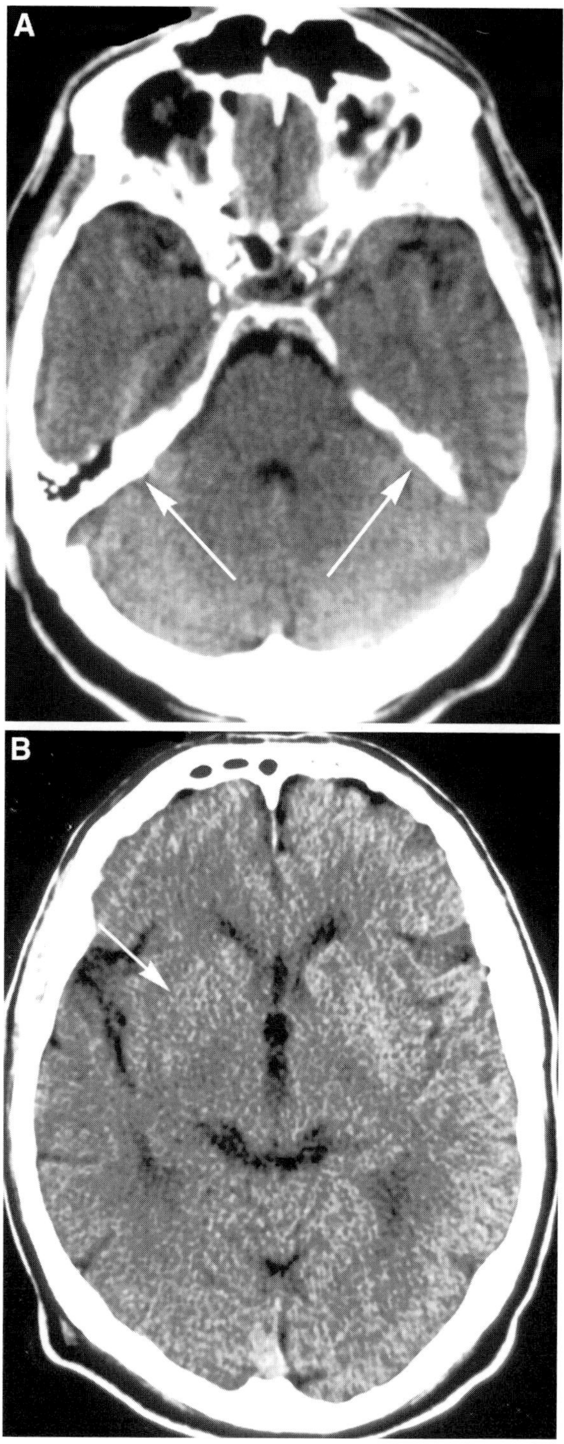
A
B

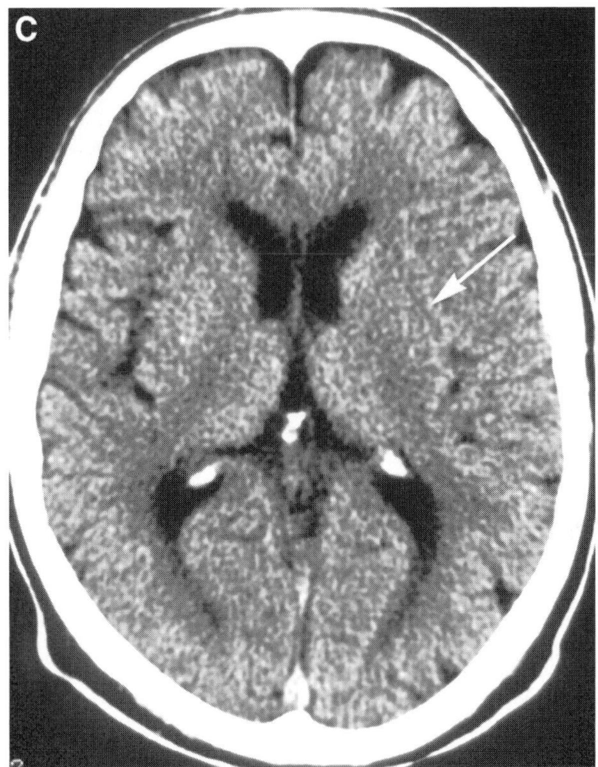

Fig. 4. The obliquity of a computed tomography scan can be recognized by comparing the upper rim of both pyramids (*arrows*). In consequence of this obliquity, the right lentiform nucleus appeared less dense in one section (**B**), and the left putamen appeared less dense in the adjacent upper section when compared to the contralateral side (**C**).

Ischemic edema and vasodilatation can cause a swelling of brain parenchyma. Ischemic edema means net uptake of water into brain tissue and is thus associated with a decline in X-ray attenuation. Brain swelling as a result of vasodilatation can develop under two conditions: (1) with low perfusion pressure, but intact cerebrovascular autoregulatory capacity, and (2) with venous obstruction *(12,13)*. This type of brain tissue is not associated with hypodensity, but can be associated with hyperdensity because of the increase in regional CBV. Brain swelling with iso- or hyperdensity is reversible, if the arterial or venous obstruction is treated successfully. CT does not reliably detect brain swelling early after ischemia onset but in some cases early swelling can be inferred because enlargement of brain tissue diminishes the CSF space. Asymmetric loss of CSF spaces might imply early tissue swelling, but because of the natural asymmetry of cerebral sulci, cisterns, and ventricles, it could be hard to decide whether the CSF space

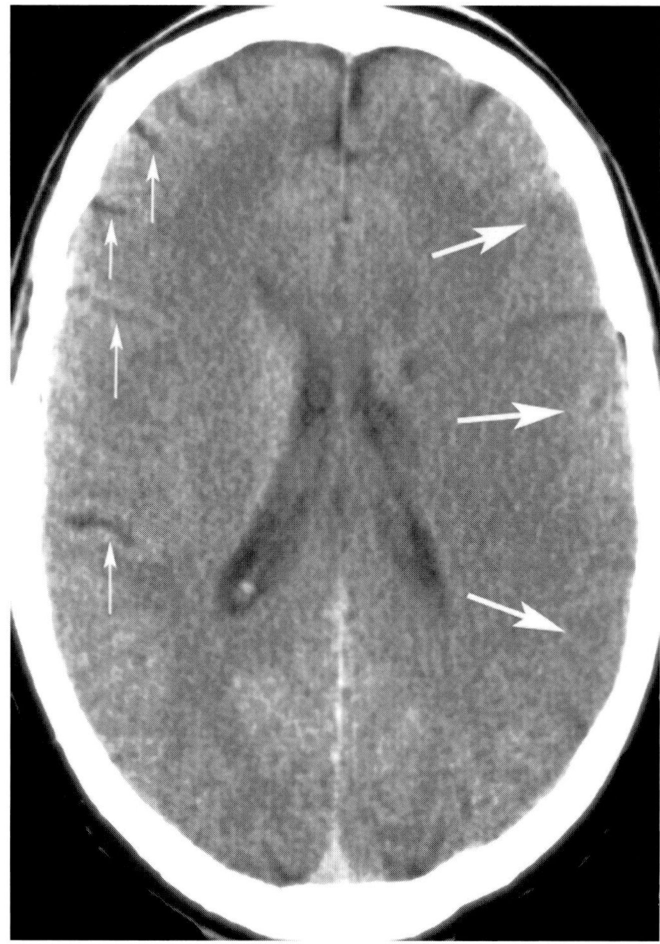

Fig. 5. Computed tomography scan obtained in a 40-yr-old man with severe rightsided hemiparesis. Effacement of the left cortical sulci in addition to hypodensity (*large arrows*). For comparison note the sulci of the right cerebral hemisphere (*small arrows*).

is unilaterally compressed or contra laterally enlarged. Clearer signs are the regional effacement of sulci, compression of the entire lateral ventricle, and in particular the combination of both (Fig. 5).

A decline in CBF below 12 mL/100 g × min causes the brain tissue to immediately take up water *(14,15)*. In experimental animals, tissue water concentration increased steadily from 80.7% to 83% within 4 hof MCA occlusion *(14)*. An increase by 1% of tissue water content causes a decrease of X-ray attenuation by 2 to 3 HU *(16)*. In our own experiments, X-ray attenuation declined by 7.5 ± 1.6 HU within 4 h of MCA occlusion and hypodensity became visible in the MCA territory of 2 of 10 animals within 2 h after MCA occlusion. Hypodensity could be differentiated from normal brain parenchyma in all 10 animals by 3 h after MCA occlusion *(17)*. The decline in attenuation at 4 h by 7.5 ± 1.6 HU corresponds to a 2.5%–3.8% increase in brain tissue water content in good agreement with the observations by Schuier and Hossmann *(14)*. Moreover, we could show that X-ray attenuation correlates inversely with the degree of ischemic edema *(18)*. Using a CT window of 80 HU or less, the contrast resolution is 4 HU or less, which corresponds with an increase in brain tissue water content of less than 1.3–2%. Hypodensity of gray matter causes a diminished contrast to adjacent white matter and thus a loss of anatomical margins. Gray matter hypodensity, thus explains negative phenomena like "obscuration of lentiform nucleus" *(19)* and "loss of the insular ribbon" *(20)*, so called "early infarct signs" (Figs. 2 and 4). Gray-matter hypodensity in its early stage causes a loss in anatomical information, which may explain why this finding is easily missed.

The delayed detection of parenchymal hypodensity after arterial occlusion has another important consequence: the CT finding of parenchymal hypodensity is highly specific for irreversible tissue damage because ischemic edema becomes irreversible within 2 h *(14,21)* and indicates irreversibly damaged brain tissue *(15)*. A CT scan without hypodensity, however, implies that at least some reversible ischemic edema may be present, and entirely irreversible ischemic tissue damage has not developed.

In contrast to the subtle changes on the CT gray scale, diffusion-weighted MR imaging (DWI) shows ischemic brain parenchyma with high signal that is easily discernible from normal brain tissue. Both imaging modalities do not show the same brain pathology, however. The reduction of CBF down to 30 mL/100g × min causes cell swelling and the reduction of the extracellular fluid space *(14)*. Exactly at this CBF value, the apparent diffusion coefficient of protons start to decline *(22,23)*. DWI is thus sensitive for much milder degrees of brain ischemia than CT. The critical CBF threshold for signal increase on DWI is even above the CBF threshold for neuronal dysfunction, whereas CT hypodensity indicates ischemic tissue damage. In other words, brain tissue with disturbed proton diffusion can recover, but brain tissue with diminished X-ray attenuation cannot recover if blood flow is restored.

Partial volume artifacts may mimic parenchymal hypodensity on CT. These artifacts occur if the CT section is in parallel to the brain's surface and includes parenchyma and CSF in same voxels. A typical location for this artifact is the temporal lobe.

Because hypoattenuating brain tissue represents ischemic edema and irreversible injury, its extent and location might be associated with the patient's prognosis and response to reperfusion therapy. The European Cooperative Acute Stroke Studies (ECASS) group, therefore, suggested excluding patients with hypoattenuating brain tissue exceeding one-third of the MCA territory from the first trial of recombinant tissue plasminogen activator (rt-PA) for stroke. Another approach is to subdivide the MCA territory into 10 regions and to subtract one point for each region being affected by ischemic edema. The Alberta Stroke Program Early CT Score (ASPECTS) thus provides information about the extent, pattern, and location of the ischemic edema. *(24)*. Neither the one-third rule nor the ASPECTS score have yet been proven to valid and reliable exclusion criteria for patient selection for thrombolysis after stroke; however, considerable further research is ongoing.

THE DETECTION OF INTRACRANIAL HEMORRHAGE AND STROKE MIMICS BY CT

In acute stroke, blood may be present in one or more of cranial compartments: brain parenchyma, ventricles, subarachnoid space, and subdural or epidural space. Clinically, an acute parenchymal hemorrhage cannot be distinguished reliably from ischemic stroke. After acute hemorrhage, blood appears as a hyperattenuated, often space-occupying mass (Fig. 6). The degree of hyperdensity depends on the amount of blood, whether it is clotted or not, and whether the blood is intermixed with CSF or brain tissue. Hemorrhages related to coagulopathies or treatment with anticoagulants or thrombolytics are often inhomogeneous with fluid levels (Fig. 7). Sensitivity of CT for the detection of parenchymal hemorrhage is nearly 100%, but small hemorrhages into the brain parenchyma or subarachnoid space can be overlooked (Fig. 8). The investigators of ECASS I and II missed two small parenchymal hemorrhages and one SAH in 1420 patients (0.1%) *(25,26)*. The detection of blood within infarcted, hypodense brain tissue is problematic, but of importance. The hemorrhagic transformation of ischemic brain tissue is normal; the extent of hemorrhage varies under the influence of thrombolytics and anticoagulants. Hemorrhagic transformation may appear on CT like normal gray matter surrounded by ischemic edema—slightly hyperattenuating spots scattered within the infarct—or it may present as a dense hematoma within the ischemic edema, with and without space occupying effect. It is unlikely that mild degrees of hemorrhagic transformation affect the neurological status of the patient. The term "symptomatic hemorrhage" for each sign of blood within ischemic infarctions is, therefore, highly problematic and may have contributed to the overestimation of the risk from these types of bleedings after thrombolytic therapy *(27)*. It was shown that only intracerebral hematomas with space occupying effect are associated with clinical deterioration and poor outcome *(28,29)*.

The location of the hematoma often provides clues about its underlying etiology (Table 2). Acute hemorrhages usually show hyperattenuation without surrounding edema. If marked edema is present under those circumstances, underlying neoplasm should be suspected. Multiple hemorrhagic lesions should suggest metastatic disease, coagulopathy, or cerebral amyloid angiopathy.

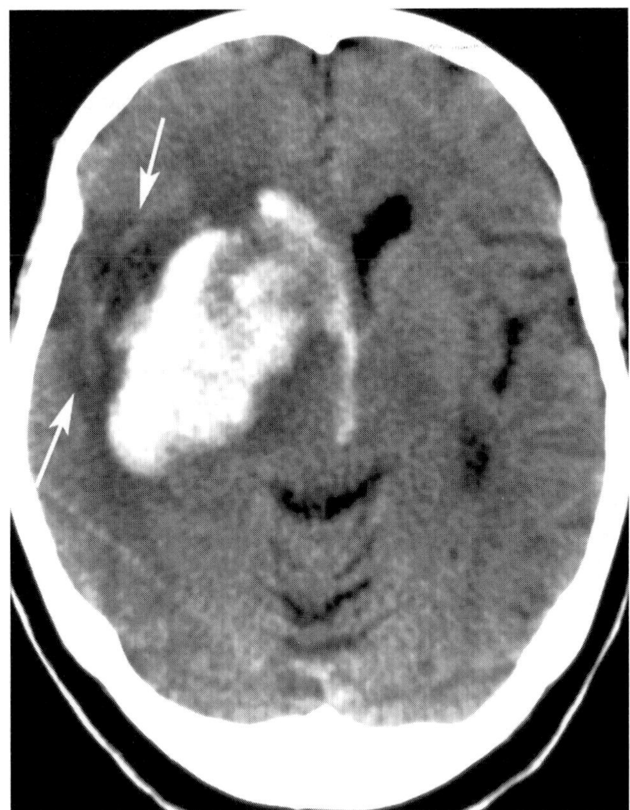

Fig. 6. Parenchymal hematoma of the right basal ganglia and intraventricular hemorrhage. The wedge-shaped hypodensity lateral of the hematoma (*arrows*) is suspicious for an underlying ischemic infarction.

CT is 90% sensitive for detection of SAH within the first 24 h of bleeding. When blood later intermixes with CSF the density will be similar to the adjacent brain and difficult to visualize. If the hemorrhage is small, it may be missed entirely by the scan, necessitating lumbar puncture for definitive diagnosis in patients with a syndrome highly suspicious for SAH. The sensitivity of CT in detecting subarachnoid blood declines to approx 50% at 1 wk after SAH *(30)*.

Regarding ICH, CT is only sensitive for fresh clotted blood, whereas MRI detects blood in all stages of hemoglobin degradation and can identify patients with the history of clinically silent brain microbleeds; the clinical significance of silent microbleeds remains to be determined. Calcification of the basal ganglia can occasionally be mistaken for deep intraparenchymal hemorrhage. It has a similar degree of attenuation as acute blood, but may be distinguished by its characteristic location and tendency to be bilateral.

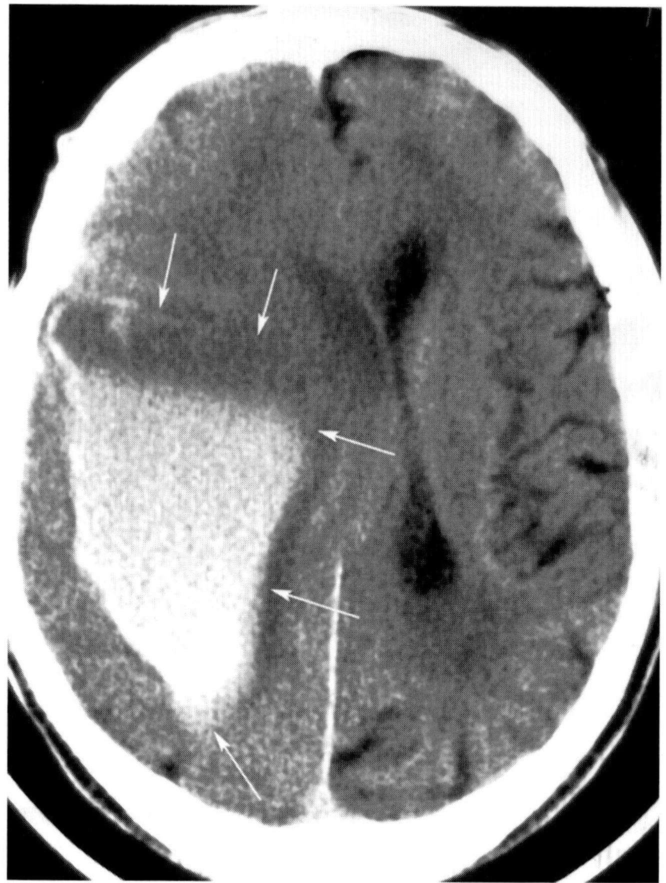

Fig. 7. Parenchymal hemorrhage after myocardial infarction and thrombolysis. Signs of unclotted blood: the upper portion is free of cells and hypodense. Increasing density in the lower portion owing to sedimentation of cellular elements (*arrows*).

Brain tumors and tumor-like lesions (e.g., acute focal demyelinations in multiple sclerosis), can cause a stroke syndrome. The characteristics of these lesions on CT are the space occupying effect on the surrounding structures, caused by cell neoplasia and/or reactive edema, and the replacement of normal anatomy by structures showing a mixture of attenuation values. *Hypo*density in this regard can be attributed to necrosis, cysts, or edema. An increased neoplastic or inflammatory cell density causes *hyper*density of these lesions on the unenhanced CT.

An approach to the interpretation of CT in the setting of acute stroke is presented in Table 3.

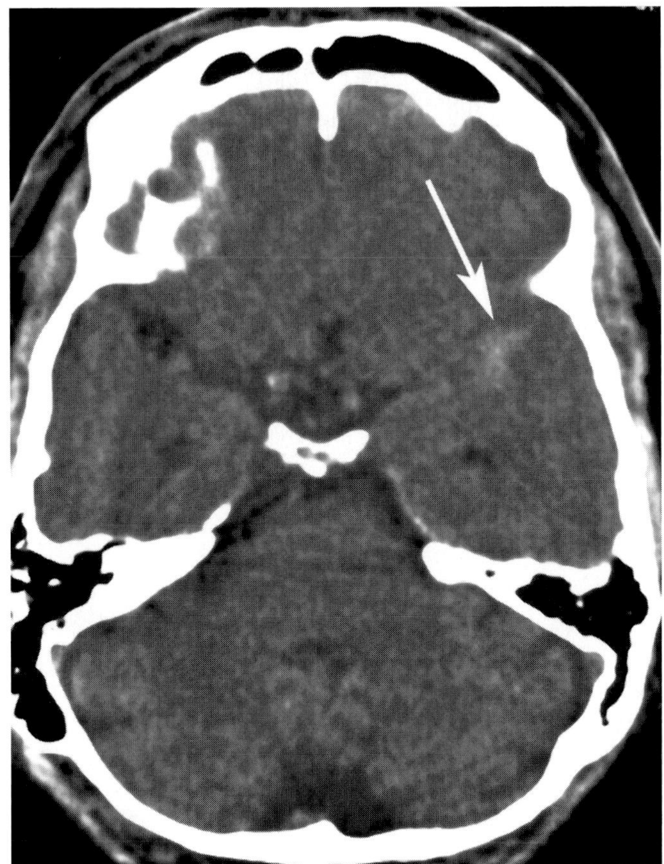

Fig. 8. Small hyperattenuated area in the left anterior Sylvian fissure (*arrow*). Low-contrast because of broad window of 160 Hounsfeld Units. The subarachnoid hemorrhage was overlooked, and the patient was randomized to recombinant tissue plasminogen activator. The hemorrhage was confirmed by the follow-up computed tomography. The patient had an excellent clinical outcome.

TYPICAL CT FINDINGS WITHIN THE FIRST 6 HOURS OF STROKE ONSET

The most relevant and highly underestimated finding in acute stroke patients is a normal CT. Figure 9A shows the CT of a man who woke up a right-sided hemiparesis and global aphasia at 6 AM. The noncontrast CT was completely normal despite severe symptoms for hours, but the CT angiography showed a long and tight stenosis of the proximal left internal carotid artery (ICA). The symptoms resolved completely within 3 d after the patient had undergone a stent-

Table 2
Common Causes of Spontaneous Cerebral Hemorrhage and their Typical Locations

Cause	*Location*
Hypertension	Basal ganglia (usually putamen) Thalamus Pons Cerebellum External capsule
Vascular malformation	All intracranial locations possible
Cerebral amyloid angiopathy	Adjacent to the brain surface Lobar
Bleeding diathesis	Lobar Multiple locations

protected angioplasty of his left ICA 8 h after stroke onset (*see* Fig. 9B for pre-stent and Fig. 9C for post-stent images). Many physicians still think that a lack of pathological CT findings in acute stroke patients reflects the low sensitivity of CT; it is widely overlooked that brain tissue appears hypoattenuating on CT only if regional CBF decreases below the threshold for ischemic damage. In some patients, ischemic edema may develop later or will never develop after the onset of stroke symptoms, because CBF can diminish below the threshold for neuronal function, but not that for structural integrity. These patients may have the best chances for functional recovery if CBF is restored.

The prejudice that CT is generally negative within the first 24 to 48 h after stroke is still handed down in review articles *(31),* although many studies have described positive findings even within the first 6 h of stroke onset: Tomura et al. studied 25 patients with embolic cerebral infarction between 40 and 340 min after the onset of symptoms. Twenty-three CT scans (92%) were positive with "obscuration of the lentiform nucleus" caused by hypodensity *(19).* Bozzao et al. observed parenchymal hypodensity in 25 of 36 (69%) patients *(32)* . A "loss of the insular ribbon" was reported in 23 of 27 (85%) patients *(20).* Horowitz et al. reported on hypodensity and mass effect in 56% of 50 scans *(33).* When comparing MRI to CT imaging in identical patients within 3 h of symptom onset, CT was positive in 19 (53%) patients and MRI in 18 (50%) patients with hemispheric stroke *(34).* We reported 17 (68%) positive CT scans performed in a series of 25 patients with MCA trunk occlusion during the first 2 h after symptom onset. The incidence of positive CT findings increased to 89% in the third hour after symptom onset and to 100% thereafter *(9).* In another series of patients with hemispheric stroke, the incidence of early CT signs of infarction was 82% *(35).* In patients selected for thrombolytic therapy, 12 of 23 (52%) patients had a parenchymal hypodensity on the CT performed within 3 h of stroke onset *(36).* In a

Table 3
Important Questions for the Interpretation of Computed Tomography (CT) in Acute Stroke

Characteristics of CT Findings				
Normal	*Tissue hypodensity*	*Hyperdensity*	*Tissue swelling*	*Arterial hyperdensity*
No subtle hypodensity or swelling in the region suspicious from the clinical findings? How severe is the stroke syndrome? Brain stem infarction?	No artifact? Extent and shape? Correspondence to arterial territory? Which artery? If no correspondence: venous infarction, astrocytoma, encephalitis?	Blood or calcification? If blood: Location? Mass effect? Blockage of cerebrospinal fluid pathways? Already edema? Abnormal vessels? Tumor?	Is it real? With hypodensity? Extent? Corresponding to arterial territory? Direct signs of vascular obstruction?	Which segment of which artery? Associated tissue hypodensity or swelling?

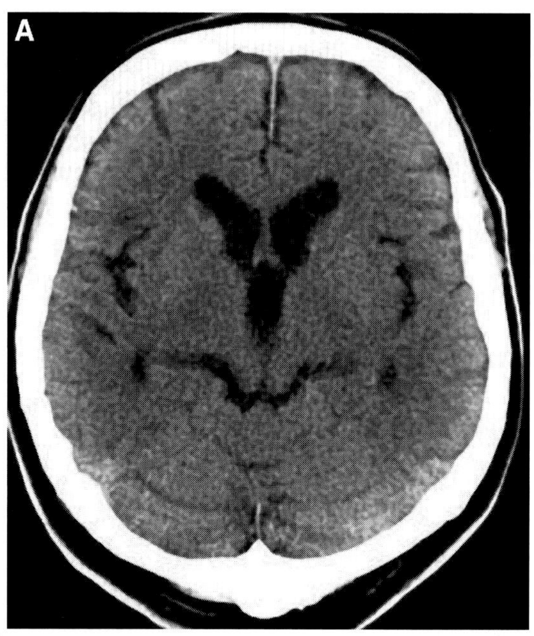
A

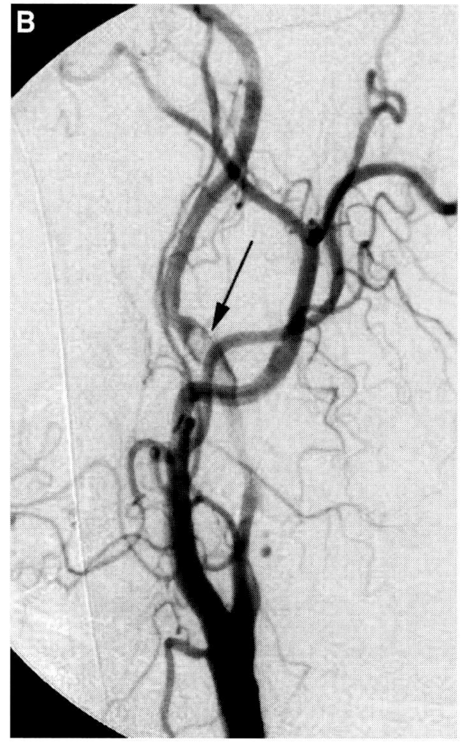
B

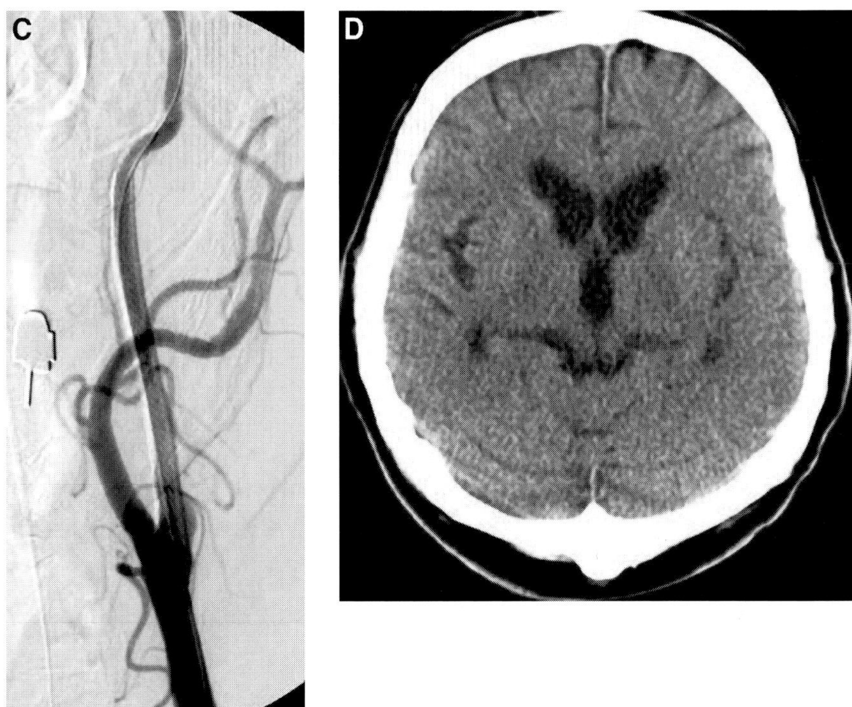

Fig. 9. Computed tomography (CT) of a 74-yr-old man who woke up with aright-sided hemiparesis and aphasia. The CT (**A**) was obtained in the morning and was completely normal, whereas CT angiography showed a tight stenosis of the left internal carotid artery that was confirmed by digital subtraction angiography (DSA) (**B**). DSA detected a thrombus within the stenosis (*arrow*). The thrombus disappeared during stent protected angioplasty (**C**). The patient recovered completely within 3 d. The follow-up CT (**D**) was normal.

series of 100 consecutive patients with MCA infarction, CT detected hypodensity of the lentiform nucleus in 48% and of the insular cortex in 59% of the patients within 14 h of stroke onset *(37)*.

To our knowledge, the incidence of early CT findings in stroke was never assessed in an unselected population of stroke patients. Varying criteria for patient selection and uncertain capability to recognize ischemic edema on CT may explain the variation in the incidence of findings among studies. The detection of parenchymal hypodensity in patients with acute stroke by neuroradiologists is possible with moderate to good interrater reliability *(37–39)*. Moreover, it was shown that special training of nonradiologists can enhance the proportion of CT findings and improve the estimation of the extent of early ischemic edema *(40)*.

Table 4
Positive Computed Tomography Findings in Trials on Thrombolytic Therapy

Study	*Time Interval*	*Findings (%)*	*Extent of Ischemic Edema*
ECASS I	6 h	54	Yes
ECASS II	6 h	66	Yes
MAST-I	6 h	12	No
MAST-E	6 h	68	No
PROACT II	6 h	83	Yes

ECASS, European Cooperative Acute Stroke Study *(17,18)*; MAST–I, Multicentre Acute Stroke Trial–Italy Group *(41)*; MAST–E,The Multicentre Acute Stroke Trial –Europe Study Group *(42)*; PROACT, Prolyse in Acute Cerebral Thromboembolism Trial *(43)*.

The incidence of early CT findings varies among the large studies on thrombolytic therapy (Table 4). In ECASS II, a panel of three neuroradiologists blinded to clinical outcome and follow-up CT prospectively evaluated all CT scans using predefined categories. This panel categorized the extent of hypodensity on baseline CT scans: normal, hypodensity of the MCA territory ≤33%/>33%, and hypodensity outside the MCA territory. These data offer the opportunity to study the clinical relevance and prospective value of 792 early CT findings with the limitation that the ECASS II investigators tried to exclude patients with MCA territory hypodensity >33%; in fact only 37 (4.6%) of these >33% patients were randomized.

The ECASS II investigators randomized 800 patients. Eight baseline CT (1%) were unavailable for the evaluation by the CT panel. No hypodensity was seen in 341 (43%) patients. Parenchymal hypodensities were associated with tissue swelling in 50% of the patients. Only one patient showed focal tissue swelling, but no hypodensity on the baseline CT. This patient was randomized to rt-PA, developed a small infarct, and had an excellent clinical outcome without functional disturbance at 90 d after stroke. Four-hundred-and-three patients (50%) had a hypodensity of 33% or less MCA territory, and 11 patients (1.4%) had a hypodensity outside the MCA territory. The National Institutes of Health Stroke Scale (NIHSS) at baseline—applied without the score for distal motor function—was different among these groups: patients with a normal CT or a hypodensity outside the MCA territory had a mean NIHSS score of 9.5 ± 5.1; patients with nore more than 33% hypodensity had an NIHSS score of 13.3 ± 6.0; and patients with larger hypodensity showed an NIHSS score of 17.1 ± 6.9 ($p <$ 0.0001, Bonferroni-Dunn) (Table 5).

The incidence of positive CT findings varied during the time between symptom onset and CT scan (Fig. 10). CT was positive in 18 of 36 (50%) patients who underwent CT within 1 h of symptom onset. The earliest positive CT was obtained

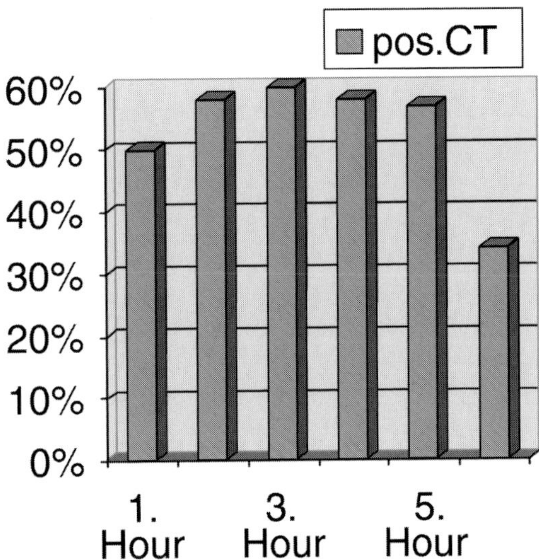

Fig. 10. Incidence of hypodensities on computed tomography at various intervals after symptom onset in European Cooperative Acute Stroke Study II. The decline in the sixth hour reflects an increased proportion of patients with small subcortical infarcts.

at 22 min after witnessed symptom onset (Fig. 11). This observation suggests that the ischemic edema may develop faster in humans than in experimental animals. The proportion of positive findings increased only slightly up to 60% after the first hour, and declined remarkably in the sixth hourafter stroke onset. The late decline in positive CT findings is best explained by a selection bias: relatively lately recruited patients were clinically less severely affected and developed smaller infarcts.

If one takes a well-demarcated infarct on CT at 1 d after stroke as the gold standard for a permanent ischemic lesion, the predictive values of the baseline CT can be calculated (Table 6). In ECASS II, the baseline CT was highly predictive and specific for ischemic lesions. Eleven findings in the placebo group and four findings in the group treated with rt-PA were falsely judged as early infarct, but could retrospectively be identified as artifacts. Remarkably, no hypodense ischemic lesion on baseline CT became normal, even after rt-PA treatment. The sensitivity of early CT for permanent ischemic lesions was 66% in the placebo group and 65% in the rt-PA group, implying that one-third of permanent ischemic lesions developed after the baseline CT was performed whether the patient was treated with placebo or rt-PA.

THE IMPACT OF CT FINDINGS ON THROMBOLYTIC THERAPY

The CT data of ECASS II suggest that parenchymal hypodensity on CT within 6 h of symptom onset suggests the presence of an ischemic lesion that cannot be reversed or diminished by treatment with intravenous 0.9 mg/kg rt-PA. Moreover, rt-PA treatment in this study did not prevent delayed infarction in one-third of the patients. If this is true, treatment with rt-PA may be beneficial when only a minor proportion of an arterial territory is hypodense when treatment is initiated. When designing their trials, the ECASS investigators followed the hypothesis that treatment with rt-PA will be ineffective and probably risky in patients with large ischemic edema already present at randomization. "Large" ischemic edema was artificially defined as a volume of hypodense brain tissue exceeding one-third of the MCA territory. This definition was based on the consideration that patients with such large edema have only minor chances to recover and that they may have an increased risk for cerebral hemorrhage after thrombolysis.

In ECASS I and II, 9 of 51 patients with a MCA territory hypodensity greater than 33% died from cerebral hemorrhages after rt-PA treatment, but none after placebo ($p < 0.01$, χ^2). The absolute risk increase for fatal cerebral hemorrhage was 17.6% in these patients and only 3.3% in patients with normal CT and 1.4% in patients with small hypodensity (Table 7). The risk to die from large ischemic edema with mass effect was clearly associated with the extent of hypodense tissue on baseline CT in both treatment groups ($p < 0.0001$, χ^2) and appeared slightly reduced after treatment with rt-PA (not significant). Some of these infarcts with large ischemic edema were presumably transformed into hemorrhages and patients died then from "cerebral hemorrhage" because the hemorrhage was more obvious on follow-up CT than the ischemic changes.

This risk increase for fatal hemorrhages in patients with large volumes of hypodense brain tissue on baseline CT does not clearly influence the overall outcome analysis. The results of ECASS I and II could not prove so far that the response to 1.1 mg/kg or 0.9 mg/kg rt-PA intravenously is different if the patients have no, small, or large hypodensities on the baseline CT. Table 8 presents outcome data of both studies after stratification according to the baseline CT: a significant beneficial effect of rt-PA is seen only in patients with MCA territory hypodensity of 33% or less, whereas patients with greater than 33% hypodensity

Fig. 11. (*opposite page*) Hypodensity of the right putamen detected 22 min after the onset of left hemiparesis in a 79-yr-old woman (**A**). National Institutes of Health Stroke Scale at baseline was11. The ischemic lesion is confirmed by the follow-up computed tomography 26 h later (**B**). The patient was randomized to recombinant tissue plasminogen activator and had an excellent outcome without functional disturbance.

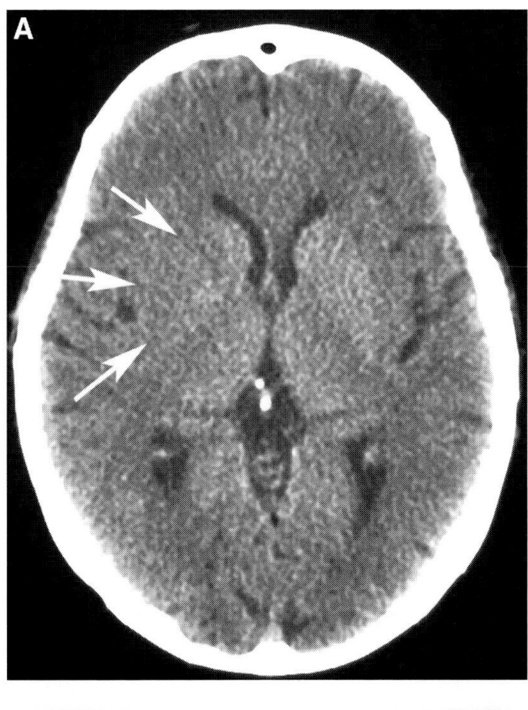
A

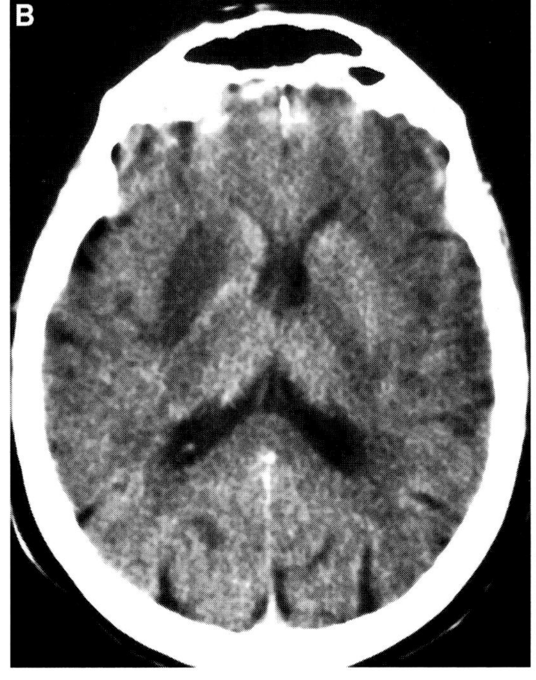
B

Table 5
Extent of MCA Territory Hypodensity on Baseline CT, Baseline Characteristics, NIHSS at Baseline and Follow-up, Symptomatic Hemorrhage, Disability, and Death in the ECASS II Placebo Group

	Hypodensity of MCA Territory			
	None	*≤33%*	*>33%*	*p*
Age (yr)	67 ± 11	65 ± 11	63 ± 14	0.168[a]
Male (%)	55	59	41	0.327[b]
NIHSS				
Baseline	9.6 ± 5.2	13.5 ± 6.6	15.1 ± 5.5	< 0.0001[a]
24 h	7.8 ± 6.6	12.5 ± 8.7	16.5 ± 9.6	< 0.0001 [a]
3 mo	6.4 ± 11.8	10.4 ± 13.3	19.4 ± 17.6	< 0.0001 [a]
Sympt. Hemorrhage (%)	3.0	8.8	0	0.072 [b]
Disability/death (%) (Rankin >2)	44	60	82	0.002 [b]
Death (%)	7.9	11.3	35.3	0.005 [b]

[a]ANOVA
[b]χ^2 test.
MCA, middle cerebral artery; CT, computed tomography; NIHSS, National Institutes of Health Stroke Scale; ECASS, European Cooperative Acute Stroke Study.

Table 6
Predictive Values of Baseline CT in ECASS II

	Placebo		*rt-PA*	
	n (%)	*95% CI*	*n (%)*	*95% CI*
Positive predictive value	211/222 (95)	91–97	218/222 (98)	95–99
Negative predictive value	48/158 (30)	24–38	63/180 (35)	28–42
Sensitivity	211/321 (66)	60–71	218/335 (65)	60–70
Specificity	48/59 (81)	69–90	63/67 (94)	85–98
Accuracy	259/380 (68)	63–73	281/402 (70)	65–74

CT, computed tomography, ECASS, European Cooperative Acute Stroke Study; rt-PA, recombinant tissue plasminogen activator; CI, confidence interval.

show a trend for deterioration with rt-PA *(44)*. The 95% confidence intervals of the three subgroups overlap each other, however, so any difference among them could be caused by chance. The view that patients with extended ischemic edema on CT do not respond well to reperfusion therapy was recently supported by the observation that patients with an ASPECTS of less than 8 did not benefit from IA infusion of pro-urokinase, whereas patients with an ASPECTS of more than 7 did *(45)*.

Table 7

ECASS I and II: Parenchymal Hypodensity of the MCA Territory on Baseline CT and Response to Treatment With rt-PA

	No Hypodensity *n = 688*				*Hypodensity ≤33% MCA Territory* *n = 618*				*Hypodensity >33% MCA Territory* *n = 89*			
Outcome Events	*rt-PA* *n = 354*	*Placebo* *n = 334*	*Difference* *%*	*OR* *95%CI*	*rt-PA* *n = 304*	*Placebo* *n = 314*	*Difference* *%*	*OR* *95%CI*	*rt-PA* *n = 51*	*Placebo* *n = 38*	*Difference* *%*	*OR* *95%CI*
Rankin: 0–1	170	144		1.22	97	75		1.49	6	6		0.71
	(48.0)	(43.1)	4.9	0.90–1.65	(31.9)	(23.9)	8.0	1.05–2.13	(11.8)	(15.8)	–4.0	0.21–2.41
Fatal edema	3	4		0.71	15	18		0.85	11	10		0.77
	(0.8)	(1.2)	–0.4	0.16–3.17	(4.9)	(5.7)	–0.8	0.42–1.73	(21.6)	(26.3)	–4.7	0.28–2.06
Fatal hemorrhage	16	4		3.91	11	7		1.65	9	0		–
	(4.5)	(1.2)	3.3	1.29 – 11.80	(3.6)	(2.2)	1.4	0.63–4.30	(17.6)	(0)	17.6	

Note. Percentages in brackets. ECASS, European Cooperative Acute Stroke Study; MCA, middle cerebral artery; CT, computed tomography; rt-PA, recombinant tissure plasminogen activator; OR, odds ratio; CI, confidence interval.

SUMMARY: MAIN COMPUTED TOMOGRAPHY FINDINGS AND ITS CONSEQUENCES

According to the combined results of all randomized rt-PA trials, patients with different types of ischemic stroke benefit from treatment with rt-PA within the first 270 min after stroke onset, if CT had excluded ICH *(46)*. CT detects ischemic edema if the tissue water content has increased by about 2% after arterial occlusion and is highly specific for a permanent ischemic lesion, which cannot be diminished by thrombolysis.

The ECASS and Prolyse in Acute Cerebral Thromboembolism Trial results suggest that patients with hypodensity exceeding one-third of the MCA territory corresponding to an ASPECTS of less than 8 do not benefit from treatment with thrombolytics and have a higher risk for symptomatic cerebral hemorrhage. The number of patients with large hypodensity studied so far is rather small, however, and no definite conclusions can be drawn for other types of stroke treatment. In patients with acute stroke and no or only small volumes of hypodensity, additional information is needed to find out whether an arterial obstruction and relevant hypoperfusion is present when treatment is initiated.

REFERENCES

1. von Kummer R, Bourquain H, Bastianello S, et al. Early prediction of irreversible brain damage after ischemic stroke by computed tomography. *Radiology* 2001;219:95–100.
2. von Kummer R, Bozzao L, Manelfe C. *Early CT Diagnosis of Hemispheric Brain Infarction. 1st Ed.* Heidelberg:Springer; 1995.
3. Brooks R. A quantitative theory of the Hounsfield unit and its application of dual energy scanning. *J Comput Assist Tomogr* 1977;1:487–493.
4. Rieth KG, Fujiwara K, Di Chiro G, et al. Serial measurements of CT attenuation and specific gravity in experimental cerebral edema. *Radiology* 1980;135:343–348.
5. Knauth M, Brandt T, Jansen O, von Kummer, Wildermuth S, Sartor K. CT-Angiographie bei Basilaristhrombose. *Radiologe* 1996;36:855–858.
6. Koenig M, Klotz E, Luka B, Venderink D, Spittler J, Heuser L. Perfusion CT of the brain: Diagnostic approach for early detection of ischemic stroke. *Radiology* 1998;209:85–93.
7. Hoeffner E, Case I, Jain R, et al. Cerebral Perfusion CT: Technique and clinical applications. *Radiology* 2004;231:632–644.
8. Tomsick T. Commentary. Sensitivity and prognostic value of early CT in occlusion of the middle cerebral artery trunk. *AJNR* 1994;15:16–18.
9. von Kummer R, Meyding-Lamadé U, Forsting M, et al. Sensitivity and prognostic value of early computed tomography in middle cerebral artery trunk occlusion. *AJNR* 1994;15:9–15.
10. Kirchhof K, Welzel T, Mecke C, Zoubaa S, Sartor K. Differentiation of white, mixed, and red thrombi: Value of CT in estimation of the prognosis of thrombolysis-Phantom study. *Radiology* 2003;228:126–130.
11. Tomsick T, Brott T, Olinger C, et al. Hyperdense middle cerebral artery: incidence and quantitative significance. *Neuroradiology* 1989;31:312–315.
12. Gibbs J, Wise R, Leenders K, Jones T. Evaluation of cerebral perfusion reserve in patients with carotid-artery occlusion. *Lancet* 1984;8372:310–314.
13. Yuh W, Simonson T, Wang A, et al. Venous sinus occlusive Disease: MR Findings. *AJNR* 1994;15:309–316.

14. Schuier FJ, Hossmann KA. Experimental brain infarcts in cats. II. Ischemic brain edema. *Stroke* 1980;11:593–601.
15. Hossmann KA. Viability thresholds and the penumbra of focal ischemia. *Ann Neurol* 1994;36:557–565.
16. Unger E, Littlefield J, Gado M. Water content and water structure in CT and MR signal changes: Possible influence in detection of early stroke. *AJNR* 1988;9:687–691.
17. von Kummer R, Weber J. Brain and vascular imaging in acute ischemic stroke: The potential of computed tomography. *Neurology* 1997;49(Suppl 4):S52–S55.
18. Dzialowski I, Weber J, Doerfler A, Forsting M, von Kummer R. Brain Tissue Water Uptake After Middle Cerebral Artery Occlusion Assessed With CT. *J Neuroimaging* 2004;14:42–48.
19. Tomura N, Uemura K, Inugami A, Fujita H, Higano S, Shishido F. Early CT finding in cerebral infarction. *Radiology* 1988;168:463–467.
20. Truwit C, Barkovich A, Gean-Marton A, Hibri N, Norman D. Loss of the insular ribbon: Another early CT sign of acute middle cerebral artery infarction. *Radiology* 1990;176:801–806.
21. Ianotti F, Hoff J. Ischemic brain edema with and without reperfusion: An experimental study in gerbils. *Stroke* 1983;14:562–567.
22. Perez-Trepichio A, Xue M, Ng T, et al. Sensitivity of magnetic resonance diffusion-weighted imaging and regional relationship between the apparent diffusion coefficient and cerebral blood flow in rat focal cerebral ischemia. *Stroke* 1995;26:667–675.
23. Wang Y, Hu W, Perez-Trepichio A, et al. Brain tissue sodium is a ticking clock telling time after arterial occlusion in rat focal cerebral ischemia. *Stroke* 2000;31:1386–1392.
24. Barber P, Demchuk A, Zhang J, Buchan A. Validity and reliability of a quantitative computed tomography score in predicting outcome of hyperacute stroke before thrombolytic therapy. *Lancet* 2000;355:1670–1674.
25. Hacke W, Kaste M, Fieschi C, et al. Intravenous thrombolysis with recombinant tissue plasminogen activator for acute hemispheric stroke. The European Cooperative Acute Stroke Study (ECASS). *JAMA* 1995;274:1017–1025.
26. Hacke W, Kaste M, Fieschi C, et al. Randomised double-blind placebo-controlled trial of thrombolytic therapy with intravenous alteplase in acute ischaemic stroke (ECASS II). *Lancet* 1998;352:1245–1251.
27. The NINDS t-PA Stroke Study Group. Intracerebral hemorrhage after intravenous t-PA therapy for ischemic stroke. *Stroke* 1997;28:2109–118.
28. Berger C, Fiorelli M, Steiner T, et al. Hemorrhagic transformation of ischemic brain tissue: Asymptomatic or symptomatic? *Stroke* 2001;32:1330–1335.
29. Fiorelli M, Bastianello S, von Kummer R, et al. Hemorrhagic Transformation within 36 hours of a cerebral infarct: Relationships with early clinical deterioration and 3-month outcome in the European Cooperative Acute Stroke Study I (ECASS I) Cohort. *Stroke* 1999;30:2280–2284.
30. Schievink W. Intracranial aneurysms. *N Engl J Med* 1997;336:28–40.
31. Gilman S. Imaging of the brain. *N Engl J Med* 1998;338(12):812–820.
32. Bozzao L, Bastianello S, Fantozzi LM, Angeloni U, Argentino C, Fieschi C. Correlation of angiographic and sequential CT findings in patients with evolving cerebral infarction. *AJNR*1989;10:1215–1222.
33. Horowitz SH, Zito JL, Donnarumma R, Patel M, Alvir J. Computed tomographic - angiographic findings within the first five hours of cerebral infarction. *Stroke* 1991;22:1245–1253.
34. Mohr J, Biller J, Hilal S, et al. Magnetic resonance versus computed tomographic imaging in acute stroke. *Stroke* 1995;26:807–812.
35. von Kummer R, Nolte PN, Schnittger H, Thron A, Ringelstein EB. Detectability of hemispheric ischemic infarction by computed tomography within 6 hours after stroke. *Neuroradiology* 1996;38:31–33.
36. Grond M, von Kummer R, Sobesky J, Schmülling S, Heiss W-D. Early computed-tomography abnormalities in acute stroke. *Lancet* 1997;350:1595–1596.

37. Moulin T, Cattin F, Crépin-Leblond T, et al. Early CT signs in acute middle cerebral artery infarction: Predictive value for subsequent infarct locations and outcome. *Neurology* 1996;47:355–375.
38. von Kummer R, Holle R, Grzyska U, et al. Interobserver agreement in assessing early CT signs of middle cerebral artery infarction. *AJNR* 1996;17:1743–1748.
39. Marks M, Holmgren E, Fox A, Patel S, von Kummer R, Froehlich J. Evaluation of early computed tomographic findings in acute ischemic stroke. *Stroke* 1999;30:389–392.
40. von Kummer R. Effect of training in reading CT scans on patient selection for ECASS II. *Neurology* 1998;51 (Suppl 3):S50–S52.
41. Multicentre Acute Stroke Trial-Italy (MAST-I) Group. Randomised controlled trial of streptokinase, aspirin, and combination of both in treatment of acute ischaemic stroke. *Lancet* 1995;346:1509–1514.
42. The Multicenter Acute Stroke Trial - Europe Study Group. Thrombolytic therapy with streptokinase in acute ischemic stroke. *N Engl J Med* 1996;335:145–150.
43. Furlan A, Higashida R, Wechsler L, et al. Intra-arterial Prourokinase for acute ischemic stroke. *JAMA* 1999;282:2003–2011.
44. von Kummer R, Allen K, Holle R, et al. Acute stroke: usefulness of early CT findings before thrombolytic therapy. *Radiology* 1997;205:327–333.
45. Hill MD, Rowley HA, Adler F, et al. for the PROACT-II-Investigators. Selection of acute ischemic stroke patients for intra-arterial thrombolysis with pro-urokinase by using ASPECTS. *Stroke* 2003;34:1925–1931.
46. The ATLANTIS, ECASS, and NINDS rt-PA Study Group Investigators. Association of outcome with early stroke treatment: pooled analysis of ATLANTIS, ECASS, and NINDS rt-PA stroke trials. *Lancet* 2004;363:768–774.

17 Using Magnetic Resonance Imaging to Select and Manage Patients for Treatment

Peter D. Schellinger, MD, PhD,
Chelsea S. Kidwell, MD, *and Steven Warach,* MD, PhD

Contents

INTRODUCTION

Thrombolysis is the treatment of choice for eligible acute stroke within 3 h after symptom onset. However, in the United States, only 2–5% of acute stroke patients receive this therapy, and among those patients who are treated there remains a risk of developing a symptomatic intracerebral hemorrhage (ICH) *(1–3)*. Moreover, no treatment beyond 3 h has been approved by regulatory agencies. Thus, there is an urgent need to optimize safety and efficacy of throm-

From: *Current Clinical Neurology: Thrombolytic Therapy for Acute Stroke, Second Edition*
Edited by: P. D. Lyden © Humana Press Inc., Totowa, NJ

bolytic therapy in the early time window (<3 h from onset), and identify selection criteria for therapies that can be safely extended into later time windows. Multimodal neuroimaging techniques are now available in the clinical setting and may provide an opportunity to meet both these needs.

Neuroimaging in the acute stroke setting plays a number of important roles: to confirm or exclude the diagnosis of cerebrovascular disease (ischemia or hemorrhage), to provide insight into the underlying stroke mechanism (embolic, hemodynamic), or to provide important information regarding prognosis based on size and location of the injury. In clinical trials, imaging can serve as an outcome measure of treatment effects. However, one of the most promising roles for neuroimaging in the acute stroke setting is the potential to select patients for acute therapies, particularly beyond the 3-h window. Multiparametric magnetic resonance imaging (MRI) has the potential to extend the time window for treatment by basing therapy on individual pathophysiology by identifying those patients most likely to benefit from therapy (those with an ischemic penumbra) as well as those most likely to suffer complications (e.g., hemorrhagic transformation).

MRI STROKE PROTOCOLS

A multiparametric MRI protocol generally includes the following sequences:

- Diffusion-weighted imaging (DWI) to identify early ischemic injury and bioenergetic compromise.
- Perfusion-weighted imaging (PWI) to identify regions of hemodynamic compromise.
- T2*-weighted imaging (T2*-WI), which are sensitive to tissue differences in magnetic susceptibility, to identify both acute and chronic hemorrhage based on the paramagnetic properties of iron found in hemoglobin and its breakdown products. By convention, standard T2*-WI is termed gradient echo (GRE) and echo planar T2*-WI is termed susceptibility-weighted imaging (SWI).
- Neck and intracranial MR angiography (MRA) to identify large vessel stenoses and occlusions (some centers omit the neck MRA acutely to minimize the duration of the study).
- A T2-WI or fluid attenuated inversion recovery (FLAIR) sequence to provide an anatomical brain image that depicts microangiopathic changes, edema, old infarcts, and other, nonischemic, pathology.

Until recently, there had been doubts regarding the feasibility and practicality of performing stroke MRI in the clinical setting *(4)*. However, recent reports confirmed the widespread availability of advanced MRI techniques for acute stroke evaluation in the United States *(5)*. A survey of physicians involved in acute stroke care (including 37% respondents from community hospitals) indicated that 90% currently have acute MRI capability. A second survey from Illinois found that 74% of acute-care medical facilities had MRI availability for stroke diagnosis *(6)*. Thus, in a majority of hospitals in the United States, the infrastructure to use MRI for acute stroke diagnosis is already in place.

In addition, several groups have demonstrated that logistic obstacles can be overcome *(7,8)*. Practice and experience with stroke MRI—and a dedicated stroke team—significantly reduces the time and effort for a complete stroke MRI protocol that need not exceed 15 min including patient transfer and positioning; such turn around times should facilitate 24-h availability *(9)*.

DIAGNOSIS: ISCHEMIA

On T2-WI ischemic infarction appears as a hyperintense lesion. Definite signal changes, however, are seen—at the earliest—by 2 h after stroke onset in animal experiments and 6–8 h after stroke onset in patients *(10)*. Neither a diagnosis of parenchymal ischemia nor the differentiation of ischemic core from penumbral tissue is possible with T2-WI.

The introduction of echo planar imaging, including DWI, in the 1990s revolutionized the role of MRI in acute stroke evaluation. DWI detects the Brownian molecular motion of water, a phenomenon first described in 1965, and demonstrates ischemic tissue changes within minutes after vessel occlusion *(11)*. In acute ischemia, there is a net shift of extracellular water into the intracellular compartment (cytotoxic edema) with a consecutive reduction of free water diffusion. The rate of diffusion can be measured quantitatively in the form of the apparent diffusion coefficient (ADC). Acute ischemic lesions appear hyperintense on diffusion-weighted sequences and hypointense of ADC maps.

In order to interpret changes on DWI correctly, true acute ischemic changes must be differentiated from other causes of hyperintensity on DWI (e.g., anisotropy, susceptibility artifact near brain–air interface, T2-WI hyperintensity shine-through). In the hyperacute stroke setting, a lesion seen on strongly DWI and not seen on T2-WI is more likely to reflect acute ischemia (i.e., less than 3 h from onset), than any of the mentioned other causes (Fig. 1). Even greater specificity is assured when ADC-parameter maps are calculated in addition to DWI and T2-WI. Acute ischemic lesions will appear hyperintense on DWI and hypointense on ADC. Newer DWI techniques, such as FLAIR-DWI to reduce cerebrospinal fluid contamination *(12)*, diffusion tensor imaging and high field (3 Tesla) imaging may further improve the diagnostic yield of DWI.

DWI is superior to computed tomography (CT) in the diagnosis of acute ischemic stroke *(13–16)*. A blinded comparison of MRI (including GRE and DWI) to CT in a broad spectrum of patients with suspected stroke provided conclusive evidence for the superior sensitivity of DWI for diagnosis of acute ischemic stroke (Fig. 2) *(17)*. A representative sample of patients ($N = 356$) was drawn from among patients who presented to a hospital emergency department over an 18-mo period; the emergency physician diagnosed possible acute stroke,

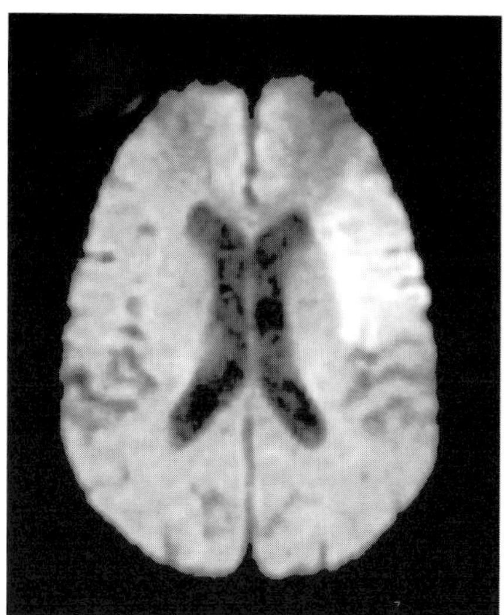

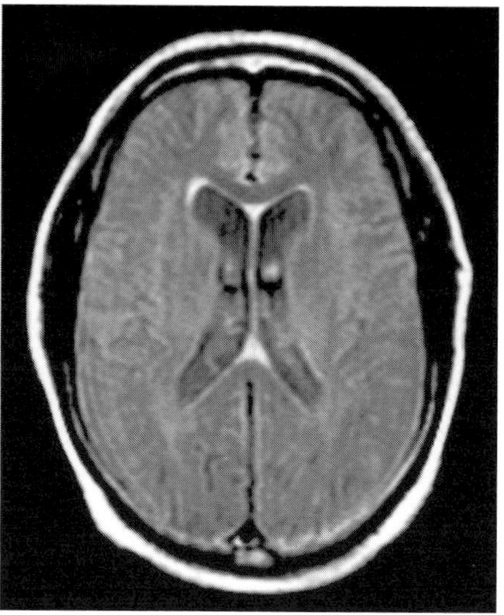

Fig. 1. Diffusion-weighted imaging (DWI) (*left*) and fluid attenuated inversion recovery (FLAIR) (*right*) of an acute stroke patient less than 3 h after symptom onset. DWI shows a hyperintensity in the left middle cerebral artery territory, whereas FLAIR is without pathological findings.

thus including a representative proportion of patients with not only ischemic strokes, but also non-ischemic strokes and stroke mimics. Patients with the suspected diagnosis of acute stroke were imaged at a median of 33 min earlier by MRI than by CT. Four reviewers (two neuroradiologists and two stroke neurologists) interpreted all scans blinded to clinical information, independently of each other and of CT–DWI pairings; and the final diagnosis was defined as the majority opinion. Overall ischemic stroke was diagnosed from DWI in 46% and from CT in 10% of patients (46% and 7% in the subset of 90 patients scanned within 3 h from onset). Relative to hospital discharge diagnosis of acute ischemic stroke (219 of 356 patients), the sensitivity, specificity, and accuracy were 83%, 97%, 89% for MRI and 17%, 98%, 54% for CT, respectively. In the under-3-h subgroup, the sensitivity, specificity and accuracy were 73%, 92%, 81% for MRI and 12%, 100%, 49% for CT, respectively. False-negative DWI were associated with mild strokes (National Institutes of Health Stroke Scale [NIHSS] score <4), brainstem strokes, and early strokes (<3 h). Other studies have reported higher sensitivities for DWI and CT, but these studies lacked a cohort of non-stroke controls and had samples with more severe deficits than an unselected sample presenting to emergency departments (Fig. 2).

Compared to CT, DWI is particularly useful in identifying small cortical, subcortical, or posterior fossa lesions, particularly in the acute phase. In addition, numerous studies showed that initial diffusion lesion volumes correlate well

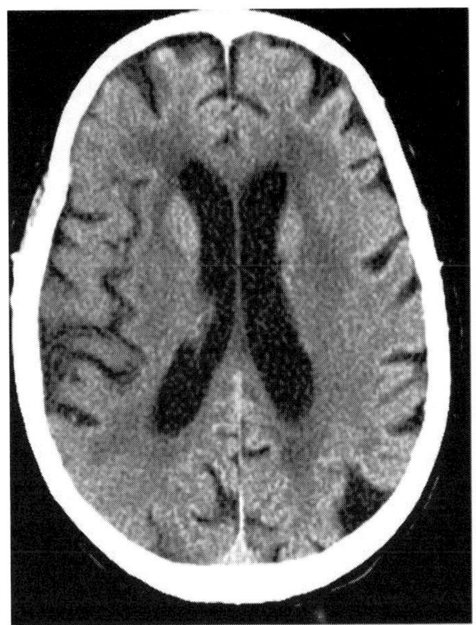
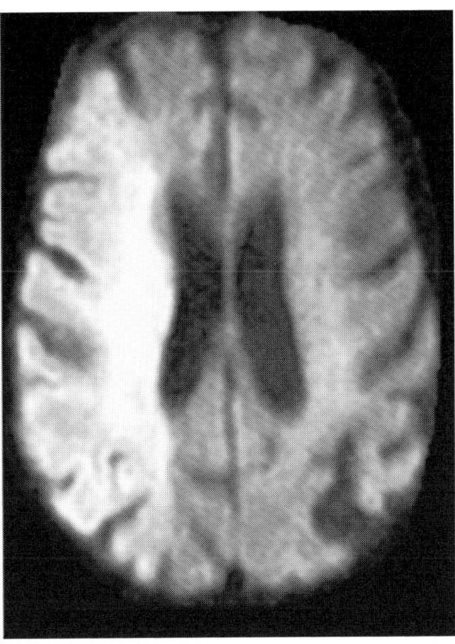

Fig. 2. Computed tomography and diffusion-weighted imaging (DWI) images from a patient presenting at 2 h after onset of left hemiparesis and hemisensory loss. Ischemia within right middle cerebral artery territory is more evident of DWI image.

with final infarct volumes as well as neurological and functional outcomes in acute stroke patients, suggesting that diffusion MR can provide important early prognostic information *(18–20)*. Diffusion imaging provides new insights into the underlying pathophysiology of transient ischemic attacks (TIAs). Aggregate data from seven observational studies reported in abstract or manuscript format demonstrated that almost one-half of patients with clinical TIA syndromes have a DWI abnormality *(21–27)*. Although the majority of these studies suggest that the likelihood of a positive DWI increases with longer symptom duration, this relationship is not absolute. Although these lesions may resolve in some cases, the majority of patients have imaging evidence of permanent ischemic injury *(21)*. Based on these findings, the term "acute ischemic cerebrovascular syndrome" (AICS) may be used to describe a spectrum of clinical presentations that share a similar underlying pathophysiology: cerebral ischemia *(28,29)*.

DIAGNOSIS: HEMODYNAMIC COMPROMISE

PWI allows the measurement of capillary perfusion with the dynamic susceptibility contrast-enhanced technique. A paramagnetic contrast agent is injected as an intravenous bolus and the signal change within the brain is tracked by ultrafast MR sequences *(30)*. The vascular hemodynamic parameters that are calculated from the MR-derived contrast-bolus-over-time-curve include mean transit time, cerebral blood volume, relative cerebral blood flow, and time-to-peak measures. The contrast bolus passage causes a signal loss that increases with the perfused cerebral blood volume (CBV). In ischemic brain tissue with reduced perfusion or zero perfusion, less (or no) contrast agent is present and the T2*-WI signal remains hyperintense.

It is not yet clear which PWI parameter gives the optimum measure of critical hypoperfusion, nor which provides the best differentiation between infarct core and penumbra or penumbra and benign oligemia. Many researchers believe that, in clinical practice, a mean transit time or TTP measures provides the best prognostic information *(31,32)*. Calculation of quantitative cerebral blood flow (CBF) requires knowledge of the arterial input function, which in clinical practice is estimated from a major artery such as the middle cerebral artery or the internal cerebral artery. However, quantitative CBF perfusion measures have not rigorously been validated against gold standards.

DIAGNOSIS: HEMORRHAGE

Noncontrast CT has been the standard imaging modality of choice for the initial evaluation of patients presenting with acute stroke symptoms because of its ability to accurately identify acute hemorrhage *(33,34)*. Accurate early detection of blood is crucial because acute hemorrhage is a contraindication to the use of thrombolytic agents in the acute stroke setting.

Whereas conventional T1- and T2-weighted MRI sequences are highly sensitive for the detection of subacute and chronic blood, they are less sensitive to parenchymal hemorrhage under 6 h. Over the past few years, a growing body of data demonstrated that both hyperacute and chronic parenchymal blood can be accurately detected using GRE sequences or SWI *(35)*. These sequences detect the paramagnetic effects of deoxyhemoglobin, methemoglobin and ultimately hemosiderin.

The appearance of ICH depends on several factors such as the MRI sequence, field strength, and the oxygen saturation of hemoglobin and its degradation. Other factors are protein concentration, hydration, form and size of red blood cells, hematocrit, clot retraction and clot structure. In the very first minutes after symptom onset, the center of the lesion appears heterogeneous on all images (T2-WI, T2*WI, T1-WI), because of a local predominance of oxyhemoglobin. On GRE or SWI, the periphery of the hematoma appears as a hypointense rim (Fig. 3). Over time, this hypointensity expands into the core of the hematoma due to a progressive centripetal increase in concentration of deoxyhemoglobin. There is often a surrounding rim, which appears hyperintense on T2-WI and T2*-WI but hypointense on T1-WI and represents perifocal vasogenic edema.

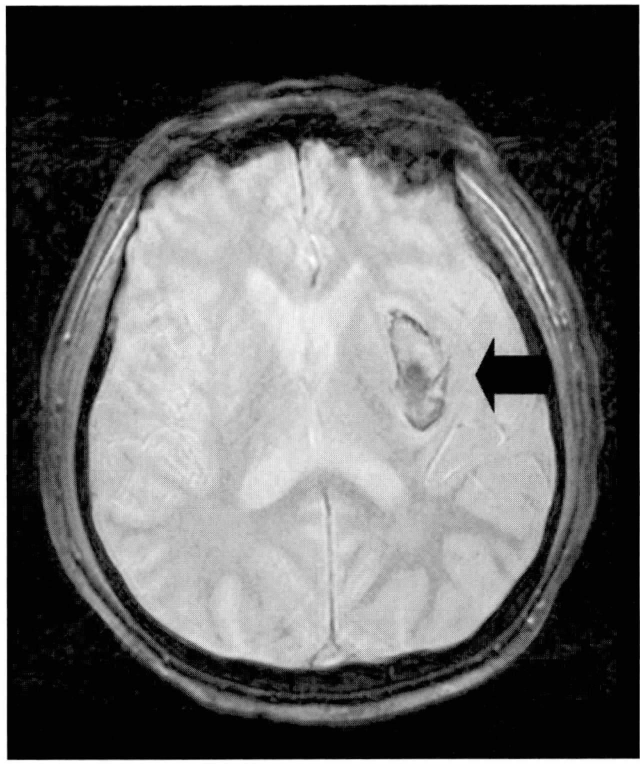

Fig. 3. Gradient echo appearance of hyperacute hemorrhage in left basal ganglia image less than 3 h from symptom onset. Rim of hematoma appears hypointense, whereas core of hematoma has mixed signal intensities.

Recently, two multicenter studies evaluated the accuracy of stroke MRI for the detection of hyperacute ICH *(36,37)*. In the German Collaborative study, images from 62 ICH patients and 62 nonhemorrhagic stroke patients—all imaged within the first 6 h after symptom onset (mean 3 h 18 min)—were scanned with CT and MR after randomization for the order of presentation. The images were read blind to clinical presentation. Three experienced readers identified ICH with a 100% sensitivity (confidence interval [CI]: 97.1–100 %) and a 100% overall accuracy.

In the Hemorrhage Early MRI Evaluation (HEME) study, 200 patients with acute stroke symptoms within 6 h of onset were imaged with MRI prior to CT. The overall accuracy of MRI and CT for acute hemorrhage was 98%. However, several cases of hemorrhagic transformation not visualized at all on CT were detected on MRI. The HEME study also demonstrated the superiority of gradient echo MRI sequences for the identification of chronic hemorrhage. In 49 patients, GRE demonstrated chronic blood not apparent on CT. The majority of these chronic hemorrhages were categorized as microbleeds—clinically silent, small, punctate lesions appearing as round hypointense regions on GRE sequences (Fig. 3) *(38)*. Microbleeds are most commonly associated with microangiopathy as a result of hypertension, cerebral amyloid angiopathy, or prior ischemic injury, and are presumably caused by weakening of the vessel walls. Although the role of microbleeds in determining patient eligibility for thrombolytic therapy remains unknown, prior studies suggest that the presence of microbleeds may be an independent risk factor for hemorrhage in patients treated with anti-thrombotic or thrombolytic therapy *(39–41)*. In combination, these studies suggest that MRI may be acceptable as the sole imaging technique for acute stroke patients at centers with expertise in interpreting these findings (Fig. 4).

A question remains, however, about the sensitiviy of MRI for subarachnoid hemorrhage (SAH): prior studies suggested that both GRE and FLAIR images may be accurate in identifying SAH, but a prospective, confirmatory study must be done *(42–44)*. Because neither CT nor MRI can exclude SAH with 100% reliability, it is important to stress for the clinician that in any patient in whom SAH is contemplated, an extensive evaluation should be pursued, including CT as well as lumbar puncture if CT is negative.

DIAGNOSIS: VASCULAR PATHOLOGY

Three types of MRA are in clinical use. Time-of-flight (TOF) MRA depends on the movement of blood into the imaging field. The magnetization of protons in stationary tissue are saturated by repeated low-flip angle radiofrequency pulses, whereas protons in the vessels flowing into the tissue remain unsaturated appear and relatively bright. The data are then post-processed using a maximum intensity projection algorithm for angiographic reconstruction. In practice, inspection of the source images is often necessary to evaluate subtle or ambiguous findings. Three dimensional rather than two-dimensional TOF MRA is the most common implementation of MRA in clinical practice because it gives superior spatial resolution and is less prone to signal loss from turbulent flow at sites of stenoses, although two-dimensional TOF may be more sensitive to slower flow. Phase contrast MRA is another technique for generating angiographic-style images based on the velocity and direction of flow. Phase-contrast MRA is based on the principle that moving spins develop a phase shift relative to stationary spins in the presence of a pair of opposing magnetic field gradients. There is superior background suppression with phase contrast MRA, but acquisition times tend to be longer and more prone to artifacts.

The most promising new approach is contrast-enhanced MRA of the carotid arteries, in which a more rapid MR acquisition is timed to a bolus injection of

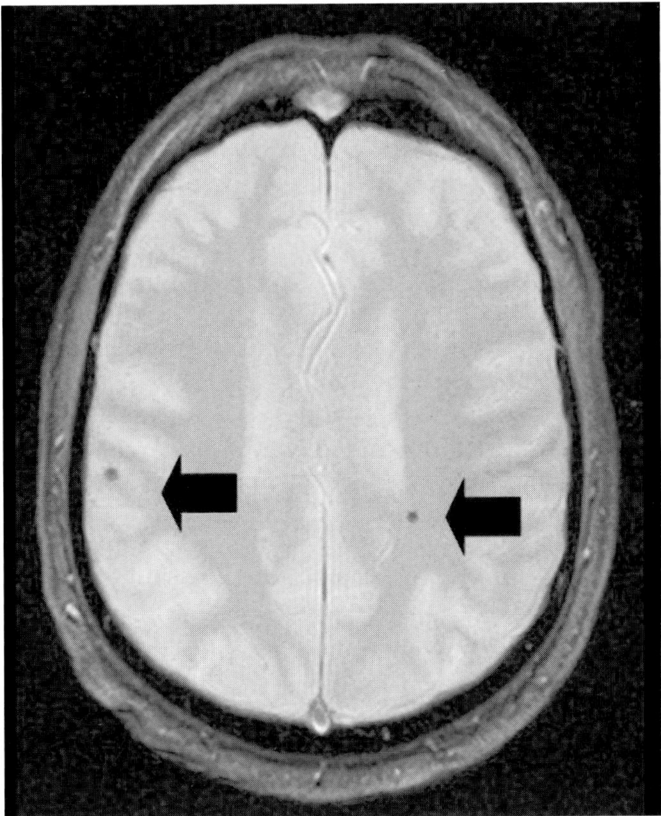

Fig. 4. Example of bilateral microbleeds (*black arrows*) on gradient echo imaging.

contrast over a larger field of view; carotid MRA with contrast compares favorably to conventional angiography for the diagnosis of carotid stenosis. The accuracy of contrast-enhanced MRA for detecting vascular disease in vertebral artery origins and the aortic arch is being investigated.

MRA rivals conventional angiography for the detection of arterial stenoses and occlusions, although there is a tendency of MRA to overestimate the degree of stenosis because turbulent flow causes proton de-phasing; also calcifications at the site of the stenosis may cause interference, and the smaller intracranial vessels are not well visualized. A normal screening MRA is reliable in excluding hemodynamically significant stenoses. False-positive results can arise when the degree of carotid stenosis is overestimated or when the carotid artery is kinked or changes direction abruptly, distally in the carotid artery as it enters the carotid canal because of susceptibility artifact between vessel and bone, and in the presence of surgical clips. Sensitivity and specificity for carotid occlusion has been found to be 100% in most studies. In the intracranial vasculature, MRA is useful in identifying acute proximal large vessel occlusions and stenoses, but is not currently reliable in identifying distal or branch occlusions.

SELECTION: IDENTIFYING THE ISCHEMIC PENUMBRA AND PATIENTS AT INCREASED RISK FROM THERAPIES

The target for most therapeutic interventions for focal cerebral ischemia should be ischemic tissue that can respond to treatment and is not irreversibly injured. The characterization of potentially reversible loss of function vs irreversible tissue damage is based on the concept of the ischemic penumbra *(45)*. Until recently, only positron emission tomography and single-photon emission computed tomography imaging could approximately define ischemia and penumbra thresholds. However, it is not feasible to routinely perform these imaging studies in the acute stroke clinical setting.

Novel MRI techniques including PWI and DWI add another dimension to diagnostic imaging of the ischemic penumbra *(46–48)*. In a simplified approach, it has been hypothesized that DWI, in the absence of reperfusion, more or less reflects the irreversibly damaged infarct core and PWI the complete area of hypoperfusion *(49–52)*. The volume difference between these two regions is termed diffusion–perfusion mismatch (Fig. 5) (i.e., PWI minus DWI volume—sometimes also as ratio: PWI/DWI volume). The diffusion–perfusion mismatch volume could measure the ischemic penumbra (i.e., tissue at risk of infarction); the natural history of early diffusion abnormalities in untreated patients is to grow over time into the area of the initial perfusion abnormality *(49)*. In addition, a number of groups demonstrated that DWI lesion volume growth can be interrupted with early recanalization *(32,52,53)*. It should be noted that the qualitative identification of more than 20% mismatch has been 95% accurate as a selection criterion in a clinical trial *(54)*.

Overall, this simple model of diffusion–perfusion mismatch appears to be acceptably accurate in most acute stroke patients and the findings of stroke MRI are consistent with our pathophysiological understanding *(32,48)*. Using the mismatch concept, it may become possible to categorize patients into two groups: those who may profit from a specific penumbral salvage therapy and those in whom little ischemic tissue remains to benefit.

The two-zone diffusion–perfusion mismatch model, however, has two limitations. The visually identified PWI lesion includes not only at-risk tissue, but also regions of benign oligemia (tissue with impaired blood flow, but not in danger of infarcting). At present, the optimum PWI algorithm to differentiate oligemia from ischemia has not been established. In addition, DWI abnormalities are potentially reversible, especially with early reperfusion (Fig. 6) *(55)*. Therefore, in some patients, the penumbra includes a portion of the DWI abnormality.

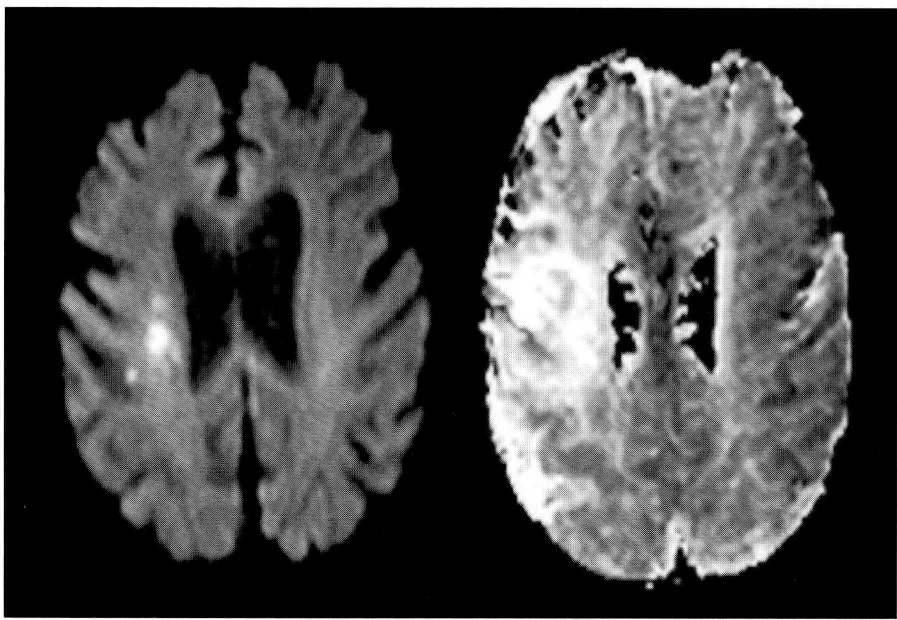

Fig. 5. Example of diffusion–perfusion mismatch in a patient imaging with magnetic resonance imaging at 4 h after symptom onset. Diffusion-weighted image *(left)* shows small region of periventricular hyperintensity. Mean transit time perfusion map *(right)* shows much larger perfusion deficit.

These findings have led to a modified model of the MRI-defined penumbra (Fig. 7) *(56)*. Despite these limitations, the mismatch model may provide an approximation of the penumbra that is clinically useful; this model has the advantage of simplicity. A further discussion of alternative penumbra models may be found in Chapter 3. Alternative multivariate approaches that incorporate data from multiple MRI sequences are under development and have the potential to more accurately predict the ischemic penumbra *(57,58)*.

Another potential use of stroke MRI is the identification of patients at high risk for symptomatic ICH after thrombolytic or other treatment. Preliminary studies suggest that very low-ADC values may be predictive of subsequent HT *(59)*. Other biomarkers such as early blood–brain barrier disruption may also identify patients at risk for reperfusion injury and/or hemorrhagic transformation at a time when therapeutic intervention is still possible *(60)*.

FROM THEORY TO PRACTICE

In a stroke center organized for immediate access to MRI acquisition and interpretation, MRI is often used instead of CT as the neuroimaging screen prior

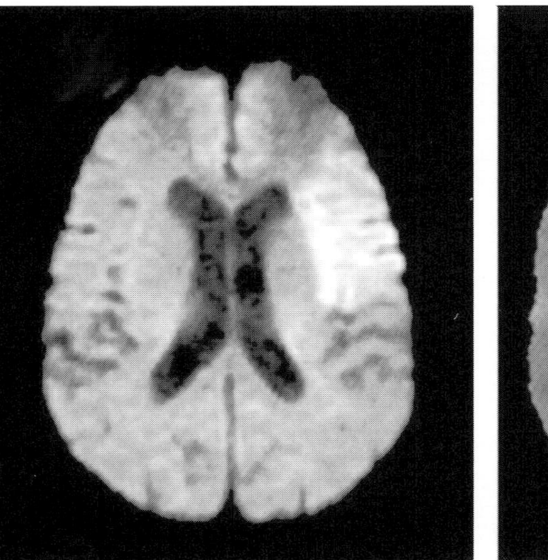

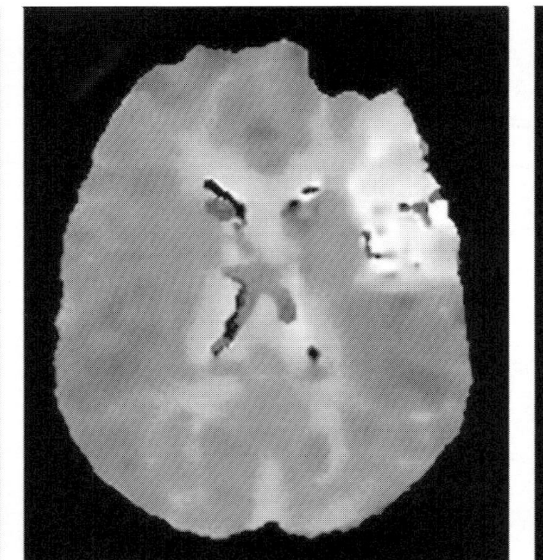

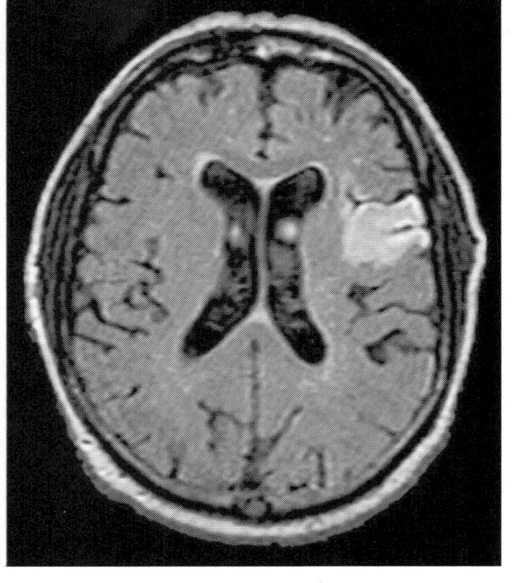

Fig. 6. A 74-yr-old man with a history of hypertension, diabetes, and new onset atrial fibrillation presented with nonfluent aphasia and right hemiparesis (NIHSS score= 7). He was treated with intravenous alteplase starting 2 h and 42 min after symptom onset. Pretreatment diffusion-weighted imaging (DWI) obtained 2 hs 5 min after symptom onset is displayed on the left of the figure, and the concurrent perfusion-weighted imaging in the middle. Follow-up fluid attenuated inversion recovery (FLAIR) image obtained 108 d after stroke onset are displayed on the right. The initial DWI lesion volume was 54.1 cc, and the follow-up FLAIR lesion volume 23.5 cc (reversal of 57% of acute ischemic lesion). The patient recovered with occasional word finding difficulty and modified Rankin score = 1.

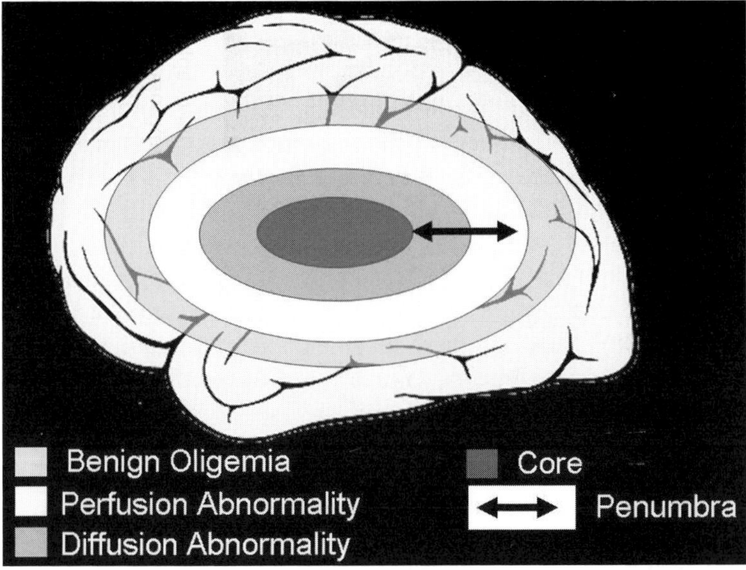

Fig. 7. Modified view of ischemic penumbra as defined by magnetic resonance imaging. *See* color insert following p.110.

to standard intravenous thrombolytic therapy, with times to treatment within published benchmarks. The potential advantages include greater diagnostic accuracy for ischemic and nonischemic pathology, facilitating thrombolysis in patients with uncertain clinical diagnoses, but definite AICS by MRI criteria, and excluding patients with normal CT but confirmed non-ischemic pathology by MRI. MRI may also serve to screen patients for possible intra-arterial thrombolysis *(8)*.

A growing body of data is now available suggesting the utility of employing MRI to identify the ischemic penumbra and assessing response to therapies. Chalela and colleagues studied patients with MRI before and after standard intravenous alteplase therapy and found that perfusion defect reduction by more than 30% within 2–4 h after treatment predicted good outcome (median Rankin score (mRS) 0–1) more reliably than age, pretreatment NIHSS score, or other imaging variables *(61)*. Parsons and colleagues reported a comparison of imaging and clinical outcomes in a group of 16 patients with diffusion/perfusion mismatch treated with intravenous tissue plasminogen activator (t-PA) between 3 and 6 h from onset, compared to a group of 16 historical controls *(53)*. They found that the intravenous t-PA-treated patients had a substantially greater rate of recanalization, smaller infarct volume, greater penumbral salvage, and greater clinical improvement.

Kuelkens et al. used an imaging-based algorithm to make intravenous t-PA treatment decisions in the 3–6-h time window ($N = 48$) *(13)*. Compared to patients treated 0–3 h employing standard National Institute of Neurological Disorders and Stroke criteria, there was no difference in the rate of symptomatic ICH (5.2 vs 4.2%) but there were significantly more asymptomatic ICH and hemorrhagic conversions in the late thrombolysis group (1.7 vs 10.4%, $p = 0.03$). There was a trend toward a lower mortality in the stroke MRI group (16.5% vs 6.3%, $p = 0.08$). Interestingly, the outcome (independent vs dependent or dead, mRS 0–2 vs mRS 3–6) of the stroke MRI group was nominally better than that of the early group, but this difference was not statistically different (47% vs 62.5%, odds ratio 0.54, CI 0.27–1.06). These numbers suggest that by employing imaging-based selection criteria, the time window for treating stroke with thrombolytic therapy might be widened without increased risk of adverse outcomes. However, this will need to be demonstrated in a prospective, randomized clinical trial.

CLINICAL TRIALS

A future role of stroke MRI will be in facilitating clinical trials *(62)*. To demonstrate the clinical utility of an MRI-based acute stroke imaging protocol, randomized, controlled clinical trials employing MRI must be performed. At present, there are a number of roles for MRI in acute stroke trials. In phase II "proof-of-concept" trials, MRI is increasingly being employed as an outcome measure. Stroke MRI parameters such as "lesion growth" or "tissue-at-risk saved" have been and are currently used as markers for drug efficacy in acute stroke studies *(20)*. Trends toward benefit using clinical scales at phase II have been notoriously poor predictors of clinical outcomes in phase III trials that use much larger samples. Proof of pharmacological activity in phase II would be advantageous and efficient before embarking on lengthy, expensive, labor-intensive, and potentially risky phase III clinical trials without evidence of target therapeutic effects. Image-guided phase II studies may identify target biological activity in fewer than 200 patients.

In addition to exploring MRI as an outcome marker, a number of clinical trials are underway that are designed to validate various MRI models for identifying the ischemic penumbra, and in turn, with the goal of identifying the best candidates for reperfusion therapies, even in later than 3-h time windows. In addition, a number of clinical trials are already using MRI criteria to select patients for trial enrolment. The goal of these image-based patient selection studies is to narrow the range of patient characteristics leading to a more homogeneous sample, reducing within-group variance, and increasing the statistical power (lowering sample size requirement) of the experimental design to demonstrate efficacy.

One of these trials has now completed enrollment with promising preliminary results. The Desmoteplase in Acute Stroke investigators reported the results of a dose-escalation trial of the novel thrombolytic Desmoteplase, derived from saliva of the vampire bat (*Desmodus rotundus*) *(54)*. Patients were treated 3–9 h from symptom onset. Diffusion–perfusion mismatch was required for study enrollment. The investigators found a dose-related response both on early reperfusion rates as well as clinical outcome

ALTERNATIVE APPROACHES AND FUTURE DEVELOPMENTS

Acute stroke is not only treated at specialized academic medical centers; indeed, the majority of patients present first in local general hospitals that have no MRI facilities. New CT protocols including noncontrast CT (exclusion of ICH), CT angiography (vessel status) using a source image analysis, and perfusion CT may significantly improve the diagnostic yield when compared to noncontrast CT alone *(63–65)*. Modern CT scanners are more widely available and less expensive than MRI scanners. However, although most community hospitals are capable of performing noncontrast CT scans, advanced CT imaging software and hardware as well as neuroradiological expertise required for multimodal CT imaging with angiography or perfusion is not currently widely available. Perfusion CT probably is as reliable as PWI in detecting regions of hemodynamic compromise *(66)*. However, as with PWI, quantification of cerebral blood flow measures has not been validated. Furthermore, the maximum brain area that can be imaged with current technology is a 2-cm wide slab at the base of the brain; apical infarctions in the most cephalad territories may not be detected. This disadvantage may eventually be overcome with the next generation of CT scanners with larger detector rows.

In the future, it is likely that individual hospitals will adopt either a CT or MRI approach incorporating multimodal techniques that provide detailed individual pathophysiological information assisting in treatment decision making.

CONCLUSIONS

At present, thrombolytic therapy for acute ischemic stroke is underutilized. Among the major problems are that relatively few candidates meet the clinical and time criteria. As the probability of a favorable response to intravenous alteplase decreases with the time from onset of symptoms *(67,68)* and the probability of stroke patients having a penumbra decreases with time from onset *(69)*, selection of patients with neuroimaging signatures of penumbra may prove to be a rational approach to expanding the indications for thrombolytic therapy. New imaging technologies such as DWI and PWI in a multiparametric stroke protocol may help to identify patients eligible for recanalization therapies who would otherwise be untreated using standard criteria. Investigations are underway to determine whether MRI selection beyond established time windows may be beneficial or carry less risk. Furthermore, these novel techniques can be used for and implemented in the design of pharmaceutical trials and thereby help to reduce the study size and make the study sample more homogeneous. This may reduce the number of negative trials while increasing the number and quality of positive studies and therefore be beneficial for developing and establishing new therapies for acute ischemic stroke.

REFERENCES

1. NINDS rt-PA Stroke Group. Tissue plasminogen activator for acute ischemic stroke. *N Engl J Med* 1995;333:1581–1587
2. Reed SD, Cramer SC, Blough DK, Meyer K, Jarvik JG. Treatment with tissue plasminogen activator and inpatient mortality rates for patients with ischemic stroke treated in community hospitals. *Stroke* 2001;32:1832–1840
3. Johnston SC, Fung LH, Gillum LA, et al. Utilization of intravenous tissue-type plasminogen activator for ischemic stroke at academic medical centers: the influence of ethnicity. *Stroke* 2001;32:1061–1068
4. Powers WJ, Zivin J. Magnetic resonance imaging in acute stroke: not ready for prime time [editorial; comment]. *Neurology* 1998;50:842–843
5. Liebeskind DS, Yang CK, Sayre J, Bakshi R. Neuroimaging of cerebral ischemia in clinical practice (abstract). *Stroke* 2003;34:255.
6. Ruland S, Gorelick PB, Schneck M, Kim D, Moore CG, Leurgans S. Acute stroke care in Illinois: a statewide assessment of diagnostic and treatment capabilities. *Stroke* 2002;33:1334–1339
7. Schellinger PD, Jansen O, Fiebach JB, et al. Feasibility and practicality of MR imaging of stroke in the management of hyperacute cerebral ischemia. *AJNR* 2000;21:1184–1189
8. Sunshine JL, Tarr RW, Lanzieri CF, Landis DM, Selman WR, Lewin JS. Hyperacute stroke: ultrafast MR imaging to triage patients prior to therapy. *Radiology* 1999;212:325–332
9. Schellinger PD, Jansen O, Fiebach JB, et al. Monitoring intravenous recombinant tissue plasminogen activator thrombolysis for acute ischemic stroke with diffusion and perfusion MRI. *Stroke* 2000;31:1318–1328
10. Mohr JP, Biller J, Hilal SK, et al. Magnetic resonance versus computed tomographic imaging in acute stroke. *Stroke* 1995;26:807–812
11. Moseley ME, Cohen Y, Mintorovitch J, et al. Early detection of regional cerebral ischemia in cats: comparison of diffusion- and T2-weighted MRI and spectroscopy. *Magn Reson Med* 1990;14:330–346
12. Latour LL, Warach S. Cerebral spinal fluid contamination of the measurement of the apparent diffusion coefficient of water in acute stroke. *Magn Reson Med* 2002;48:478–486
13. Kuelkens S, Schwark C, Schellinger PD, Fiebach JB, Ringleb PA, Hacke W. Systemic thombolysis in ischemic stroke 3 to 6 hours after onset of symptoms using a MR-based algorithm. *Stroke* 2003;34:247A.
14. Fiebach JB, Schellinger PD, Jansen O, et al. CT and diffusion-weighted MR imaging in randomized order: diffusion-weighted imaging results in higher accuracy and lower interrater variability in the diagnosis of hyperacute ischemic stroke. *Stroke* 2002;33:2206–2210
15. Berger C, Fiorelli M, Steiner T, et al. Hemorrhagic transformation of ischemic brain tissue : asymptomatic or symptomatic? *Stroke* 2001;32:1330–1335.
16. Saur D, Kucinski T, Grzyska U, et al. Sensitivity and interrater agreement of CT and diffusion-weighted MR imaging in hyperacute stroke. *AJNR Am J Neuroradiol* 2003;24:878–885
17. Chalela JA, Latour LL, Jeffries N, Warach S. Hemorrhage and Early MRI Evaluation from Emergency Room (HEME-ER): a prospective, single center comparison of MRI to CT for the emergency diagnosis of intracranial hemorrhage in patients with suspected acute cerebrovascular disease. *Stroke* 2003;34:239–240

18. L^vblad KO, Laubach HJ, Baird AE, et al. Clinical experience with diffusion-weighted MR in patients with acute stroke. *AJNR*1998;19:1061–1066
19. Barber PA, Darby DG, Desmond PM, et al. Prediction of stroke outcome with echoplanar perfusion- and diffusion-weighted MRI. *Neurology* 1998;51:418–426
20. Warach S, Pettigrew LC, Dashe JF, et al. Effect of citicoline on ischemic lesions as measured by diffusion-weighted magnetic resonance imaging. Citicoline 010 investigators. *Ann Neurol* 2000;48:713–722.
21. Kidwell CS, Alger JR, Di Salle F, et al. Diffusion MRI in patients with transient ischemic attacks. *Stroke* 1999;30:1174–1180
22. Engelter ST, Provenzale JM, Petrella JR, Alberts MJ. Diffusion MR imaging and transient ischemic attacks [letter; comment]. *Stroke* 1999;30:2762-2763
23. Ay H, Oliveira-Filho J, Buonanno FS, et al. "Footprints" of transient ischemic attacks: a diffusion-weighted MRI study. *Cerebrovasc Dis* 2002;14:177–186
24. Takayama H, Mihara B, Kobayashi M, Hozumi A, Sadanaga H, Gomi S. [usefulness of diffusion-weighted MRI in the diagnosis of transient ischemic attacks]. *No To Shinkei* 2000;52:919–923.
25. Bisschops RHC, Kappelle LJ, Mali W, van der Grond J. Hemodynamic and metabolic changes in transient ischemic attack patients. *Stroke* 2001;33:110–115.
26. Rovira A, Rovira-Gols A, Pedraza S, Grive E, Molina C, Alvarez-Sabin J. Diffusion-weighted MR imaging in the acute phase of transient ischemic attacks. *AJNR* 2002;23:77–83.
27. Kamal AK, Segal AZ, Ulug AM. Quantitative diffusion-weighted MR imaging in transient ischemic attacks. *AJNR* 2002;23:1533–1538.
28. Warach S, Kidwell CS. The redefinition of TIA: the uses and limitations of dwi in acute ischemic cerebrovascular syndromes. *Neurology* 2004;62:359–360.
29. Kidwell CS, Warach S. Acute ischemic cerebrovascular syndrome: diagnostic criteria. *Stroke* 2003;34:2995–2998.
30. Rosen BR, Belliveau JW, Vevea JM, Brady TJ. Perfusion imaging with NMR contrast agents. *Magc Res Med* 1990;14:249–265.
31. Baird AE, Lovblad KO, Dashe JF, et al. Clinical correlations of diffusion and perfusion lesion volumes in acute ischemic stroke. *Cerebrovasc Dis* 2000;10:441–448.
32. Schellinger PD, Fiebach JB, Jansen O, et al. Stroke magnetic resonance imaging within 6 hours after onset of hyperacute cerebral ischemia. *Ann Neurol* 2001;49:460–469.
33. Broderick JP, Adams HP, Jr., Barsan W, et al. Guidelines for the management of spontaneous intracerebral hemorrhage: a statement for healthcare professionals from a special writing group of the Stroke Council, American Heart Association. *Stroke* 1999;30:905–915.
34. Adams HP, Jr., Adams RJ, Brott T, et al. Guidelines for the early management of patients with ischemic stroke: a scientific statement from the Stroke Council of the American Stroke Association. *Stroke* 2003;34:1056–1083.
35. Atlas SW, Thulborn KR. MR detection of hyperacute parenchymal hemorrhage of the brain. *AJNR* 1998;19:1471–1477.
36. Fiebach JB, Schellinger PD, Gass A, et al. Stroke magnetic resonance imaging is accurate in hyperacute intracerebral hemorrhage: a multicenter study on the validity of stroke imaging. *Stroke* 2004;35:502–506.
37. Kidwell CS, Chalela JA, Saver JL, Davis S, Starkman S, Warach S. Hemorrhage Early MRI Evaluation (HEME) study: preliminary results of a multicenter trial of neuroimaging in patients with acute stroke symptoms within 6 hours of onset (abstract). *Stroke* 2003;34:239.
38. Fazekas F, Kleinert R, Roob G, Kleinert G, Kapeller P, Schmidt R, Hartung HP. Histopathologic analysis of foci of signal loss on gradient-echo T2*-weighted MR images in patients with spontaneous intracerebral hemorrhage: evidence of microangiopathy-related microbleeds. 1999;20:637–642.

39. Fan YH, Zhang L, Lam WW, Mok VC, Wong KS. Cerebral microbleeds as a risk factor for subsequent intracerebral hemorrhages among patients with acute ischemic stroke. *Stroke* 2003;34:2459–2462.
40. Kidwell CS, Saver JL, Villablanca JP, et al. Magnetic resonance imaging detection of microbleeds before thrombolysis: an emerging application. *Stroke* 2002;33:95–98.
41. Chalela JA, Kang DW, Warach S. Cerebral microbleeds: MRI marker of a diffuse hemorrhage prone state. *J Neuroimaging*2004;14:454–457.
42. Wiesmann M, Mayer TE, Yousry I, Medele R, Hamann GF, Bruckmann H. Detection of hyperacute subarachnoid hemorrhage of the brain by using magnetic resonance imaging. *J Neurosurg* 2002;96:684–689.
43. Singer MB, Atlas SW, Drayer BP. Subarachnoid space disease: diagnosis with fluid-attenuated inversion-recovery MR imaging and comparison with gadolinium-enhanced spin-echo MR imaging—blinded reader study. *Radiology*. 1998;208:417–422.
44. Mitchell P, Wilkinson ID, Hoggard N, et al. Detection of subarachnoid haemorrhage with magnetic resonance imaging. *J Neurol Neurosurg Psychiatry* 2001;70:205–211.
45. Astrup J, Siesjo BK, Symon L. Thresholds in cerebral ischemia—the ischemic penumbra. *Stroke* 1981;12:723–725.
46. Warach S. Tissue viability thresholds in acute stroke: the 4-factor model. *Stroke* 2001;32: 2460–2461.
47. Fisher M, Prichard JW, Warach S. New magnetic resonance techniques for acute ischemic stroke. *JAMA* 1995;274:908–911.
48. Schellinger PD. MRI-guided therapy in acute stroke. *Expert Rev Cardiovasc Ther* 2003;1:569–580.
49. Baird AE, Benfield A, Schlaug G, et al. Enlargement of human cerebral ischemic lesion volumes measured by diffusion-weighted magnetic resonance imaging. *Ann Neurol* 1997;41:581–589.
50. Warach S, Dashe JF, Edelman RR. Clinical outcome in ischemic stroke predicted by early diffusion-weighted and perfusion magnetic resonance imaging: a preliminary analysis. *J Cereb Blood Flow Metab* 1996;16:53–59.
51. Warach S, Gaa J, Siewert B, Wielopolski P, Edelman RR. Acute human stroke studied by whole brain echo planar diffusion-weighted magnetic resonance imaging. *Ann Neurol* 1995;37:231–241.
52. Jansen O, Schellinger P, Fiebach J, Hacke W, Sartor K. Early recanalisation in acute ischaemic stroke saves tissue at risk defined by MRI [letter]. *Lancet* 1999;353:2036–2037.
53. Parsons MW, Barber PA, Chalk J, et al. Diffusion- and perfusion-weighted MRI response to thrombolysis in stroke. *Ann Neurol* 2002;51:28–37.
54. Warach S, Investigators FTD. Early reperfusion related to clinical response in dias. *International Stroke Conference, San Diego, CA*. 2004.
55. Kidwell CS, Saver JL, Mattiello et al. Thrombolytic reversal of acute human cerebral ischemic injury shown by diffusion/perfusion magnetic resonance imaging. *Ann Neurol* 2000;47:462–469.
56. Kidwell CS, Alger JR, Saver JL. Beyond mismatch: evolving paradigms in imaging the ischemic penumbra with multimodal magnetic resonance imaging. *Stroke* 2003;34:2729–2735.
57. Wu O, Koroshetz WJ, Ostergaard L, et al. Predicting tissue outcome in acute human cerebralischemia using combined diffusion- and perfusion-weighted MR imaging. *Stroke* 2001;32:933–942.
58. Jacobs MA, Mitsias P, Soltanian-Zadeh H, et al. Multiparametric MRI tissue characterization in clinical stroke with correlation to clinical outcome: part 2. *Stroke* 2001;32:950–957.
59. Tong DC, Adami A, Moseley ME, Marks MP. Relationship between apparent diffusion coefficient and subsequent hemorrhagic transformation following acute ischemic stroke. *Stroke* 2000;31:2378–2384.

60. Latour LL, Kang DW, Ezzeddine MA, Chalela JA, Warach S. Early blood–brain barrier disruption in human focal brain ischemia. *Ann Neurol* 2004;56(4):468–477.
61. Chalela JA, Kang DW, Luby M, et al. Early magnetic resonance imaging findings in patients receiving tissue plasminogen activator predict outcome: insights into the pathophysiology of acute stroke in the thrombolysis era. *Ann Neurol* 2004;55:105–112.
62. Warach S. Use of diffusion and perfusion magnetic resonance imaging as a tool in acute stroke clinical trials. *Curr Control Trials Cardiovasc Med* 2001;2:38–44.
63. Schramm P, Schellinger PD, Klotz E, et al. Comparison of perfusion computed tomography and computed tomography angiography source images with perfusion-weighted imaging and diffusion-weighted imaging in patients with acute stroke of less than 6 hours' duration. *Stroke* 2004;35:1652–1658.
64. Lev MH, Segal AZ, Farkas J, et al. Utility of perfusion-weighted CT imaging in acute middle cerebral artery stroke treated with intra-arterial thrombolysis: prediction of final infarct volume and clinical outcome. *Stroke* 2001;32:2021–2028.
65. Wintermark M, Reichhart M, Thiran JP, et al. Prognostic accuracy of cerebral blood flow measurement by perfusion computed tomography, at the time of emergency room admission, in acute stroke patients. *Ann Neurol* 2002;51:417–432.
66. Koenig M, Kraus M, Theek C, Klotz E, Gehlen W, Heuser L. Quantitative assessment of the ischemic brain by means of perfusion- related parameters derived from perfusion CT. *Stroke* 2001;32:431–437.
67. Marler JR, Tilley BC, Lu M, et al. Early stroke treatment associated with better outcome: the NINDS rt-PA Stroke Study. *Neurology* 2000;55:1649–1655.
68. Hacke W, Donnan G, Fieschi C, et al. Association of outcome with early stroke treatment: pooled analysis of ATLANTIS, ECASS, and NINDS rt-PA Stroke trials. *Lancet* 2004;363: 768–774.
69. Darby DG, Barber PA, Gerraty RP, et al. Pathophysiological topography of acute ischemia by combined diffusion- weighted and perfusion MRI. *Stroke* 1999;30:2043–2052.

18 The rt-PA for Acute Stroke Protocol

John Marler, MD *and Patrick D. Lyden,* MD

CONTENTS

INTRODUCTION

To successfully identify, triage, diagnose, and treat an acute stroke victim in time requires a coordinated, multidisciplinary effort that is organized around a predefined protocol. The protocol assures that all needed action will occur in a timely fashion. Also, the ratio of stroke to stroke-mimics may be one to four or five, which mandates the presence of an efficient, skilled procedure for eliminating the mimics (e.g., Todd's paralysis, transient ischemic attack, hysteria, migraine, and carpal tunnel syndrome). Stroke patients must be stabilized according to basic protocols (*A*irway, *B*reathing, *C*irculation) before the neurological evaluation begins; this process should require no more than 1 or 2 min. Stroke management then includes diagnosis and possibly treatment. All of the above is best accomplished with a institutionalized stroke team, comparable to a code blue team that rehearses, monitors performance, and uses feedback to continually improve care.

HISTORY AND RATIONALE FOR THROMBOLYTIC STROKE THERAPY PROTOCOLS

The current tissue plasminogen activator (t-PA) for acute stroke protocol reflects considerable development efforts. Departing for this protocol is unwise, as has been confirmed in several studies. The published guidelines grew slowly

From: *Current Clinical Neurology: Thrombolytic Therapy for Acute Stroke, Second Edition*
Edited by: P. D. Lyden © Humana Press Inc., Totowa, NJ

over the course of several National Institutes of Neurologic Disorders and Stroke (NINDS)-sponsored trials *(1–8)*. At each step in the development of the protocol, a team of investigators evaluated the clinical utility of each item in the protocol. Specific trials were done to determine the best, safest dose of t-PA (*see* Chapters 4–7). The final version of the protocol is contained in the Food and Drug Administration approved package insert, based on the definitive US trial.

The NINDS Stroke Trial investigators published the US study of thrombolysis for stroke in December 1995 *(6)*. Patients received 0.9 mg/kg of t-PA within 3 h of stroke symptom onset. There was scrupulous attention to blood pressure (BP) management prior to thrombolysis: patients were not treated if BP remained elevated above 185/110 after gentle anti-hypertensive treatment. After thrombolysis, patients received sufficient BP management to maintain their BP below those limits. Subsequent analysis of the NINDS data revealed that all subgroups of patients responded to t-PA including patients with different subtypes of stroke, patients with a range of stroke severity, and patients of all ages *(7)*. As a result of this success, the research protocol developed for these trials has become the approved protocol for clinical use of t-PA.

PATIENT SELECTION AND PROTOCOL

Shortly after the publication of the NINDS study, practice guidelines for the use of t-PA in stroke patients were promulgated by the American Academy of Neurology, and the American Heart Association *(9,10)*. These were recently updated *(11)*. Any physician contemplating thrombolytic stroke therapy should study these guidelines carefully, and a continuing medical education course may be helpful as well. A plethora of vital information, including protocols, guidelines, sample orders, and relevant summaries are available on the Web to any physician. Table 1 lists three starting pages. In addition, many stroke research centers have published websites containing their orders and protocols. These sites can generally be accessed via one of the sites listed in Table 1. Prior to the first use of any thrombolytic drug, physicians should rehearse the Code Stroke with a team consisting of, at a minimum, an emergency department (ED) nurse, and a radiologist. Health care systems may need to be changed to allow rapid identification, triage, and treatment of acute stroke patients, and guidelines for this are available *(12,13)*.

Potential stroke victims must be identified as early as possible. Ideally, bystanders and witnesses will learn to recognize strokes, although further education efforts are needed from large, voluntary health organizations, such as the American Stroke Association (AHA) and National Stroke Association, to enhance public awareness. It is unlikely, however, that the complexity of stroke presentation will ever be fully appreciated by the lay public. There are simplified lists of stroke warning signs that may assist in this process.

Table 1
Important Websites Containing Useful Stroke Therapy Protocols

Site	*Sponsor*	*Contents*	*Links to other sites?*
www.stroke-site.org	NINDS Stroke Division	Protocols, scales, guidelines, sample Consensus statements	Yes; very complete, very simple to use
www.stroke.org	National Stroke Association	Consensus statements, general information	Yes. Not oriented to physicians
www.strokeassociation.org	American Stroke Association	Consensus statements NIHSS certification	No.

Patients may be examined first by prehospital providers (paramedics and emergency medical technicians), and considerable advance work should be done by them (*see* Chapter 15) *(14)*. Patients will arrive in the hospital ED by ambulance, or as a walk-in. By whichever route, the next step should be activation of the code stroke system. In some communities, this could include radio activation of the stroke team by medics in the field. The stroke team must be prepared at all times to respond immediately to the ED. In busy neurology practices this preparedness will mandate an on-call schedule with reduced clinic schedules to facilitate immediate response. In medical centers with hospitalists, it may be better for the neurologists to train ED or hospitalist physicians to handle the early phases of the code stroke. Prior to arrival of the code team, department staff should begin the code stroke protocol. This process is facilitated by standing orders that can be initiated by department nursing staff without physician authorization.

It is critical to first establish the time of stoke onset because thrombolysis must begin within 3–6 h. The physician should be suspicious of any secondhand estimates of onset time; it is critical to obtain corroboration from other witnesses. In many cases, the code team physician should telephone the home or scene and try to obtain information from a direct witness. Questions such as these should be asked: When did this happen? What did you first notice? If you returned from an errand to find the victim symptomatic, when was the last time you knew the victim was symptom free? Often using a "time anchor," a term coined by the Cincinnati Stroke Team, is useful: find an event with a known time, such as a television program or the time the call was made to 911, and relate the stroke onset to that event *(15)*. If the patient awoke with symptoms, the onset time is pushed back to the bedtime or last time the victim was known to be at baseline.

Although it is important to carefully set the onset time, there is a risk in overemphasizing some statements from well-meaning friends and family. It is human nature to revisit memory, and try to "explain" a tragedy: often witnesses will embellish with statements like "well, now that you mention it, he was feeling poorly last evening." Versions of "She seemed different last night" have frequently been encountered. These statements must be vigorously pursued: Was there weakness? Were there speech or language deficits? Unless a relatively clear-cut description of definite neurological impairments can be elicited, such vague statements should not be used to set the onset time.

After setting the onset time, a brief past medical history is needed. A thorough history and review of symptoms will be obtained after the code is over; at this point the focus is on stroke risk factors, emphasizing potential sources of cardiac embolism. Knowledge of the medications is essential, especially anti-thrombotics such as Coumadin and aspirin. Next, a brief but thorough examination must be done to elicit focal neurological findings consistent with acute stroke. Until later, time-consuming assessments such as a detailed mental status assessment or prolonged sensory battery should be avided. At this point, the sole purpose is to confirm the presence of focal findings and perform enough examination to preliminarily localize the occluded artery.

Next, specific laboratory studies must be drawn to search for conditions that mimic stroke, such as hypoglycemia, or that may confound therapy, such as a prolonged prothrombin time. The full list of tests is included in the standard orders and is contained in Tables 2–4. A 12-lead electrocardiogram (EKG) must be done to rule out a simultaneous myocardial infarction, which is present in about 5% of all stroke patients *(16)*. Finally, the patient must be taken to radiology for a brain computed tomography (CT) scan to rule out hemorrhage.

Because time is critical, the above sequence must be amended as needed to maintain speed. The physician in charge of the code stroke must ask for status updates, and amend the sequence of events accordingly. For example, if the CT scanner is ready for the patient, but the EKG has not been done, it would be better to go the scanner first and get the EKG upon returning from CT. A frequent source of delay is the transportation of the specimens or the patient. Neurologists are not generally accustomed to worrying about such details, but in the course of analyzing stroke teams at many medical centers, we have found this area problematic. The physician must specify that the STAT specimens from the code stroke must be walked over to the laboratory specifically, even in hospitals that have an established code stroke system. Similarly, medical center policy usually mandates the use of escorts to physically transport a patient to radiology for a brain CT scan; this delays the scan. In our experience, quicker results will obtain if the stroke team members personally move the patient.

Prior to administration of thrombolytics, BP must be less than 185/110. A gentle anti-hypertensive, such as labetolol, may be used but if this fails then the patient must not receive thrombolysis. Recently, nicardipine was added by the AHA to their guidelines for acute BP management after stroke *(11)*. This calcium

Table 2
Sample Physician's Orders for Preliminary Evaluation of a Stroke Patient After Arrival at Emergency DepartmentWhen rt-PA Treatment is Being Considered

Date	*Physician's order*
_______	1. Record time of stroke onset (last time patient seen without stroke symptoms)
_______	2. Activate stroke response system
_______	3. Complete vital signs once, then blood pressure every 15 min
_______	4. STAT noncontrast computed tomography scan of head
_______	5. STAT blood draw for:
_______	a. Complete blood count with platelet count
_______	b. PT and aPTT
_______	c. Glucose (can be done by fingerstick)
_______	6. IV Access: NS or 0.45 NS keep open at 50 cc/h
_______	7. No heparin, warfarin, or aspirin.
	Physician signature _______________________

These orders are available for public copying from the NINDS Stroke Division website at www.stroke-site.org. rt-PA, recombinant tissue plasminogen activator; PT, prothrombin time; aPTT, activated partial thromboplastin time; IV, intravenous; NS, normal saline.

channel blocker will gently lower BP, and may have neuroprotective effects *(17)*. After thrombolysis, however, aggressive therapy must be used to keep the pressure below those limits. Detailed laboratory studies confirmed that elevations of BP predispose to hemorrhage after thrombolysis *(18–20)*. Analysis of the patients in the National Institute of Neurological Disorders and Stroke (NINDS) study for deleterious effects of anti-hypertensive therapy revealed none *(21)*. The patient should be admitted to an observation area where frequent vital signs and neurological checks can be performed.

The selection criteria for thrombolytic stroke therapy are listed in Table 5. These selection criteria are based on the NINDS Trial, and are listed here with minor modification. The criteria reflect primarily a concern for patient safety; therefore, some of the restrictions may seem over-cautious. Current studies will evaluate some of the more restrictive criteria, such as the prohibition of heparin for 24 h following thrombolysis. Physicians who depart from the guidelines should do so only after careful consideration and discussion with the patient and family. Clear documentation should detail the reasons for departing from the criteria. For example, a physician may judge that a patient with a platelet count of 95,000 could safely be treated. Such a decision is well within the purview of an individual physician's judgment, but the thoughts and decision-making process should be well documented. Also, the physician should document concur-

Table 3
Sample Physician's Orders for Treatment of Acute Ischemic Stroke With rt-PA After Preliminary Evaluation

Date	*Physician's order*
______	1. Second IV Access: saline lock with NS flush in opposite arm
______	2. Record results for CT scan, CBC, platelet count, glucose
______	3. If patient has been on warfarin or heparin, record results for PT or PTT
______	4. Give t-PA ____ mg IV over 1 min as a 10% bolus
______	Followed immediately by ____ mg IV by continuous infusion over 60 min for a total dose of ____ mg. Dose calculation:
	Choose the smallest of the following two total stroke treatment doses:
______	a. Maximum total dose 90 mg
______	b. Estimated patient weight in kilograms _____ × 0.9 mg/kg. = _____ mg.
	Total stroke dose = ______ mg, prepared as a 1:1 dilution.
	10% of total dose. Total dose _____ × 0.1 = ______ mg.
	Total dose ____ mg – bolus _____ mg + ______ mg. continuous infusion
______	5. Vital signs and neurological checks every 15 min. for 2 h after start of rt-PA infusion
______	6. No heparin, warfarin, or aspirin for 24 h from start of rt-PA infusion
______	7. Maintain systolic BP <185 and diastolic BP <110 as per protocol.
______	8. Transfer to acute stroke or intensive care unit for monitoring.
	Physician signature ______________________________

Note: These orders represent only one potential approach to the management of patients with ischemic stroke. For each patient, physicians and institutions must determine treatment appropriate for their own situation. These orders are available for public copying from the NINDS Stroke Division website at www.stroke-site.org. rt-PA, recombinant tissue plasminogen activator; IV, intravenous; NS, normal saline; CT, coputed tomography; CBC, complete blood count; PT, prothrombin time; PTT, partial thromboplastin time; BP, blood pressure.

rence of the patient and family, and their understanding of increased risks with protocol deviations.

There are no special subgroups of patients that are particularly likely to respond to t-PA. A complete discussion of targeting subgroups for thrombolytic therapy is presented in Chapter 8. As presented there, extensive analysis failed to identify subgroups that fail to respond to thrombolysis or are particularly likely to hemorrhage*(7,8)*. Thus, the criteria listed in Table 5 are the best guide to patient selection.

The t-PA is administered as an intravenous infusion of 0.9 mg/kg; a 10% bolus is given over 1 min and the remainder is infused over 60 min. The laboratory values may be checked after the bolus; that is, the bolus should not be delayed

Table 4
Sample Physician's Orders for Treatment of Acute Ischemic Stroke in Acute Care Unit After Infusion of rt-PA

Date	*Physician's order*
________	1. Continue emergency department orders for rt-PA infusion and monitoring vital signs and neurological checks until 2 h after start of rt-PA infusion
________	2. Vital signs (BP, P, R) and neurological checks (LOC and arm/leg weakness) every 30 min for 6 h, then every 60 min for 16 h after start of rt-PA.
________	3. Bleeding precautions: check puncture sites for bleeding or hematomas. Apply digital pressure or pressure dressing to active compressible bleeding sites. Evaluate urine, stool, emesis, or other secretions for blood. Perform hemoccult testing if there is evidence of bleeding
________	4. Call Dr. _______, pager # ________ immediately for evidence of bleeding, neurologic deterioration, or vital signs outside the following parameters:
________	a. Systolic BP >185 or Systolic BP <110
________	b. Diastolic BP >105 or Diastolic BP <60
________	c. Pulse <50
________	d. Respirations >24
________	e. Decline in neurological status or worsening of stroke signs
________	5. 0.45 NS or NS IV to keep open at 50 cc/h × 24 h
________	6. O_2 at 2 L/min by nasal cannula (if needed)
________	7. Continuous cardiac monitoring (if needed)
________	8. I's and O's.
________	9. Diet: NPO except meds for 24 h
________	10. Bed rest
________	11. Medications: Acetaminophen 650 mg po. PRN for pain every 4–6 h
________	12. Patient's regular medications previously prescribed, if appropriate
________	13. No heparin, warfarin, or aspirin for 24 h
________	14. After 24 h: CT to exclude ICH before any anticoagulants.

Physician signature ____

Note: These orders represent only one potential approach to the management of patients with ischemic stroke. For each patient, physicians and institutions must determine treatment appropriate for their own situation. These orders are available for public copying from the NINDS Stroke Division website at www.stroke-site.org. rt-PA, recombinant tissue plasminogen activator; BP, blood pressure; P, pulse; R, respirations; LOC, loss of consciousness; NS, normal saline; IV, intravenous; NPO, nothing by mouth; PRN; as needed; CT, computed tomography; ICH, intracerebral hemorrhage.

Table 5
Selection Criteria for Thrombolytic Therapy for Stroke

Patient selection:

Patients must be treated within 3 h of ischemic stroke symptom onset[a]
Obtain baseline computed tomography (CT) to rule out intracranial hemorrhage (ICH), subarachnoid hemorrhage (SAH)

Contraindications:

Greater than 3 h from acute ischemic stroke symptom onset [a]
Rapidly improving minor or major stroke (i.e., transient ischemic attack)
ICH on CT or by history
Suspicion of SAH despite negative head CT
Recent intracranial surgery or serious head trauma or recent previous stroke (in last 3 mo)
Uncontrolled hypertension at time of treatment (e.g., >185 mmHg systolic or >105 mmHg diastolic)
Seizure at the onset of stroke
Active internal bleeding (e.g., gastrointestinal, urinary) within 21 d
Intracranial neoplasm, arterial-venous malformation, aneurysm
Glucose <50 or >400 mg/dL
Lumbar puncture within 7 d, major surgery within 14 d
Arterial puncture at noncompressible site
Acute myocardial infarction (MI) or post-MI pericarditis
Known bleeding diathesis, including but not limited to:
    Current use of oral anticoagulants (e.g., warafin sodium) with prothrombin time >15 s
    Administration of heparin within 48 hpreceding the onset of stroke and have an elevated activated partial thromboplastin time at presentation
Platelet count over 100,000/mm^3
Warning: Carefully consider patients with major early infarct signs on a CT scan (e.g., substantial edema, mass effect, or midline shift)
Warning: Carefully consider risks/benefits in patients with severe neurological deficit (e.g., National Institutes of Health Stroke Scale score >22) at presentation. An increased risk of ICH may exist.

[a]Occasional patients may be treated over 3 h; *see* the text. (Adapted from the NINDS t-PA Stroke Trial Protocol and the Activase Package Insert, Genentech, South San Francisco.)

pending the laboratory results unless the patient is known to be taking Coumadin or is at risk for thrombocytopenia. During the infusion, BP must be carefully maintained below 180/105; serial neurological checks are used to assess the patient's progress. During this hour a more detailed history and neurological examination are preformed, noting any risk factors that may indicate etiology for the stroke. Ancillary investigations, including carotid ultrasound or cardiac echocardiography are considered. After the infusion is ended, the patient should be observed for evidence of response to therapy, or complications, in an observation or intensive care unit.

A number of research groups have now published data showing that community-based neurologists can deliver the drug with statistics that mirror the original study. A full meta-analysis of the community experience since 1996 was recently published *(22)*. For example, in Houston, Chiu and colleagues found a hemorrhage rate of 7% in two community hospitals and one university hospital *(23)*. Full recovery was seen in 37%, mirroring the data seen in the original study. Time to treatment (door-to-needle) was about 100 min, and there was no significant difference between the community and university settings. In a very large survey of 389 successfully treated patients, the rate of good outcomes was the same as in the NINDS trial, and the hemorrhage rate was lower *(24)*. This survey included patients from 57 medical centers, of which only 24 were academic. All of these reports of community experiences are limited by the unavoidable fact that they cannot be blinded or placebo-controlled. Also, unless cases are collected prospectively, there is the risk of biased case selection. At this time, however, it is fair to conclude that if the NINDS protocol is followed scrupulously, then outcome results identical to the original study can be obtained in community hospitals.

FUTURE STRATEGIES

Alternatives to thrombolysis will be necessary for a variety of reasons. Only half of all evaluated patients presented within 3 h of stroke symptoms beginning in the NINDS Stroke Study. Few patients are admitted to the hospital within 3 h, mainly because witnesses and patients do not recognize the warning signs of stroke. Delay in seeking care is attributable to the attitudes of patients, witnesses, and the health care system *(25–27)*. Organizing community stroke networks, including stroke teams, may help in this regard *(27–29)*. The success of public education efforts cannot be predicted, so it must be assumed that there will be many acute stroke patients who present beyond the time window needed for t-PA treatment. Neuroprotection may provide an alternative for reducing damage after stroke. Additionally, neuroprotection may prolong the window for safe use of thrombolysis (*see* Chapter 3). The pathophysiology of brain hemorrhage after thrombolysis is not clearly known, but it appears related to the volume of brain damage that occurs *(30)*. If this is true, and if the volume of brain damage can be limited with a neuroprotectant, then it is reasonable to think that the time window for thrombolysis could be extended. Thus, if paramedics were summoned to evaluate a patient and it did not appear that there was time to get to the hospital for thrombolysis, then a neuroprotectant could be given in the field, which might salvage enough brain that thrombolysis could be given at a later time point *(31)*.

Without doubt, stroke treatment in the future will involve combination chemotherapy *(32)*. No one drug is likely to be successful in all patients and for all strokes. The challenge is to determine which drugs to use in what doses in the combination. An important limitation in this area is that combination trials are difficult. Considerable work is needed in the laboratory to develop criteria for evaluating combination treatments. A logical and efficient strategy is also needed because there are an infinite variety of drugs and different doses to try in combination *(33)*.

Tremendous hope still holds for imaging (*see* Chapters 16 and 17). In the future, an imaging battery will likely document both the vascular occlusion and the brain at risk—region and quantity. Much validation work remains to be done, and for the time being clinical selection criteria are preferred. There is now doubt, however, that eventually imaging criteria will replace the clinical selection criteria described in Table 5.

REFERENCES

1. Brott TG, Haley EC, Jr., Levy DE, et al. Urgent therapy for stroke: part 1. Pilot study of tissue plasminogen activator administered within 90 minutes. *Stroke* 1992; 23:632–640.
2. Brott T, Haley EC, Levy DE, et al. Very early therapy for cerebral infarction with tissue plasminogen activator (tPA). *Stroke* 1988; 19:8.
3. Haley EC, Jr., Levy DE, Brott TG, et al. Urgent therapy for stroke: part II. Pilot study of tissue plasminogen activator administered 91-180 minutes from onset. *Stroke* 1992; 23:641–645.
4. Haley EC, Brott TG, Sheppard GL, et al. Pilot randomized trial of tissue plasminogen activator in acute ischemic stroke. *Stroke* 1993; 24:1000–1004.
5. Kwiatkowski TG, Libman RB, Frankel M, et al. Effects of tissue plasminogen activator for acute ischemic stroke at one year. *N Engl J Med* 1999; 340:1781–1787.
6. NINDS rt-PA Stroke Study Group. Tissue plasminogen activator for acute ischemic stroke. *N Engl J Med* 1995; 333(24):1581–1587.
7. NINDS rt-PA Stroke Study Group. Generalized efficacy of t-PA for aAcute stroke. *Stroke* 1997; 28:2119–2125.
8. NINDS rt-PA Stroke Study Group. Intracerebral hemorrhage after intravenous t-PA therapy for ischemic stroke. *Stroke* 1997; 28:2109–2118.
9. Report of the Quality Standards Subcommittee of the American Academy of Neurology. Thrombolytic therapy for acute ischemic stroke—summary statement. *Neurology* 1996; 47:835–839.
10. Adams HP, Jr., Brott TG, Furlan AJ, et al. Guidelines for thrombolytic therapy for acute stroke: a supplement to the guidelines for the management of patients with acute ischemic stroke. *Circulation* 1996; 94:1167–1174.
11. Adams HP, Jr., Adams RJ, Brott T, et al. Guidelines for the early management of patients with ischemic stroke: a scientific statement from the Stroke Council of the American Stroke Association. *Stroke* 2003; 34(4):1056–1083.
12. Tilley BC, Lyden PD, Brott TG, et al. Total quality improvement method for reduction of delays between emergency department admission and treatment of acute ischemic stroke. *Arch Neurol* 1997; 54:1466–1474.
13. Lyden PD, Rapp K, Babcock T, Rothrock J. Ultra-rapid identification, triage, and enrollment of stroke patients into clinical trials. *J Stroke Cerebrovasc Dis* 1994; 4:106–113.

14. Saver JL, Kidwell C, Eckstein M, Starkman S. Prehospital neuroprotective therapy for acute stroke: results of the Field Administration of Stroke Therapy-Magnesium (FAST-MAG) pilot trial. *Stroke* 2004; 35(5):e106–e108.
15. Timerding BL, Barsan WG, Hedges JR, et al. Stroke patient evaluation in the emergency department before pharmacologic therapy. *Am J Emerg Med* 1989; 7:11–15.
16. Myers MG, Norris JW, Hachinski VC, Weingert ME, Sole MJ. Cardiac sequelae of acute stroke. *Stroke* 1982; 13:838–842.
17. Grotta J, Spydell J, Prettigrew LC, Ostrow P, Hunter D. The effect of nicardipine on neuronal function following ischemia. *Stroke* 1986; 17:213–219.
18. Fagan SC, Bowes MP, Lyden PD, Zivin JA. Acute hypertension promotes hemorrhagic transformation in a rabbit embolic stroke model: effect of labetalol. *Exp Neurol* 1998; 150:153–158.
19. Bowes MP, Zivin JA, Thomas GR, Thibodeaux H, Fagan SC. Acute hypertension, but not thrombolysis, increases the incidence and severity of hemorrhagic transformation following experimental stroke in rabbits. *Exp Neurol* 1996; 141:40–46.
20. Levy DE, Brott TG, Haley EC, Jr., et al. Factors related to intracranial hematoma formation in patients receiving tissue-type plasminogen activator for acute ischemic stroke. *Stroke* 1994; 25:291–297.
21. Brott T, Lu M, Kothari R, et al. Hypertension and its treatment in the NINDS rt-PA stroke trial. *Stroke* 1998; 29:1504–1509.
22. Graham GD. Tissue plasminogen activator for acute ischemic stroke in clinical practice: a meta-analysis of safety data. *Stroke* 2003; 34(12):2847–2850.
23. Chiu D, Krieger D, Villar-Cordova C, et al. Intravenous tissue plasminogen activator for acute ischemic stroke feasibility, safety, and efficacy in the first year of clinical practice. *Stroke* 1998; 29:18–22.
24. Tanne D, Bates V, Verro P, et al. Initial clinical experience with IV tissue plasminogen activator for acute ischemic stroke: a multicenter survey. *Neurology* 1999; 53:424–427.
25. Lacy CR, Suh D-C, Bueno M, Kostis JB. Delay in presentation and evaluation for acute stroke. *Stroke* 2001; 32:63–69.
26. Harper GD, Haigh RA, Potter JF, Castleden CM. Factors delaying hospital admission after stroke in leicestershire. *Stroke* 1992; 23:835–838.
27. Alberts MJ, Perry A, Dawson DV, Bertels C. Effects of public and professional education on reducing the delay in presentation and referral of stroke patients. *Stroke* 1992; 23:352–356.
28. Pancioli AM, Broderick J, Kothari R, et al. Public perception of stroke warning signs and knowledge of potential risk factors. *JAMA* 1998; 279(16):1288–1292.
29. Bratina P, Greenberg L, Pasteur W, Grotta JC. Current emergency department management of stroke in Houston, Texas. *Stroke* 1995; 26:409–414.
30. Lyden PD, Zivin JA. Hemorrhagic transformation after cerebral ischemia: mechanisms and incidence. *Cerebrovasc Brain Met Rev* 1993; 5:1–16.
31. Lapchak PA. Hemorrhagic transformation following ischemic stroke: significance, causes, and relationship to therapy and treatment. *Curr Neurol Neurosci Rep* 2002; 2(1):38–43.
32. Hallenbeck JM, Frerichs KU. Stroke therapy. It may be time for an integrated approach. *Arch Neurology* 1993; 50:768–770.
33. Lyden P, Jackson-Friedman C, Shin C, Hassid S. Synergistic combinatorial stroke therapy: a quantal bioassay of a GABA agonist and a glutamate antagonist. *Experimental Neurology* 2000; 163:477–489.

IV Illustrative Cases*

*Cases prepared by Drs. Yu D. Cheng and Lama Al-Khoury.

Case 1

A 76-yr-old Hispanic woman with atrial fibrillation on warfarin, and end-stage renal disease required 3 d of hemodialysis per week. On the day of admission at 16:50 PM she was almost done with dialysis, when she suddenly became unresponsive, with left-sided weakness and sensory loss. The patient was brought to the emergency room at 17:20 PM by paramedics, where the University of California San Diego (UCSD) stroke team was consulted via a web-based telemedicine system. Neurological examination via videocamera (with a nurse assistant guiding the patient) revealed slurred speech, dense left hemianopsia, left hemiparesis, hemianesthesia, and hemineglect. The total National Institutes of Health Stroke Scale (NIHSS) was 17. Computed tomography (CT) of the head read by on the on-call radiologist was reported negative. At this point, you would:

1. Cancel the code stroke because you cannot personally examine patient at the bedside.
2. Cancel the code stroke because patient was on warfarin, and will not be a candidate for thrombolytic therapy anyway.
3. Cancel the code stroke because the patient may have a metabolic encephalopathy secondary to electrolyte disturbance.
4. Continue the code stroke because the patient may be a tissue plasminogen activator (t-PA) candidate.

With further questioning, the patient's daughter revealed that the warfarin was discontinued recently because the patient suffered significant rectal bleeding 28 ds previously: she was hospitalized and required transfusion of 6 U of packed red blood cells. Work-up with flexible sigmoidoscopy found a rectal ulcer, which was laser cauterized. The patient had another less severe rectal bleed a week after the first event; repeat flexible sigmoidoscopy found another ulcer, which was also treated the same way. The patient has had no hematochezia or melena since then. At this time, laboratory examination results showed: platelets 211,000, hemoglobin 11.5, hematocrit 34.7, glucose 105, partial thromboplastin time (PTT) 34, prothrombin time (PT) 11.9, international normalized ratio (INR) 1.0. Considering all information obtained thus far, you would consider this patient:

1. Definitely not a t-PA candidate because of multiple recent gastrointestinal (GI) bleeds.
2. Possibly not a t-PA candidate because of multiple medical problems, and mild anemia.
3. A candidate for intravenous thrombolysis.

From: *Current Clinical Neurology: Thrombolytic Therapy for Acute Stroke, Second Edition*
Edited by: P. D. Lyden © Humana Press Inc., Totowa, NJ

Following lengthy discussion regarding risks and benefits of intravenous thrombolytic therapy, including the risk of significant GI bleeding, the patient and her family members elected to go with t-PA treatment. Intravenous t-PA was given at 2 h and 10 min after the onset of symptoms. The patient was transferred to UCSD Medical Center by helicopter shortly after t-PA treatment. Upon arrival in the stroke unit, she was found to have some bright red blood on digital rectal examination, but the hematocrit did not significantly change, and the patient required no transfusion during her hospital stay. Serial neurological examinations after the patient arrived at UCSD up to 48 h showed no significant improvement, but no deterioration either. The follow-up CT and magnetic resonance imaging scans are shown in Figs. 1–3.

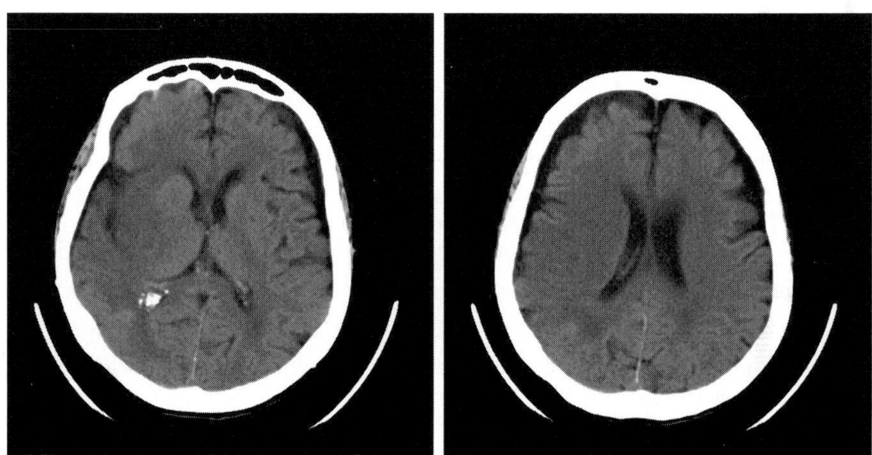

Fig 1. Repeat computed tomography of head without contrast about 15 h after symptom onset showed mild hypodensity in the area of right middle cerebral artery distribution.

COMMENT

There are many lessons illustrated by this case. First, there is an anecdotal association between warfarin cessation and acute stroke. The association derives from the very impressive case—illustrated here—of massive embolic stroke in a patient off warfarin a short time. Clinicians tend to remember such cases, and of course we never see the patients who do *not* embolize off of warfarin. Epidemiological surveys report mixed findings, and there is some evidence to support the safety of brief periods of warfarin cessation. This case illustrates the imperative to *check the history* many times. If the physician had excluded this patient from thrombolysis because of the warfarin history, an opportunity would be missed. Anytime the stroke patient presents with a history of warfarin use, the code stroke should be continued until the PT is reported back from the lab. Even

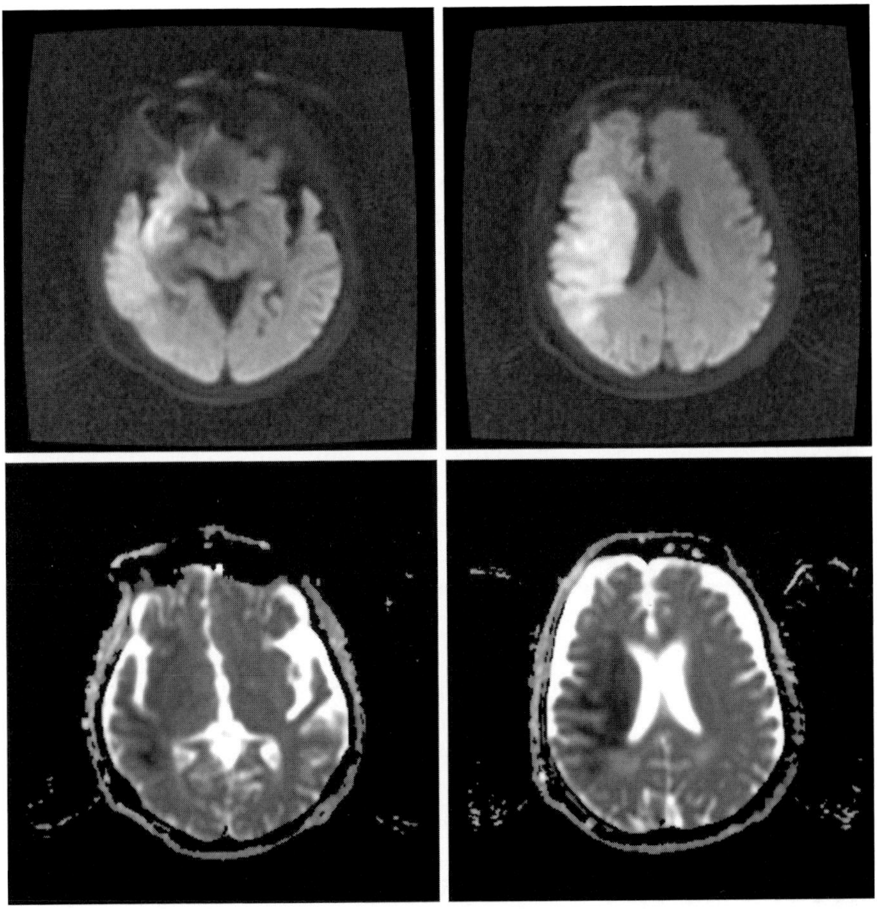

Fig. 2. Magnetic resonance imaging diffusion-weighted image and apparent diffusion coefficient scan showed acute ischemic stroke in the area of right middle cerebral artery distribution.

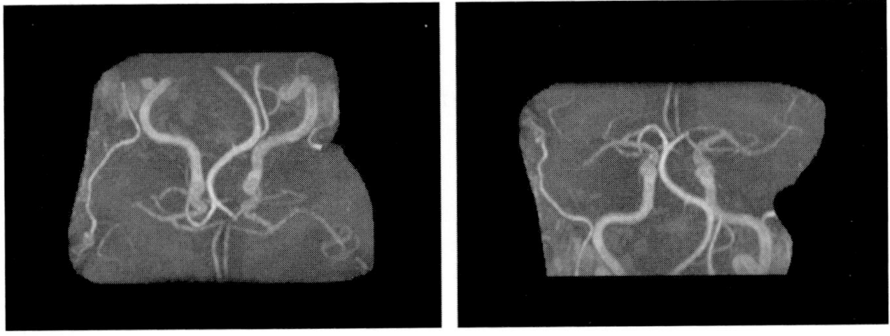

Fig. 3. Magnetic resonance angiography of circle of Willi showed truncated right middle cerebral artery.

patients on a stable dose may develop a subtherapeutic INR—and present with embolization—caused by clotting factor induction, dietary indiscretion, dehydration, and many other factors.

According to the package insert, a GI bleed within the previous 14 d excludes a patient from thrombolytic treatment. For the most part, most physicians should adhere to this rule. In this case, the patient was past the 14-d requirement, but the bleed was of such severity as to require transfusion. Without the history of successful laser cauterization, a physician could reasonably decide against thrombolysis, even if the 14 d were past. On the other hand, many patients would rather not suffer the long-term disability of a large stroke, and are willing to take the risk of thrombolysis understanding that a resulting GI bleed could require intervention. Such risk should not be taken lightly, and only in a center that is equipped for immediate arterial catheterization or stat exploratory laparotomy, or both. Telemedicine is in its infancy, and is not proven reliable. In this case, the patient was part of a clinical trial designed to measure the validity of telemedicine consultation and signed a consent form. Such consultation should not be used outside of a clinical trial, at the time of this writing (2004). The case illustrates how telemedicine might be used in the future. However, therapy was administered in a challenging case, and the patient was transferred by helicopter to a comprehensive stroke center. According to the Brain Attack Coalition Guidelines, most communities will require several basic stroke centers, equipped to administer routine intravenous thrombolysis, and a few comprehensive centers with state-of-the-art advanced care. Had there been a complication of the rt-PA therapy, it would have developed near the end of the flight (45 min). Upon arrival at UCSD, the stroke team met the patient along with the on-call general surgery fellow, just in case bleeding began during the flight. In addition, the flight team was briefed before departure about the possible complications, and was in communication with the UCSD team during the flight. A well-rehearsed transfer system was already in place, and pre- and post-flight procedures were well practiced at both the sending and receiving medical centers; such a transfer would be ill advised in the absence of such preparation.

CASE 2

An emergency department (ED) physician calls you at 17:15 PM regarding a 40-yr-old white man who was found in bed with obtundation and poor movement on the right side.

There was no history of trauma, and no recent or remote history of any cardiac symptoms. He has no prior medical problems except for low back pain for which he takes ibuprofen and very recent complaints of nausea and dizziness over the past 2 wk. For the first time, he complained of headache the morning of presentation; the headache was not severe according to his wife. Despite the headache, he went swimming with his son the same afternoon and was doing fine when he returned home at 16:15 PM, but did not make it back downstairs after he went to his room to change. His wife checked on him and found him; paramedics were called.

On presentation to the ED, his blood pressure was 130/70, pulse was regular at 70 beats per minute. Pulse oximetry was normal. The patient was intubated immediately to protect his airways before you see him. Upon your arrival, your assessment is limited because of the sedation and paralytic agents used.

Computed tomography (CT) of the brain is done and shows a linear dense middle cerebral artery (MCA) sign and a dense dot MCA sign on the left side (Fig. 1A). Moreover, there is loss of the cortical insular ribbon on the left side (Fig. 1B), with a very subtle hypodensity (Fig. 1C) in the MCA distribution as portrayed with the arrows in the figure.

Your options for management after initial assessment and review of the CT are the following:

1. Cancel the code stroke because of the dense MCA sign and its association with poor prognosis.
2. Cancel the code because you cannot get a good neurological examination because of the sedation and paralytic agents on board.
3. Re-evaluate the patient and order further work-up.

You return back from CT, and you get more detailed history from the wife: there are no historical contraindications for thrombolysis. You examine the patient after the effect of sedation and paralytic agents resolves. He is intubated, stuperous, and moves his left arm and left leg occasionally, spontaneously to pain but not to commands. Language cannot be assessed. His NIHSS score is 28.

You order an ultrasound of the neck and it confirms your suspicions, the diagnosis of arterial dissection in the left carotid artery. What would you do next?

1. Cancel the code stroke excluding the patient from thrombolysis because of the evidence of carotid dissection, admit the patient, and do nothing else.

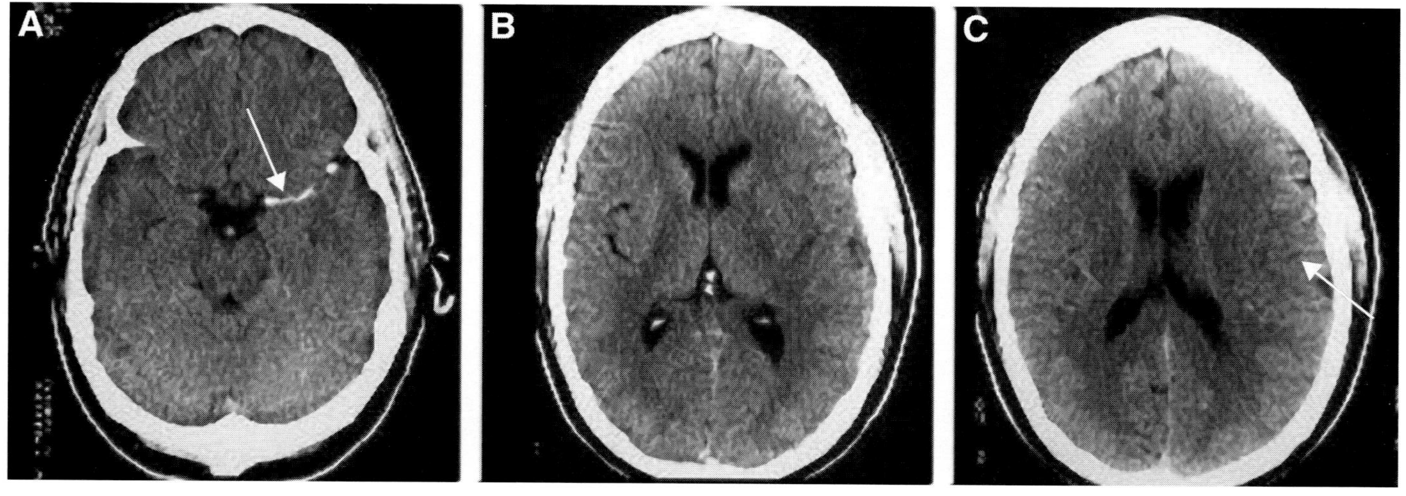

Fig. 1. Computed tomography (CT) of the brain is done and shows a linear dense middle cerebral artery (MCA) sign and a dense dot MCA sign on the left side (**A**). Moreover, there is loss of the cortical insular ribbon on the left side (**B**), with a very subtle hypodensity (**C**) in the MCA distribution as portrayed with the arrows in the figure.

2. Call the interventional specialist and arrange for an angiogram and stenting/local thrombolysis if the lesion is accessible.
3. Start the patient on anticoagulation and admit him.

The patient's wife is given the option of intravenous tissue plasminogen activator (t-PA) vs tenecteplase (TNK)-type t-PA, the latter being part of the research protocol at University of California San Diego, as dissection is not an exclusion criterion for thrombolysis in stroke. A total dose of 0.2 mg/kg TNK-rt-PA is given by intravenous push as part of the phase I trial of TNK in acute stroke treatment.

Follow-up CT of the brain at 48 h done as part of the research protocol of TNK (not for any worsening of symptoms) shows progression of the ischemic changes in the left MCA territory stroke (Fig. 2A,B). There is an island of intact brain tissue within the ischemic bed (Fig. 2B); based on Hounsfield units, this island is not an intracerebral hemorrhage.

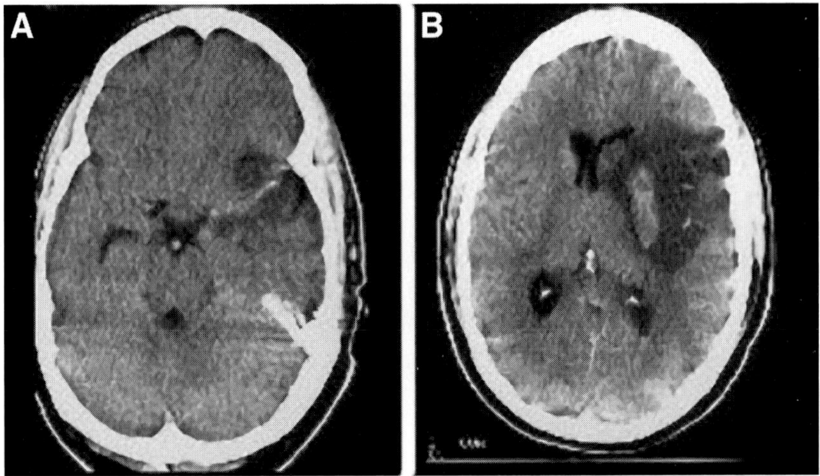

Fig. 2. Noncontrast CT brain scan done 48 h after thrombolysis.

During hospitalization, the patient slightly improves, becomes extubated in a few days and is started on speech, physical, and occupational therapies and eventually is transferred to rehabilitation. On the third month of follow-up he has regained some partial movement in the right upper extremity and right lower extremity, has residual receptive and expressive dysphasia for a residual NIHSS score of 15. He is able to walk with help using a walker.

COMMENT

Stroke in the young is one of the fast growing problems for neurologists; recent data show that stroke incidence in the 45–60 yr age group has risen faster than in any other age group. Carotid and vertebral dissection account for a large proportion of strokes in the younger age groups, but the reason for this is not clear. One consideration is that as the population ages, more individuals remain physically more active to a later age. In this case, the patient's symptoms of nausea and dizziness for 2 wk, and headache for 1 d, are difficult to reconcile with a carotid dissection. It seems reasonable to suspect the dissection was present before he went swimming, and that an embolization occurred during or after the swimming, but there is no evidence.

Dissection is *not* a contraindication to thrombolytic therapy, and indeed, many of the most impressive successes with thrombolysis occur in younger patients with embolization distal to a dissection. Patients respond to intravenous or intra-arterial therapy, but time is crucial; it is best to institute whatever therapy can start soonest and a delay for the neuro-interventional team to assemble is unacceptable. In centers with a well-rehearsed neuro-interventional team, sometimes the delay is minimal, but in a typical setting the intravenous thrombolytic should begin first, while the angiography suite is prepared. Stenting of carotid dissections has no proven benefit yet, and could possibly promote further distal embolization; such procedures should only be performed in the context of a controlled clinical trial after informed consent.

Many new thrombolytic agents will provide a better alternative to recombinant t-PA (rt-PA) (*see* Chapter 1). The TNK-mutated form of rt-PA has many putative advantages, including a longer serum half-life and greater fibrin selectivity, which should result in fewer peripheral hemorrhages, compared to native rt-PA. The natural molecule desmoteplase, derived from vampire bat saliva is even more fibrin selective than TNK, and may show less neuronal toxicity than native rt-PA. None of these agents was approved by the Food and Drug Administration as of 2004 and they should not be used outside of a clinical trial until such approval.

Embolization distal to a carotid or vertebral dissection may be prevented with anticoagulation, although rigorous data is lacking. Based on clinical experience and anecdote, most stroke specialists now consider heparin to be standard therapy for dissection patients, with conversion to long-term (3–6 mo) warfarin typical. Anticoagulation is *not* a substitute for thrombolysis, however, if the patient presents within 3 h of symptom onset. This unfortunate patient suffered a severe stroke, and made a modest recovery. It is not clear whether thrombolysis improved his ultimate recovery or not.

CASE 3

This patient is a 68-yr-old male with hypertension, peripheral vascular disease, coronary artery disease (CAD) who is status post-coronary artery bypass 6 mo ago. The patient returned for a repeat cardiac catheterization after an exercise treadmill imaging study revealed anterolateral and inferior reversible ischemia. He was brought into the cardiac angiography unit at 8:00 AM, received 1 mg of Versed immediately before the procedure, and was able to communicate with physicians and nurses without any difficulty. However, at 10:00 AM, the patient suddenly became unresponsive, and ceased moving the right side of his body. The procedure was terminated and a code stroke was activated.

The initial examination reveals a patient who is unresponsive to verbal as well as painful stimulation: the right pupil is 2 mm, left pupil 5 mm and unresponsive to bright light; there is no Doll's eye response. No spontaneous movements occur on the right side of the body, deep tendon reflexes are hyperactive bilaterally, and Babinski's sign is present bilaterally. The total NIHSS score is 26.

Based on the information available so far, what would be the most appropriate next step?

1. Cancel the code stroke because the patient is having a cardiac catheterization and thrombolytic therapy may cause bleeding from the site of the arterial puncture.
2. Cancel the code because the patient is sedated and his neurological examination may not be reliable.
3. Cancel the code because the patient has significant CAD and the presentation may represent myocardial infarction.
4. Continue the code stroke because the patient may be a candidate for intravenous thrombolytic therapy.

During assessment, the patient remains unresponsive. There is no improvement on neurological examination. His laboratory studies return with serum glucose 104, prothrombin time 10.2, partial thromboplastin time 27, international normalized ratio (INR) 1.1, and platelets 157,000. Computed tomography (CT) of head is shown (Fig. 1).

With this information should you:

1. Cancel the code stroke: this patient is not a tissue plasminogen activator (t-PA) candidate because the CT of head suggests subarachnoid hemorrhage (SAH).
2. Continue but patient is unlikely to be an intravenous thrombolytic candidate because dense artery sign suggests a low likelihood of good response to intravenous t-PA.

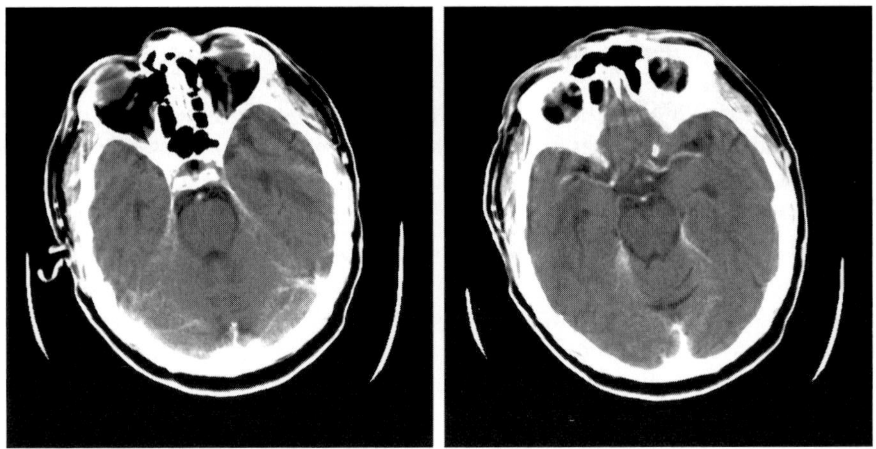

Fig. 1. Computed tomography of head obtained 60 min after symptom onset.

3. Obtain magnietic resonance image/angiography (MRI/A) of the brain and if vascular occulusion is found consider intravenous t-PA.
4. Administer intravenous t-PA now.

The patient is admitted to the stroke unit for intravenous t-PA; a dose of 0.9 mg/kg (10% intravenous bolus, 90% intravenous infusion within 1 h) is administered 1 h and 43 min after symptom onset. About 45 min after t-PA bolus, the patient wakes up, NIHSS score improves to 4 (with mild slurred speech, right facial droop, and drift on right arm and leg). However, 1 h later, the patient drifts into coma again with all his symptoms recurring. At this point, you think:

1. I knew it! It must be intracranial hemorrhage (ICH). Call neurosurgeon now.
2. Start heparin now, the basilar artery may be re-occluded.
3. No heparin, because patient just received intravenous t-PA, and may have a big stroke, heparin may significantly increase the risk of ICH.
4. CT of head STAT.

STAT MRI/A of brain is ordered. However, before the patient is transported to the MRI center, he wakes up again and neurological deficits again resolve. The MRI and MRA of brain show two small infarcts in the right cerebellar hemisphere (*arrows*), absent right vertebral artery, and a truncated left posterior cerebral artery (Fig. 2).

The patient is next given intravenous heparin without bolus, to target PTT at 1–1.5 times of normal. The patient does well throughout his hospital stay; the heparin is discontinued after 24 h and he is discharged home on clopidogrel and Verapmil. He is neurologically intact 2 wk after hospital discharge in a stroke clinic follow-up.

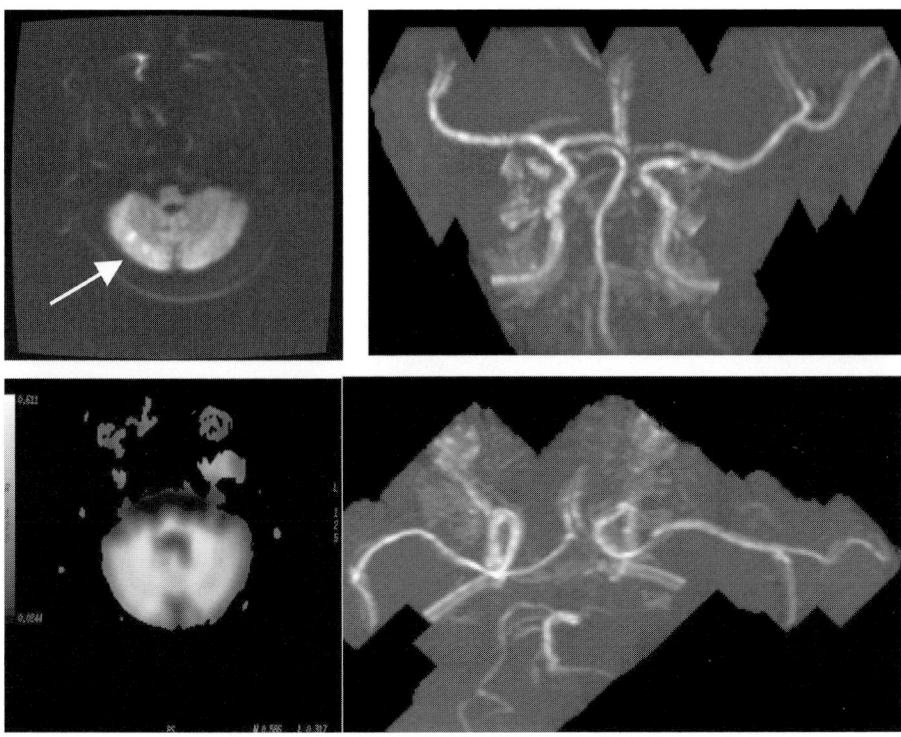

Fig. 2. MRI and MRA of brain obtained 3 h and 45 min after stroke onset.

COMMENT

This patient presumably suffered an embolization to the basilar artery during cardiac catheterization. The altered mental status was initially mistaken for medication effect, until the cardiologist realized he was obtunded 2 h after receiving a single dose of a short-acting sedative. At the moment of this realization, the examination revealed focal findings, confirming that the situation was not a result of medications.

The initial CT scan does not show SAH, although the tentorium has been volume averaged in the posterior fossa slices creating an impression of blood in the cerebellar sulci. This distinction is difficult, but the key observation is the absence of hyperintensity in between the central cerebellar folia. Furthermore, the clinical presentation is not suggestive of SAH.

Management of basilar embolization is challenging. The package insert for rt-PA prohibits the use of anticoagulants for 24 h after thrombolysis, yet most stroke specialists can repeat anecdotes of basilar re-thrombosis after successful thrombolysis. In this case, the gratifying initial response was followed by symptom recurrence, followed by remission. The presence of infarcts in the peripheral cerebellum, and the occluded left posterior cerebral artery, together suggest that the embolus was fragmented by the thrombolytic and migrated distally into multiple territories; there is no conclusive proof of this, however. Given the possibility of further thrombosis, however, the team decided to institute heparin anticoagulation anyway, despite the package insert. Such a choice may be prudent, but should be clearly explained to the family—and patient if possible—and consent documented. Further studies of combined thrombolysis and anti-thrombotic therapy are continuing, and were not considered standard care as of 2004. In certain selected cases, such as this one, however, a physician may reasonably choose to combine anti-thrombotic therapy with rt-PA.

Case 4

This 57-yr-old female is brought to the trauma center because she fell and hit the left side of her forehead on the corner of a table. Initial evaluation by a trauma surgeon found a small ecchymosis on the left forehead with some skin abrasion, significant weakness of her left upper and lower extremities, and slurred speech. You are now contacted for your opinion as to whether "this could be a stroke." You activate a code stroke and proceed to the trauma center, where you obtain the additional history that shortly after sitting down to watch a TV show the woman got up to get a soda. In the process of trying to stand up, she fell to her left because her left leg gave out and in falling, struck her head. After consulting the TV guide, you learn that the TV show she watched was scheduled to begin at noon, and she says she was sitting no more than a few minutes before deciding to get up for the soda. She denies headache, nausea, vomiting, visual or language disturbance, but speech became slurred.

Her past medical history is significant for hypertension, kidney resection in 1992 because of "kidney cancer," partial stomach resection resulting from severe peptic ulcer about 4 yr ago, and colon resection several years ago. She is not using any anticoagulation medication at the time, denied history of gastrointestinal (GI) or intracranial hemorrhage in the past.

With the history obtained, you decide to:

1. Cancel the code stroke because the patient has a head injury; she will not be a candidate for thrombolytic therapy.
2. Cancel the code because the patient has a history of severe peptic ulcer disease, thus ruling her out for thrombolytic treatment.
3. Cancel the code because the patient has history of cancer and multiple major surgeries in the past; tissue plasminogen activator (t-PA) is not safe for her.
4. Continue, she could be a t-PA candidate.

Your physical examination shows the patient to be awake, alert, oriented to person and place, but not date. Her speech is slurred, and she completely ignores her left side. She exhibits homonomous hemianopsia, her eyes deviate to the right, and she shows significant sensory and motor deficit of the left face. Her left upper extremity is flaccid, with no proximal movement; she barely moves her left lower extremity. There is a dense left hemi-anesthesia. You calculate the total NIHSS score to be 19. Laboratory studies include normal serum glucose, coagulation profiles, and platelet count. Computed tomography (CT) head scan shows a small hypodensity in the left hemisphere, a blurring of gray/white matter junctions and flattening of sulci at right parietal lobe without evidence of hemorrhage of any kind (Fig. 1). At this point, it is now 2 h and 50 min after symptom onset.

Your next decision would be to:

1. Cancel the code stroke because you probably would not have enough time to prepare t-PA anyway.
2. Cancel because the onset time is not known with certainty.
3. Cancel because early signs of right parietal lobe acute ischemia is a contraindication for t-PA therapy.
4. Call interventional neuroradiologist for intra-arterial (IA) t-PA
5. Get t-PA from pharmacy and prepare it at bedside for intravenous t-PA treatment.

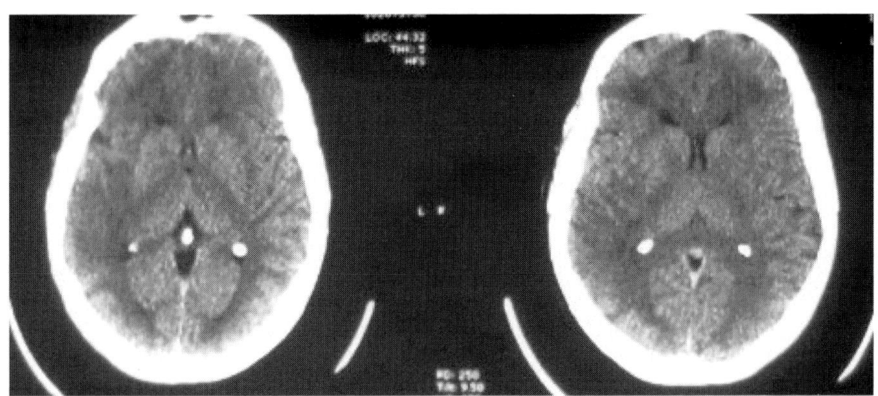

Fig. 1. Computed tomography of head taken 2 h after symptom onset.

Unfortunately, there was no t-PA in the emergency department satellite pharmacy, so you order t-PA from the main pharmacy, which is brought 20 min outside of the 3-h-window. While waiting for the rt-PA, you contact the interventional neuroradiologist, who happens to be in-house. He is able to take patient into the angiography suite within 15 min. Cerebral angiography subsequently showed a truncated right M2 branch (Fig. 2A). Thus, t-PA was slowly infused into the occlusion site over 2 h to a total of 20 mg, together with 5 mg Integrilin, to achieve partial re-canalization of the vessel (Fig. 2B) at the end of the procedure (6 hafter symptom onset).

The patient shows some improvement of slurred speech and left leg weakness immediately after the procedure and thrombolytic therapy, but the significant left arm weakness and left hemi-neglect persist. A follow-up CT of the head 24 h after the onset of symptoms shows a lucency in the right middle cerebral artery (MCA) distribution (Fig. 3). Other work up for stroke including carotid ultrasound and echocardiogram were within normal limits.

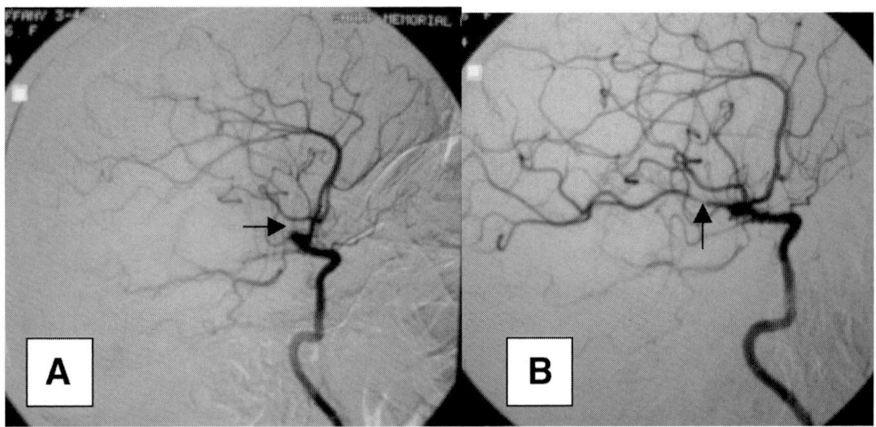

Fig. 2. **(A)** Angiogram taken before intra-arterial (IA) t-PA treatment. **(B)** Angiogram taken after IA t-PA and Integrilin infusion.

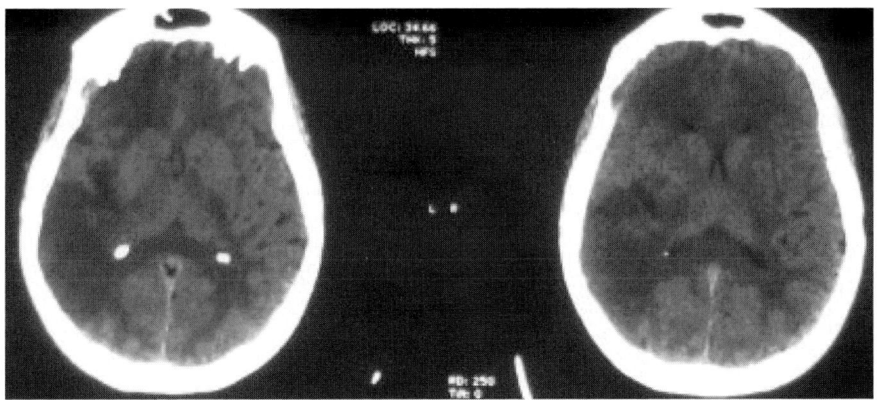

Fig. 3. Computed tomography of head obtained 24 h after symptoms onset.

COMMENT

Establishing the precise onset time is critical in all cases of thrombolytic therapy for stroke. In this case, we are fortunate that the patient was watching television, and this is a common situation. It was very helpful to know that she stood up near the beginning of the program, so the time could be further defined. There are other useful "time anchors" that you can use to refine the onset time, such as a recurring activity that always occurs at the same time every day.

Mild head trauma is common after stroke, especially severe stroke, and in some settings these patients present to the trauma unit. Only the neurologist in this case was able to decipher the sequence of events, and learn that the fall came as a result of the hemiparesis. Otherwise, there would be a suspicion of carotid dissection resulting from the fall. A skull ecchymosis or even laceration should not necessarily contraindicate thrombolytic therapy; always examine the CT head scan for evidence of hematoma or contusion. If you do elect to treat, you will need to watch the scalp injury closely, and if oozing occurs, apply a compression bandage.

The remote history of cancer surgery and peptic ulcer disease are not absolute contraindications, but should be considered. This patient should be watched carefully for any evidence of GI bleeding after thrombolytic therapy, and a GI specialist should be called in if necessary. Significant GI or gastric ulcer bleeding within the 14 d prior to the stroke would be a stronger, but still not absolute, contraindication.

The 3-h time limit for intravenous thrombolytic therapy should be absolute in most centers. In experienced centers, however, many specialists will treat over the time limit. Recent pooled analysis of the ECASS, ATLANTIS, and NINDS trial data (*see* Chapter 7) indicates that intravenous thrombolytic therapy is safe, and may have some benefit up to 4–5 h after stroke. The Food and Drug Administration approval, however, limits the therapy to only 3 h after stroke. In individual circumstances, physicians may reasonably decide to exceed the time limit, but in general the family should be informed that this use is not approved. Whether IA therapy is a reasonable alternative depends on the experience in your facility, and the availability of the team. In this case, the interventionalist was nearby, and the angiography team was already assembled. In most circumstances, however, at least an hour will be needed to bring in the team—it might be more reasonable to use the intravenous therapy.

A large acute infarction is not a contraindication to thrombolytic therapy (*see* Chapter 16), and in fact may predict and increased likelihood of benefit. A large, frank hypodensity, however, should call the onset time into question, and probably should contraindicate therapy. In this case, the degree of lucency in the MCA territory (Fig. 1) is borderline; some physicians, Dr. von Kummer included, would likely not give this patient intravenous rt-PA. The data to support this course, however, is not clear, and in many stroke centers this patient would be treated. The key steps, when subtle lucency is detected, are to: (a) re-check the time of onset and make sure it is not more than 3, (b) inform that patient or family or both that there may be an early infarct, and (c) follow the remainder of the protocol scrupulously. As shown in Chapter 13, subtle early ischemic changes may actually predict the most gratifying response to therapy. The frank hypodensity, however, would be a contraindication for all of us.

Case 5

A 57-yr-old Hispanic man presents with acute right-sided weakness that began about 1 h ago. He states that he arrived home at 3:15 PM in his usual condition. However, about 45 min later he experienced sudden onset of right-sided weakness such that he was barely able to move his right arm and leg. At the same time, patient also complained of some chest pain without nausea, vomiting, palpitation, sweating, headache, visual or speech disturbance. Paramedics were called and patient was brought to the emergency department (ED) by ambulance.

Significant past medical history includes hypertension and status post ventral abdominal wall herniation repair about one month ago; there is no history of gastrointestinal or gastric ulcer hemorrhage.

With the history obtained so far, you would like to:

1. Cancel the code stroke because the patient had a recent surgery.
2. Cancel the code stroke because the patient is having chest pain: myocardial infarction (MI) is a contraindication for tissue plasminogen activator (t-PA) therapy.
3. Continue code stroke, patient may still be a candidate for t-PA treatment.

Code stroke continues and is evaluated via an internet televideo system. On initial examination, the patient exhibits some poor effort and is not able to move either side of his face, however, there does appear to be some movement on the left side of the face intermittently but not on the right side. He barely raises his right arm and leg, but does not resist gravity. He also demonstrates some naming difficulties and dysarthria. His total NIHSS score is 10. Other physical examination shows a well-healed surgical scar on ventral abdominal wall. Laboratory studies show serum glucose of 113, INR is 1.1 and platelet count remains pending. The computed tomography of the head is read locally by the on-call neurologist, and by you over an internet imaging viewer. Both readings agree that there is no evidence of hemorrhage, mass or acute stroke. In considering thrombolytic treatment, you would like to:

1. Cancel the code stroke because you can't reliably evaluate a patient for t-PA treatment using telemedicine.
2. Cancel the code stroke because the patient exhibits poor effort on motor examination: his symptoms might be functional.
3. Wait for the result of platelet count: you can't treat the patient with t-PA without platelet count.
4. Treat the patient with t-PA because time is brain.

After discussion with the local ED physician and the patient, treatment is begun using intravenous t-PA at 0.9 mg per kg, with 10% bolus and 90% infusion over 1 h. The patient is transferred to the University of California San Diego Stroke Center by helicopter about 3 h after t-PA administration. Reassessment on arrival shows no change on NIHSS score. However, the patient's motor deficit recovers gradually over the course of hospitalization. Magnetic resonance imaging (MRI) and magnetic resonance angiography of brain performed about 16 h after the symptom onset shows no evidence of acute stroke or intracranial artery stenosis (Fig. 1). The patient receives physical and occupational therapy during the hospital stay, and is discharged with mild gait disturbance without marked motor weakness.

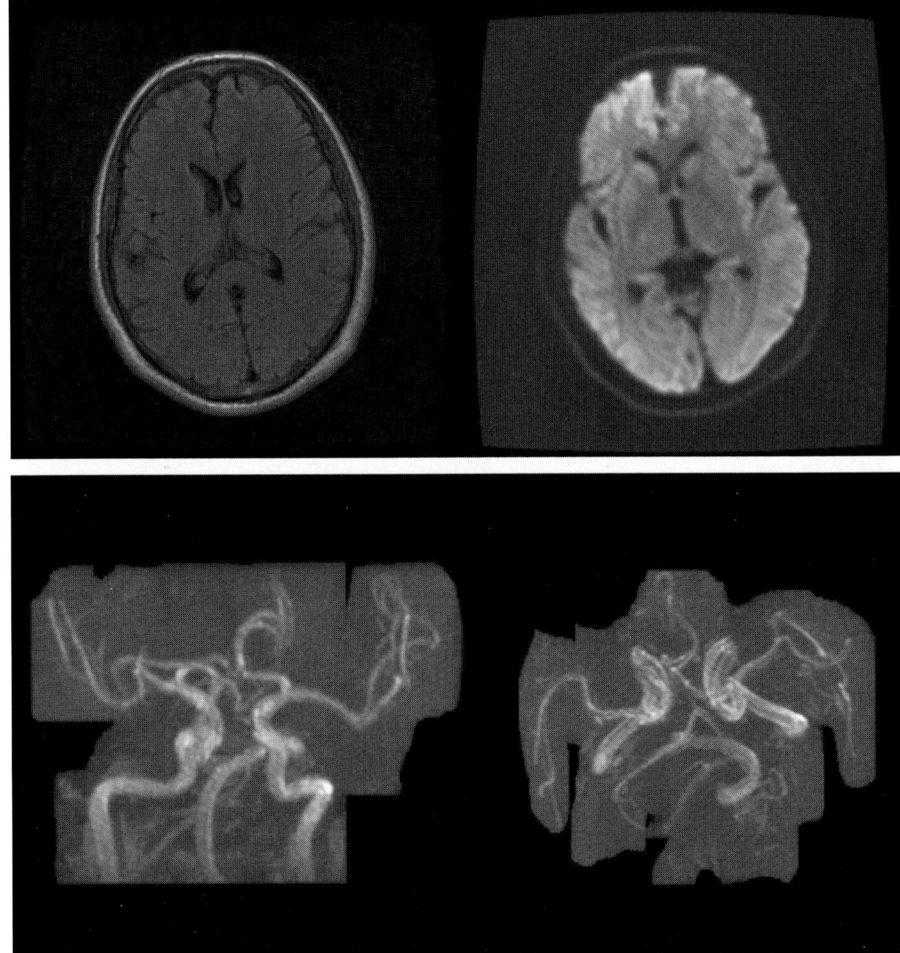

Fig. 1. Magnetic resonance imaging and magnetic resonance angiography of brain obtained 16 h after symptom onset.

COMMENT

Although acute MI is a clear contraindication to thrombolytic therapy in a stroke patient, simultaneously stroke is a contraindication to thrombolytic therapy for acute MI. Many stroke experts discuss the unique situation of a truly simultaneous acute stroke and MI; most of us would treat the patient with the dose approved for stroke (0.9 mg/kg), which is lower and theoretically safer than the cardiac dose. However, a truly simultaneous onset is rare. Much more commonly, the patient suffers an MI that is not recognized for 1 or 2 d; usually the patient is stoic, and suffers an angina equivalent such as dyspepsia or jaw pain. Finally, perhaps because of myocardial akinesia, the patient suffers an embolism and presents with stroke. In this setting, intravenous thrombolytic therapy should not be used because of the risk of hemorrhage into the weakened myocardium; cardiac rupture and pericardial tamponade have resulted.

In contrast, many patients suffer chest pain at the onset of a stroke. The clinician must proceed with caution, using history, examination, and the electrocardiogram (EKG) to evaluate the possibility of cardiac ischemia. Chest pain alone does *not* contraindicate thrombolytic therapy for stroke. If cardiac enzymes can be obtained immediately, it would be prudent to delay treatment until the results are known, but in the typical situation, the decision must be made before these tests are available. The physician should be reassured, however, by the knowledge that if the 12-lead EKG shows no frank ischemia, the risk of cardiac wall rupture owing to thrombolytic hemorrhage is very small, even if there turns out to be a small amount of subendocardial ischemia.

Telemedicine is a novel technology that was experimental as of 2004. We expect telemedicine, however, to extend the reach of consultants—including neurologists—to remote sites. It remains to be proven whether the neurological examination can be performed reliably via the internet, but it seems a reasonable hypothesis. Even if the examination proves unreliable, certainly the history can be obtained, and if the ED physician can perform the NIHSS, then the consultant may be able to render a valid decision. Much of the ongoing research should be completed by the time this book is published.

Functional embellishment clouds the neurological examination in many cases. Every experienced neurologist will recall a patient with a completely functional presentation (conversion disorder or malingering) but much more commonly, the frightened stroke patient exaggerates the findings. Among nearly 1000 thrombolytic treatments, the editor has treated a conversion disorder only once; and the literature contains precious few such reports. On the other and, it is not rare to encounter a patient who embellishes to such a degree that the clinician wonders if any true deficit underlies the presentation; usually there is indeed some underlying ischemic event. When in doubt, it is reasonable to begin treatment; thrombolytic therapy is safe in patients with no ischemia and the clock is ticking; it may be better to begin the treatment against the possibility that there is a stroke, rather than delay therapy pending clarification. Experimental studies are quite reassuring: bleeding does not occur in the brain in the absence of ischemia, so there is no serious risk to starting therapy in the ambiguous patient. In this patient, the normal diffusion weighted MRI scans argue for either a functional etiology, or successful early thrombolysis. Over the patient's hospital course, the evolution of the symptoms and the pattern of recovery strongly suggested that the patient indeed had suffered a neurological event, and the presentation was contaminated by functional overlay. Absent findings on the diffusion imaging, however, there is no way to prove this point.

Case 6

The emergency department (ED) calls a code stroke for a 71-yr-old right-handed white woman because of acute left-sided numbness and dysarthria that started 2 h prior to presentation. Her past medical history is positive for chronic atrial fibrillation (AF) on coumadin, coronary artery disease status post-coronary artery bypass surgery, and hypertension.

What would you do next?

1. Walk away and exclude the patient because she is on coumadin.
2. Accompany the patient to computed tomography (CT) scan to rule out intracranial hemorrhage (ICH).
3. Wait on the lab results and continue to evaluate the patient.

You evaluate the patient further while waiting for the CT of the brain. Her pulse is irregularly irregular at 76 beats per minute and her blood pressure is 194/74. Her electrocardiogram (ECG) shows AF and the finger-stick blood glucose check is 120. Her systemic examination shows absent bruits, no cardiac murmurs, an irregular heartbeat, and palpable and symmetric pulses. On neurological exam, she is awake and oriented, pupils are equal and reactive. Her previously reported facial weakness has apparently resolved. She has dysarthria and trace left-sided weakness in the arm and leg with no drift. The sensations are decreased to touch and pain on the left side but there is no extinction on double sensory stimulation. Cerebellar exam is normal within the level of weakness on the left side with slower rapid alternating movements on that side. The total NIHSS score is 4.

The CT scan of the brain now appears on the control room monitor, and your opinion is that it is negative except for ischemic deep white-matter changes. The patient announces that she feels much better, with clearer speech, resolving sensory symptoms and minimal residual left-sided weakness. The prothrombin time/international normalized ratio (INR) comes back as 1.6. What would you do next?

1. Give the patient an intravenous fluid bolus.
2. Exclude the patient from thrombolysis as she is on coumadin.
3. Exclude the patient from thrombolysis because of dramatic improvement.
4. Admit the patient and start on heparin and increase the dose of coumadin until the patient becomes therapeutic.

You decide against thrombolysis because the patient has dramatically improved. You admit the patient and adjust her coumadin dose to achieve therapeutic levels. The next day she wakes up with new right-sided weakness and numbness and worsening of her dysarthria. A STAT CT of the brain shows a hyperdense basilar artery, as shown in Fig. 1. Note that the patient is now almost 24 h from onset of first symptoms. As you watch, the patient's mental status starts declining. She becomes unconscious with a dilated poorly reactive right pupil, and decerebrate posturing.

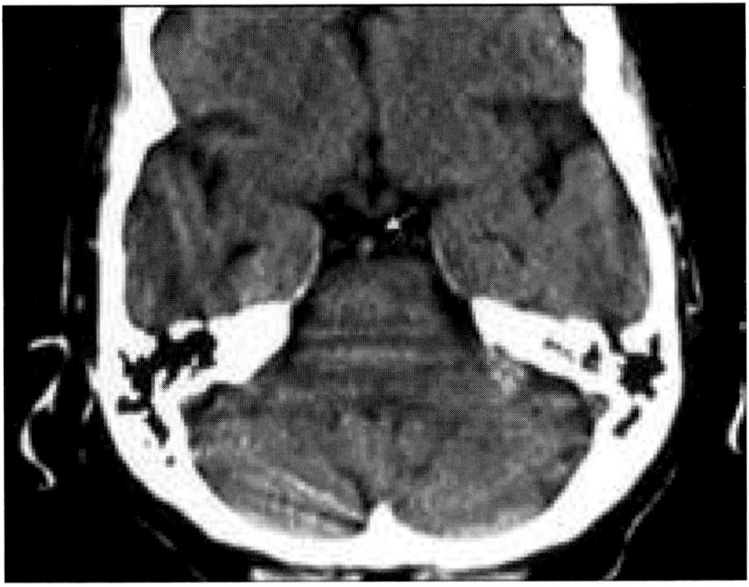

Fig. 1. Noncontrast CT brain scan after second event.

What will you do next?

1. Inform the family that the patient has a very serious and life-threatening condition with high mortality and morbidity.
2. Administer intravenous fluids and heparin, with the hope that the patient will improve.
3. Call the interventional radiologist and arrange for a STAT cerebral angiogram for possible interventional therapy.

You talk with the family and explain the diagnosis and the grim prognosis of a basilar artery thrombosis. You recommend intervention and call interventional radiology to perform a cerebral angiogram and attempt intra-arterial (IA) thrombolysis. The family members consent to the procedure.

The cerebral angiogram shown in Fig. 2 reveals a distal basilar artery thrombus with no flow distal to it (*arrow*). IA tissue plasminogen activator (t-PA) is administered with recanalization of the basilar artery and resumption of flow to the posterior cerebral arteries.

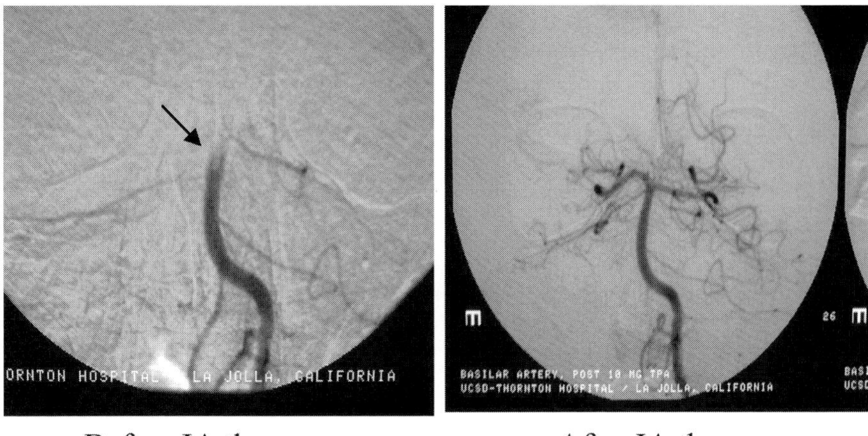

Before IA therapy After IA therapy

Fig. 2. Angiogram of the basilar artery before and after IA thrombolysis.

The patient gradually improves after the procedure. She continues to improve during the hospitalization despite pneumonia and prolonged intubation. She begins coumadin for chronic anticoagulation Eventually, she is extubated, and her final neurological exam upon discharge shows her to be awake and oriented, with only mild residual right-sided weakness. On clinic follow-up, the patient is doing very well with subtle right-sided deficit.

COMMENT

In this case, the patient was supposedly taking coumadin to prevent cardioembolic stroke from AF. The authors have seen many cases in which the patient arrives with a subtherapeutic INR, despite continuing a stable coumadin dose. Therefore, one should not exclude patients from consideration for thrombolytic therapy until the INR is obtained. On the other hand, one should generally not push intravenous t-PA until the INR has returned from the lab, an unavoidable delay in patients who say they are taking coumadin. The history suggests that this patient suffered two different embolizations; the first one resolved quickly but the second one was larger, and occluded the basilar artery. An alternative mechanism would be that the embolus occurred, and collateral flow from other sources allowed the symptoms to abate. Overnight, collateral flow waned, and new symptoms developed. There is no way to sort out these possibilities in retrospect, but *see* Chapter 12 for a more thorough explanation of the mechanisms and approaches to these sorts of cases. Basilar thrombosis is frequently fatal, so in this case, it seemed prudent to proceed to angiography when the patient worsened, even though some symptoms had been present for more than 18 h. In general, if an experienced neuro-interventionalist is available, basilar occlusions should be treated with IA therapy. Salvage has been reported up to 24 h after symptom onset, although the odds of benefit decline hourly, and early treatment has a much greater chance of benefit.

CASE 7

A code stroke is activated for a 66-yr-old man who woke up with right arm and leg aching pain and parasthesia. The patient called paramedics by himself, but before arrival in the emergency department, his right arm and leg becomes flaccidly weak. Upon arrival, the patient is very agitated, follows only simple commands, and denies headache, vertigo, or double vision. He also denies chest pain, shortness of breath, abdominal pain, neck or back pain. There was no recent trauma and the patient has no known medical problems although he admitted that he had not seen a physician for years.

Physical examination shows that the patient follows only simple commands, but was oriented to person, place, and date. His blood pressure (BP) was 240/99 on arrival, and after receiving 40 mg of intravenous labetalol, it is 198/87. The patient has no facial asymmetry but shows flaccid weakness of the right upper extremity and moderate weakness of the right lower extremity. Light touch and pinprick are diminished over the right upper and lower extremities; there is no extinction. The total NIHSS score is 9. Computed tomography (CT) of the head is shown in Fig. 1.

At this time, you decide to:

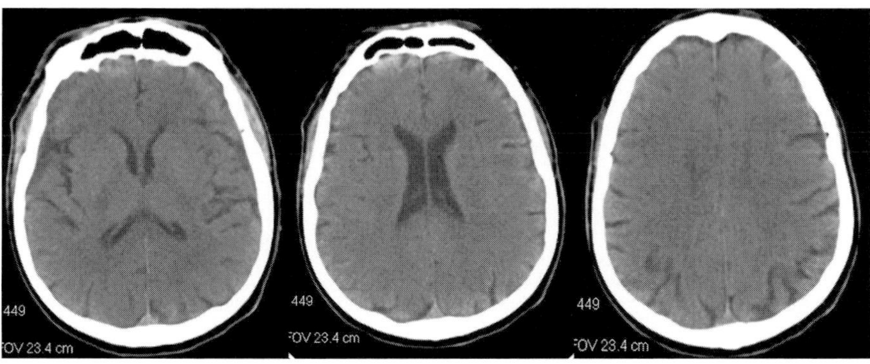

Fig. 1. Computed tomographyof head performed 20 min after the patient arrived at the emergency department.

1. Cancel the code stroke because the patient woke up with symptoms.
2. Cancel the code stroke because the patient has uncontrolled hypertension.
3. Continue.

This patient is not a candidate for tissue plasminogen activator therapy because of unknown time of onset and uncontrolled hypertension. Aggressive BP control continues; because the patient's BP continues to fluctuate, BP is also obtained from his right arm. Surprisingly, patient's BP detected from right arm was significantly lower than from left arm. With this surprise finding, you decide to:

1. Just take it easy, the patient was very agitated and because he was moving his healthy (left) arm, the BP measurements are not accurate on the left.
2. Obtain an ultrasound electively because patient may have subclavian steal or significant peripheral vascular disease in his right arm.
3. Red flag! Patient may have an aortic dissection and needs CT of chest immediately.

With arm pain, asymmetric BP and pulse, and stroke symptoms, an aortic dissection is suspected. Review of chest x-ray shows mild widening of mediastinum (Fig. 2). CT scan of neck, chest, and abdomen were performed, showing type 1 aorta dissection (Fig. 3), extending from the origin of aorta (Fig. 3C,D) to right internal carotid artery (Fig. 3E,F) and right common iliac artery (Fig. 3G).

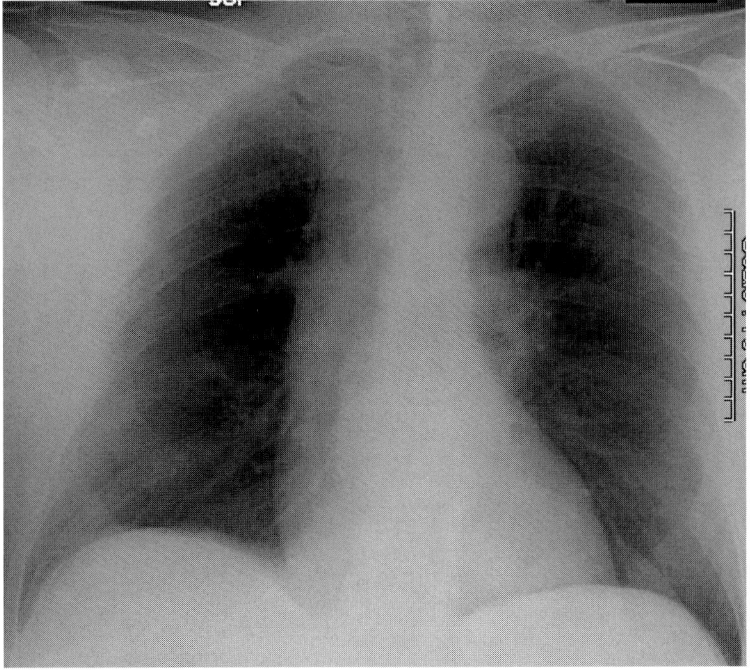

Fig. 2. Chest X-ray obtained in the emergency department during code stroke.

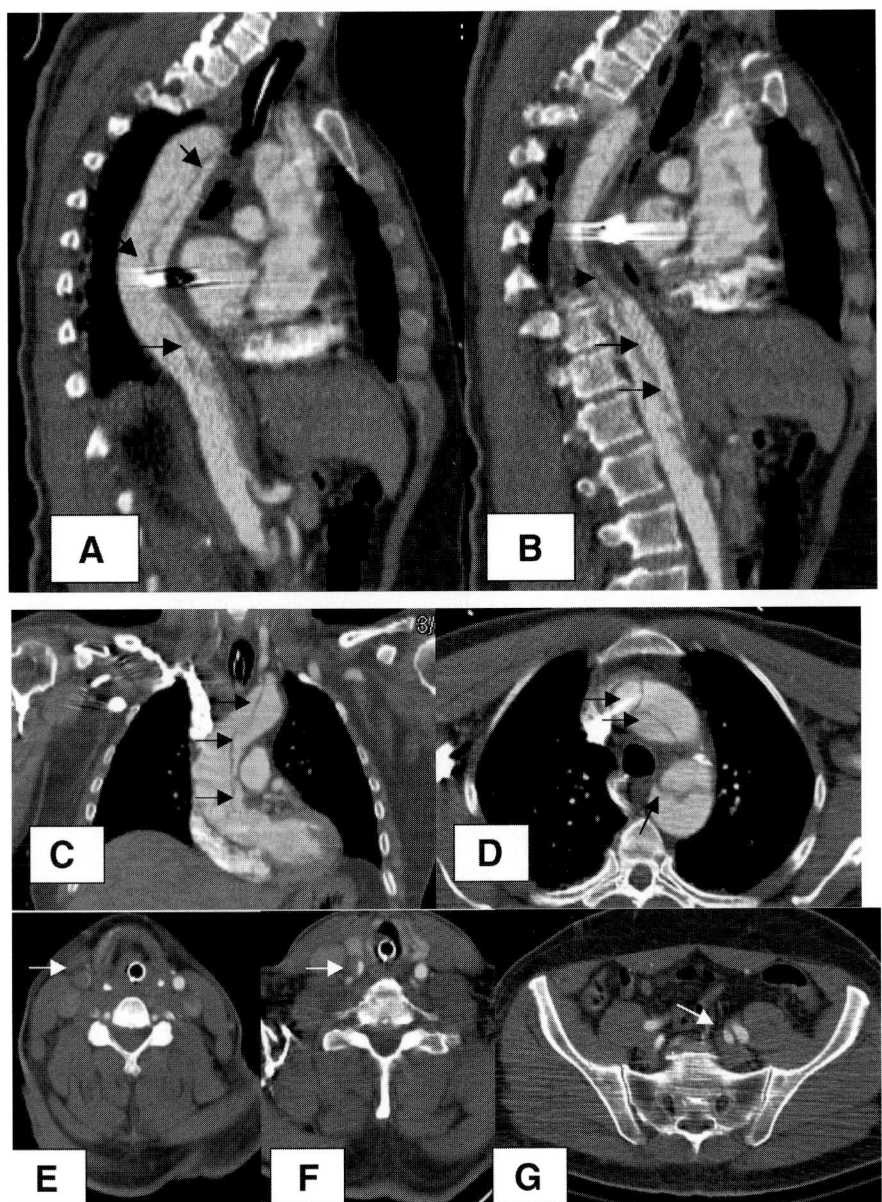

Fig. 3. Computed tomography scan of neck **(E and F)**, chest **(A–D)**, and abdomen **(G)**. *Arrows* indicate signs of aortic dissection.

The patient is immediately taken to the operating room for repair of the aortic dissection. Surgical exploration of the aorta reveals two entries for the dissection, one anterior to the take off of right coronary artery; another at the distal end of the ascending aorta opposite to the brachycephalic trunk; these are repaired. The patient is stable after surgery, showing some improvement until about 24 h later when his consciousness suddenly deteriorates. A STAT CT of the head showed multiple hypodense areas in right occipital lobe and right middle cerebral artery distribution (Fig. 4). At the same time, the patient is found to have excessive blood-like drainage from his chest tube. He is taken back to the operating room for mediastinal re-exploration and bleeding control. Large clots are evacuated from the chest cavity, and two bleeding points at anastomotic sites are repaired. The patient does very well until postoperation day 4 when he suddenly suffers uncontrolled bleeding again from the operation site. Emergency open chest at bedside finds aorta tear extending to cardiac chamber, with massive bleeding. Hemostasis and direct cardiac massage fail to revive the heart and patient expires shortly afterward.

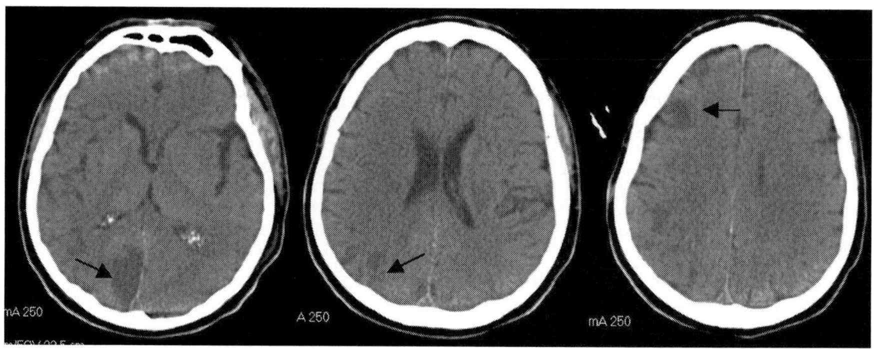

Fig. 4. Computed tomography scan of head 24 h after symptom onset.

COMMENT

Aortic dissection is not a common cause of acute stroke, but most basic stroke centers can expect a case every few years. Typically, as in this case, the presentation includes pain, and an initially missed diagnosis. Although carotid or vertebral dissections may be treated safely with thrombolytics, aortic dissection is considered to be an absolute contraindication owing to the possibility of rupture. Acute chest CT scanning is the only reliable, noninvasive diagnostic test, although eventually cardiac-gated magnetic resonance imaging scanning may become widely available. The mechanism of the infarctions in this patient were likely embolic from the aorta, but the cause of the patient's loss of consciousness remains unexplained.

CASE 8

A 73-yr-old right-handed man awoke at 6:30 AM and noticed left-sided weakness and slurred speech. He arrived at the emergency department (ED) via emergency medical service (EMS) at 7:00 am and a code stroke was activated. He went to bed at 10:00 PM the previous night, but had gotten up at 3:30 AM to use the restroom, and had no difficulties. On further questioning, he reported that 2 d prior he had the sudden onset of blindness in the right eye that completely resolved over several minutes, so he did not seek medical attention. His past medical history was notable for a remote hip fracture with resultant arthritis, for which he was taking salsalate and etodolac, and gastro-esophageal reflux disease. He was not taking antiplatelet or anticoagulant medications. He had quit smoking tobacco 13 yr prior after a 45 pack per year history.

On examination, his blood pressure is 136/80 with a pulse of 73 and respirations of 18. He is alert and appears to be resting comfortably. There is a right carotid bruit. Neurological exam showed an NIHSS score of 15: right gaze preference = 1, partial left homonymous hemianopia = 1, left facial droop = 2, flaccid left upper extremity = 4, minimal movement of left lower extremity = 3, dysarthria = 1, diminished pinprick sensation on the left = 1, visual and tactile extinction = 2. Noncontrast head computed tomography (CT) is shown in Fig. 1. Electrolytes, a complete blood count (CBC), and coagulation studies are all normal.

At this point, would you:

1. Give the patient 325 mg aspirin by mouth because he is outside the time window for intravenous tissue plaminogen activator (t-PA)?
2. Perform diffusion–perfusion magnetic resonance imaging (MRI) to identify a mismatch, indicating the patient would benefit from thrombolysis (either intravenous or intra-arterial [IA])?
3. Call the interventional team for emergency angiography and IA thrombolysis?
4. Start intravenous heparin, obtain a STAT carotid ultrasound, and call the vascular surgeon for emergency carotid endarterectomy

The patient was brought to the angiography suite and a diagnostic cerebral angiogram was started at 8:10 AM. The results are shown in Fig. 2.

At this point, you decide to arrange for the interventionalist to:

1. Stent the high-grade stenosis of the right internal carotid artery.
2. Try to pass the stenosis with a microcatheter for directed thrombolytics into the MCA occlusion.
3. Try to reach the middle cerebral artery occlusion with a microcatheter passed through the anterior communicator from the contralateral carotid.
4. Stop the procedure because the patient is already over 4.5 h from the time he was last seen normal so he will likely not benefit from thrombolytics.

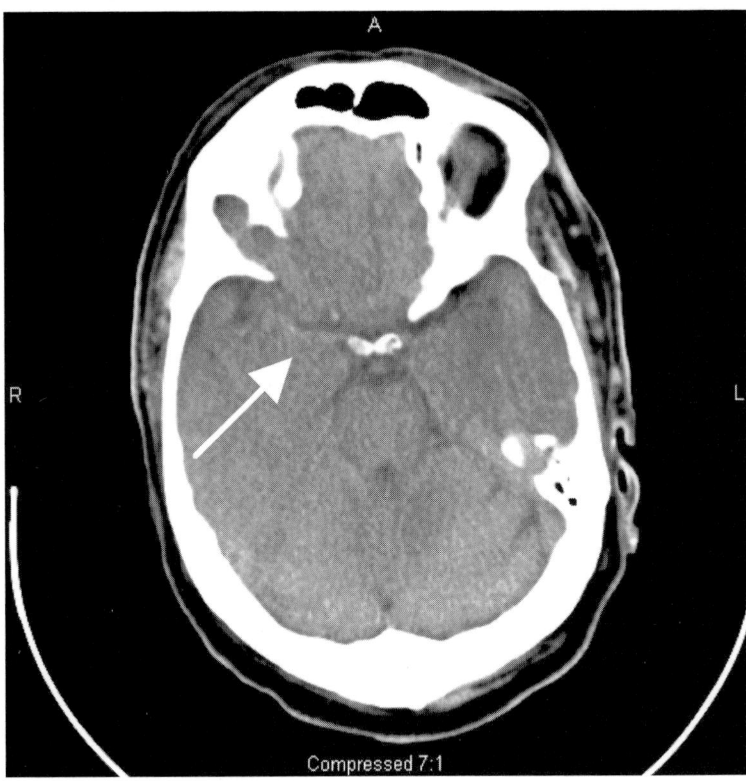

Fig. 1. Dense middle cerebral artery on the right.

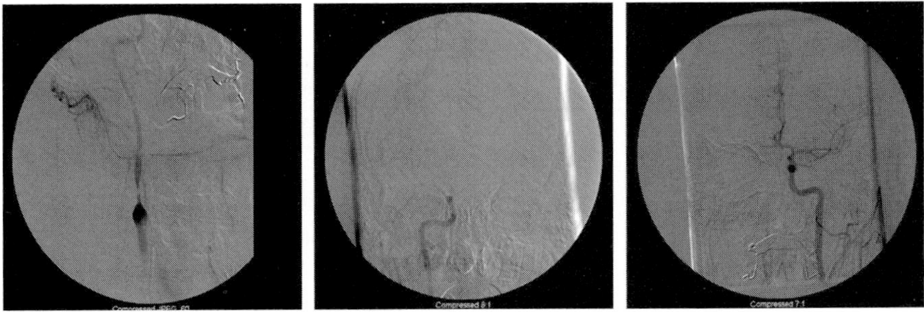

Fig. 2. High-grade proximal left intracerebral artery stenosis is seen in the left panel, a cervical view of the left carotid injection. The intracranial run, shown in the *middle panel*, shows truncated flow of the distal intracerebral artery. An intracranial view (*right panel*) is shown after injection of the contralateral carotid shows no filling or cross filling of the right middle cerebral artery.

The microcatheter was passed through the stenosis and advanced into the thrombus. IArecombinant t-PA (rt-PA) was started at 8:55 AM. Ten milligrams of rt-PA were injected into the thrombus using a pulse spray technique over 10 min, with minimal clot dissolution. Six milligrams of eptifibatide was then injected into the thrombus through the microcatheter with some improvement in flow. After repositioning the catheter, an additional 10 mg of t-PA were injected though the microcatheter using a pulse spray technique. The final angiogram is shown below. The patient began moving his left arm while still in the interventional suite and had an NIHSS score of 0 the next morning.

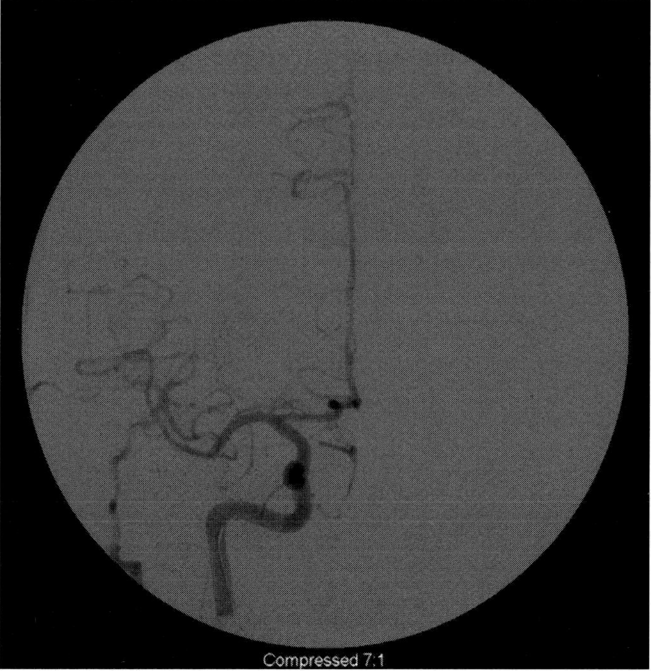

Fig. 3. Intracranial angiogram of the left distal ICA, MCA, and ACA after successful IA thrombolysis.

COMMENT

In this case, thrombolysis occurred relatively late. As reviewed in Chapter 10, the technology available for IA thrombolysis evolves by the month. Even in centers with an experienced angiography team, however, intravenous thrombolysis is still the treatment of choice in appropriate patients who present less than 3 h after symptom onset. When the patient does not qualify, IA therapy should be considered, but only if appropriate expertise is available.

Case 9

You are called for a code stroke involving a 67-yr-old right-handed white woman who was recently diagnosed with hypertension. She has a long-standing history of migraines with visual auras. In the emergency department (ED) you find the patient with her husband, who reports problems of expressive language, weakness in the right upper extremity, and to a lesser extent in the right lower extremity. Her husband states that she was normal when she woke up that day but when he came back to see her 20 min later, she had left gaze preference, was not able to speak, and was slumped over to one side in the chair. By the time he helped her to bed, her gaze deficit was completely resolved and she was able to utter a few words and short phrases. In the ED her language has improved and she denies any strength problems now. When you ask her about onset, she is able to give you the exact time the symptoms started because she was about to listen to the news but was not able to put on the radio. Based on the time the news usually begins, you deduce that she is 3.5 h from time of onset.

What would you do next?

1. Cancel the code stroke as the patient is out of the thrombolytic time window, and recommend to the ED physician intravenous fluids, admission, and stroke work-up.
2. Take further history, examine the patient, and wait on the computed tomography (CT) of the brain.

You decide to wait and evaluate the patient's history further and examine her. You go with the patient to CT, which is done, and is completely normal.

Upon probing further in her history, the patient and her husband reveal that 1 wk ago, she was not feeling well, and was brought to the ED, and was noted to have some problems with word finding that completely resolved in 20 min. She had a negative CT of the brain done at that time. The patient was started on 81 mg of enteric-coated aspirin and has been taking it daily since. You question the patient thoroughly and despite the continuing language problem she is able to communicate appropriately and she denies any symptoms that may suggest migraines or even migraine equivalent.

She denies any history of trauma or manipulation or hyperextension to the head or neck. She indicates no current headache or neck pain.

On examination, pulse is 70 per minute, regular; blood pressure is 165/90. You hear no carotid bruits, regular heart sounds, no murmers. Pulses are symmetric and palpable. The rest of the general system exam is noncontributory.

On the neurological examination, the patient is awake and oriented. She is able to communicate with you reliably but has mild expressive dysphasia and dysnomia without neglect. On her cranial nerve exam she exhibits conjugate eye movements, no gaze preference; no visual field deficits, very subtle blunting of the right nasolabial fold but otherwise normal facial movements. On motor exam, she has mild weakness in her right infraspinatus, triceps, and finger extensors, but elsewhere strength was normal. Tone and bulk are normal throughout. Sensory exam shows intact and symmetric sensation to all modalities and no sensory neglect; no agraphesthesia. Her reflexes are symmetric except for an equivocal right toe and a down-going left toe. Cerebellar exam is normal.

What do you do next?

1. You do not think that there is anything else to do and you cancel the code stroke and walk away after giving your recommendation for admission, and stroke work-up.
2. Obtain urgent radiological imaging of the extracranial carotids, and check which is quicker to obtain an ultrasound or a magnetic resonance angiogram (MRA).

You learn that the ultrasound technician is busy with other critically ill patients and will not be able to come to scan your patient before 45 min, but the magnetic resonance imaging (MRI) suite and technician are available. You accompany the patient to the magnet for an MRI of the brain, and MRA of the brain and neck. The images are shown in Figs. 1–3. You are 5 h from onset at this time.

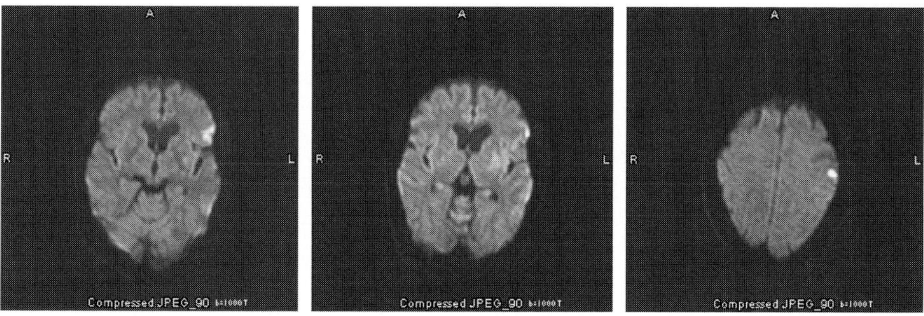

Fig. 1. Diffusion-weighted MRI about 5 h after symptom onset.

What do you do next?

1. Decide to admit the patient and start her on intravenous heparin because the MRA shows either a subtotal or total occlusion of the left internal carotid artery.
2. Call interventional radiology and request an urgent angiogram to differentiate between a total and a subtotal left internal carotid artery (ICA).
3. Consult vascular surgery.

You do all of the above: you start the patient on an intravenous drip of heparin without a bolus; meanwhile, you call the interventional radiologist who informs you that he will be able to have the angiogram suite and the interventional tech-

MRa brain

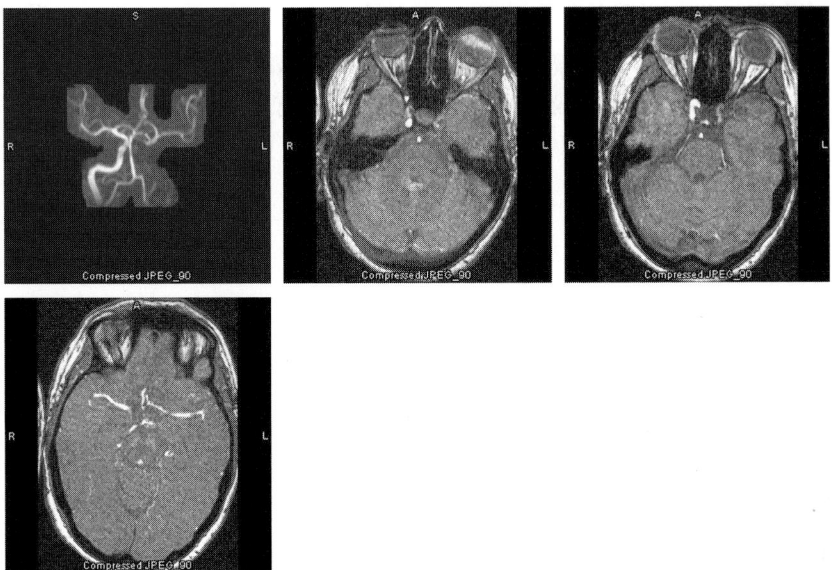

Fig. 2. MRA of the circle of Willis with selected source images.

MRa Neck

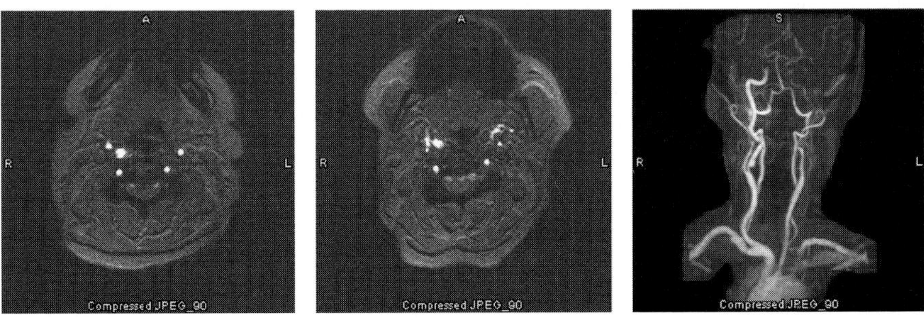

Fig. 3. MRA of the neck with selected source images.

nicians available in 1 h. You call vascular surgery and inform them about the possibility of a subtotal occlusion of the left ICA in the presence of a small branch middle cerebral artery (MCA) fresh stroke. The surgeon explains to you his hesitancy in performing a left carotid endarterectomy as there is a fresh—although small—stroke that may increase the risk of reperfusion injury.

The neck angiogram is done as shown in Fig. 4. There is a trickle of flow in the left carotid artery distal to the severe stenosis.

You inform the vascular surgeon about the findings of the angiogram: on right carotid injection there is a moderate stenosis at the bulb, good distal flow, and

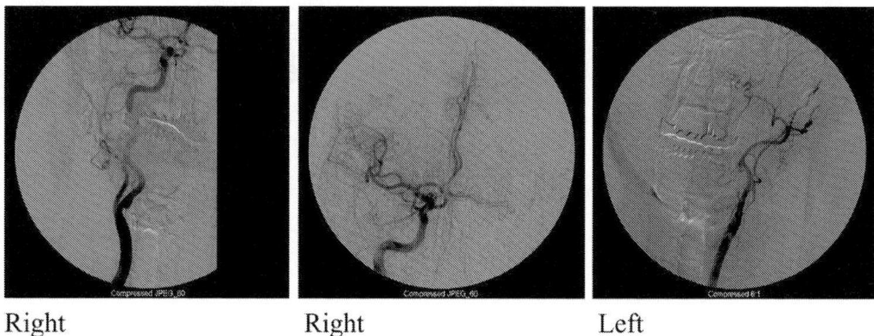

Fig. 4. Angiogram of the right ICA shows moderate stenosis and right-to-left cross-flow via the anterior communicating artery. The left ICA is severely narrowed.

some cross-flow into the left MCA via the anterior communicating artery. On left carotid injection, there is a severe stenosis with near complete occlusion. Based on these results, the surgeon recommends continuing anticoagulation for the time being with consideration of a carotid endartectomy in 4 wk. You admit the patient to the hospital, maintain anticoagulation with a target partial thromboplastin time of 1.5 times control. Over the course of her hospitalization she continues to exhibit mild residual dysphasia and mild right-sided weakness mostly in the finger extensors. Speech therapy, occupational therapy, and physical therapy are consulted.

COMMENT

This case illustrates the value of urgent vascular imaging in acute stroke cases, as eloquently outlined in Chapter 14. Her symptoms suggested rapid resolution, as if she were headed toward complete resolution (i.e., an evolving transient ischemic attack). Certainly, she was not a thrombolytic candidate, given the timing, but had she presented within the 3-hr time window, she should have been treated. However, given the extent of intravascular thrombus seen on the brain MRA source images above, it is very unlikely that intravenous tissue plasminogen activator would have helped her. On the other hand, had the ICA lesion given rise to a distal embolism, as suggested by the diffusion-weighted images, an intravenous thrombolytic may well have helped her. Therefore, until immediate vascular imaging is widespread, the best treatment guide continues to be the clinical presentation, including history, NIHSS, and noncontrast CT brain scan. Eventually, all patients will undergo prompt, multimodal imaging, including vascular imaging, so that the complex vascular lesions that can give rise to similar stroke syndromes can be differentiated.

Case 10

A 64-yr-old African-American man was brought to the emergency department (ED) by paramedics for the sudden onset of left-sided weakness and slurring of speech. At approx 9:00 AM, while walking, the patient noticed difficulty in the left upper and left lower extremity. The patient was able to continue walking but went to a friend's house and called paramedics. The patient also had experienced chest pressure early that morning which he described as intensity of 5 out of 10. These episodes were relieved with sublingual nitroglycerin, which he took himself. He arrives in the ED at 1:00 PM.

His blood pressure is 128/80, pulse 92. Motor testing reveals a left hemiparesis involving the upper and lower extremity, which are flaccid, a mild left-sided facial droop, and dysarthria. Sensory examination reveals decreased sensitivity to light touch, temperature, pinprick, and vibration on the left. Complete blood count with differential, chemistry 20 and coagulation studies are all normal. Electrocardiogram reveals normal sinus rhythm. A noncontrast computed tomography (CT) scan is performed, which is shown in Fig. 1.

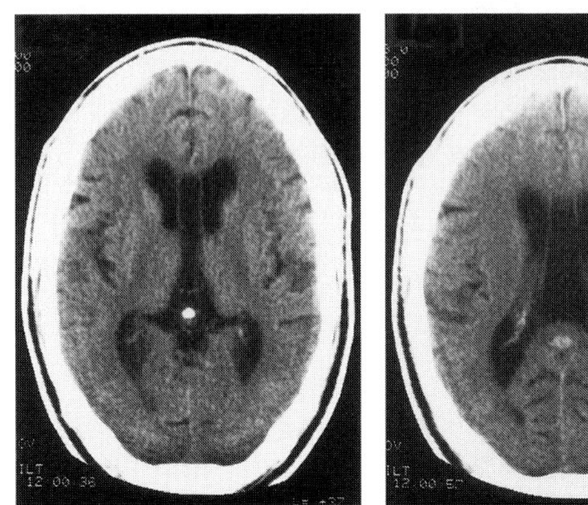
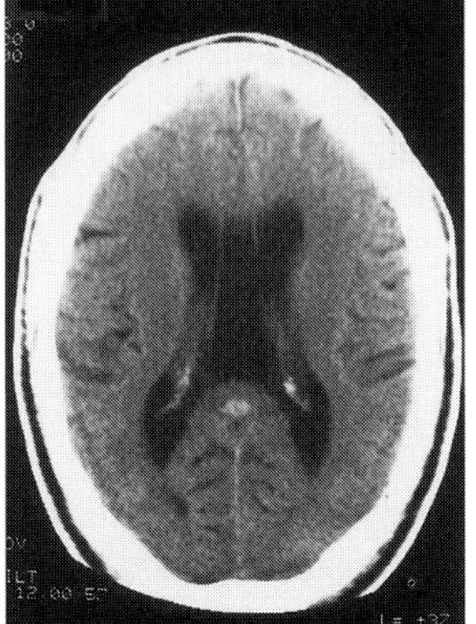
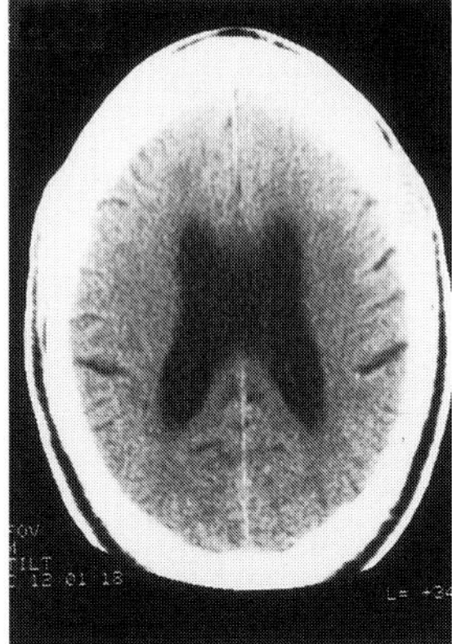

Fig. 1. Noncontrast brain CT about 6 h after symptom onset.

At this point you decide to:

1. Cancel the code stroke because the patient has presented too late.
2. Cancel the code stroke because the patient's CT scan shows no lesion.
3. Continue the code stroke and offer tissue plasminogen activator (t-PA).

The baseline films, obtained 5–6 h after onset of stroke symptoms, show no findings, other than an enlarged septum cavum pellucidum *et vergae*. In particular, there is a normal external capsule and insular ribbon, and there are normal sulci bilaterally. Since the patient is symptomatic, and the CT scan shows no evidence of early lucency (*see* Chapter 16), the patient is offered t-PA. After a thorough discussion of risks and benefits, the patient consents to treatment and receives 9 mg as a bolus, followed by 81 mg over 60 min. The left-sided numbness and weakness gradually improve over the course of admission. At the time of discharge, his hemisensory deficits are completely resolved and he is able to ambulate with the assistance of a walker demonstrating good strength and control of the walker with a slight dragging of the left lower extremity. A CT scan obtained on the second hospital day is shown in Fig. 2. The films show no definite abnormalities. A follow-up scan, obtained 3 mo later, did not reveal any ischemia related findings either.

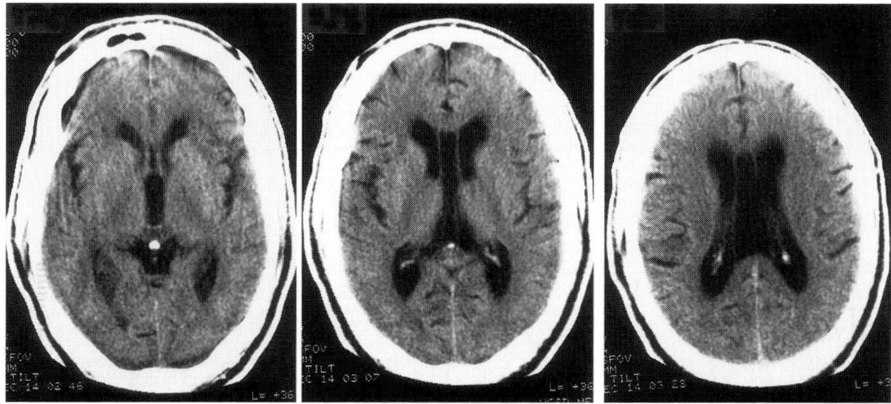

Fig. 2. Noncontrast brain CT taken 24 h after thrombolysis therapy for stroke.

COMMENT

This patient presented beyond the accepted 3-h time window for effective t-PA therapy. The decision was made to treat him with thrombolytic therapy anyway because his baseline CT scan was normal, and he was fairly young. The approved label for t-PA suggests that the drug is indicated only up to 3 h after symptom onset. Pooled analysis of the National Institute of Neurological Disorders and Stroke, the Alteplase ThromboLysis for Acute Noninterventional Therapy in Ischemic Stroke, and the European Cooperative Acute Stroke Study-2 trials suggested safety when t-PA is given as late as 6 h following stroke (*see* Chapters 7 and 16). In the pooled analysis, there was some evidence of benefit as late as 5 h, but this finding has not been confirmed in a prospective trial. In this patient, the history of hypertension and diabetes would reduce his odds of a favorable outcome with thrombolytic therapy (*see* Chapters 7 and 8). In weighing these risks and benefits, the physician should recall that no individual factor is proven to increase or decrease the risk of hemorrhage after thrombolytic stroke therapy; although this patient enjoyed a gratifying outcome, he could have suffered a hemorrhage. Based on the normal CT scan, the severity of the stroke, and the patient's relative good health, the treating physician decided to proceed with therapy after a full discussion of all the risks and benefits with the patient and family.

Case 11

You are called to the emergency department (ED) through the code stroke pager; while driving in you call the ED physician for a preliminary history: the patient is a 52-yr-old man with history of morbid obesity and hypertension. Witnesses told medics that while in a class he suddenly slumped over with right-sided weakness and slurred speech. Witnesses told medics the exact time of onset, which the ED physician estimates to be exactly 1 h ago. The ED phyician notes that the patient gave a reliable history despite his slurred speech. He denies any cardiac symptoms, history of trauma, neck manipulation, straining of the head or neck, or headache. The patient does not look in distress. His monitor shows regular sinus rhythm, and his blood pressure (BP) is 230/120 and finger stick glucose is 105.

What do you do next?

1. You decide that the patient's BP is very high and exceeds the limits for thrombolysis and therefore there is nothing that you can do; you cancel the code stroke, turn around, and drive back home.
2. You ask the ED physician to try to reduce the BP by giving BP medications.
3. You suggest an intravenous fluid bolus.
4. You proceed into the hospital and take further history, examine the patient, and require a computed tomography (CT) of the brain.

The patient receives 10 mg of labetolol as an intravenous push, and is beginning an infusion intravenous of saline at 100 mL/h when you arrive. You accompany the patient to the CT scanner, where a brain scan is performed: your reading is normal without evidence of any ischemia or hemorrhage. His 12-lead electrocardiogram (ECG) now shows regular sinus rhythm and left ventricular hypertrophy (LVH).

On return to the ED, the repeat BP is still high at 210/115, despite the 10 mg of labetolol dose given 30 min ago. You decide to give another 20 mg of labetolol intravenously. On continued physical examination, the patient has no bruits, has regular heart sounds, and a positive third heart sound, with clear lungs, a negative abdomen, and normal symmetrical pulses. Neurological exam shows the patient to be awake and oriented, without aphasia or neglect. On cranial nerve exam, he has equal and reactive pupils, no Horner, intact extraocular eye movements with conjugate gaze, no visual cuts, right central facial paresis, and mild dysarthria. Motor exam shows mild pronator drift of the right arm with orbiting around it, weak right triceps, and infraspinatus on the right side with weak right-hand interossei, but otherwise intact strength elsewhere. Sensory exam shows symmetric sensation and no extinction on double simultaneous stimulation of either cutaneous or visual stimuli. Reflexes were brisker on the right side with an upgoing right toe.

It is now 140 min from stroke onset and the patient's BP is above 200 mmHg systolic and above 100 mmHg diastolic. What do you do now?

1. Decide that the BP is hard to control with the standard BP treatment and therefore you will not give thrombolysis, to avoid the risk of hemorrhagic transformation.
2. You attempt another BP medication and see if it works before giving up on thrombolytic treatment.

The emergency department physician brings you the recent American Heart Association guidelines for managing acute BP in acute stroke patients (http://stroke.ahajournals.org/cgi/content/full/34/4/1056) and you find that intravenous nicardipine, a calcium channel blocker is another option (*see* Chapter15). You order nicardipine from the pharmacy and order the tissue plasminogen activator (t-PA) to the bedside, in order not to lose any time in case the patient's BP becomes controlled and he becomes eligible for t-PA. Nicardipine comes as an intravenous drip. He is placed on 5 mg intravenous drip perhour to be tritrated up every 15 min according to BP. After starting nicardipine, the patient's BP gradually decreased to 170/90 over 10 min, and stopped elevating.

You mix the t-PA, 100 mg in 100 cc of sterile water. The usual dose of t-PA for acute stroke treatment is 0.9 mg/kg, not to exceed 90 mg total dose. The treatment is usually given as a 10% intravenous bolus over 1 min, and the rest of the dose-90% of the total dose-is given as intravenous drip over 1 h. This patient is obese, 250 pounds, so his t-PA dose will be the maximum allowed dose of 90 mg, such that 9 mg is given intravenous push and 81 mg is given intravenous drip over 1 h after that.

After treatment, the patient does well. His strength and speech improve completely within 6 h. Speech, occupational, and physical therapy are consulted on him, and he is discharged on home on antiplatelet therapy. No cause is found after extensive workup for his stroke, other than hypertension.

COMMENT

The original protocol allowed gentle antihypertensive treatment to reduce BP prior to thrombolytic therapy (*see* Chapter 18). For example, one or two doses of labetolol (10 mg) was considered gentle. It has since become clear that elevated BP at onset of thrombolysis is a key marker of likelihood for hemorrhagic transformation (*see* Chapters 4, 8, and 18). The calcium channel blocker nifedipine was in widespread use at the time that protocol was written, but since has been replaced by a safer agent, nicardipine, which also has neuroprotective potential in experimental studies. Therefore, the American Heart Association issued a recommendation that nicardipine be used for acute blood pressure reduction in stroke patients being considered for thrombolysis. Whether intravenous nicardipine qualifies as "gentle" antihypertensive therapy is moot, because it is highly effective and generally lowers the BP quickly and smoothly. However, owing to the potential for overshoot—excessive lowering—it is important to hydrate all stroke patients, even hypertensive patients, with 100 to 300 cc normal saline upon arrival. If the physician chooses to use a nicardipine infusion, and then administers recombinant t-PA (rt-PA), it is important to keep the infusion available for later use if necessary. It is absolutely critical that the BP not increase after the thrombolytic is given, for this will likely promote hemorrhagic transformation. Some physicians will consider a nicardipine infusion as more aggressive than allowed by the rt-PA for acute stroke protocol; in this case, the need for the medication would exclude the patient from therapy with thrombolytics, including intra-arterial modalities.

The etiology of this stroke is somewhat unclear. With only a history of hypertension and obesity, and no atherosclerosis of the carotid arteries found, the most likely etiology is small vessel disease. This is consistent with his clinical presentation of pure motor hemiparesis with dysarthria and his ECG finding of LVH. At a relatively young age (52 yr), however, one must also consider other unusual causes, such as carotid dissection. A careful history and vascular imaging eliminated this possibility. Cardiac causes can present as "lacunar" syndrome, owing to small emboli, and so it would be important to arrange for echocardiography. One may challenge whether thrombolytics should be used in a patient with lacunar stroke, but from the beginning (*see* Chapters 7 and 8) it was clear that all subtypes of ischemic stroke respond to thrombolysis. In fact, the patients with lacunar syndromes on presentation have the greatest likelihood of an excellent response when given rt-PA, compared to their response if given placebo (*see* Chapter 8), as happened in this case. Furthermore, the hemorrhage risk appears to be lower in patients with lacunar syndrome, unless they also have extensive deep white-matter ischemic changes (leukoairiosis) or microbleeds (*see* Chapter 17).

Case 12

The emergency department (ED) calls a code stroke at 11:30 AM. Because your office is across the street, you arrive to evaluate the patient 5 min later, while your receptionist explains to your scheduled patients that there has been an emergency. You learn that the patient is a 63-yr-old white man with history of a hypercoagulable state, diagnosed 2 yr ago when he had a cerebral venous occlusion; he was placed on coumadin, which he has taken regularly ever since. The patient had also developed seizures since his stroke for which he is on dilantin.

The patient was doing fine this morning and went to surf with his daughter at 9:30 am; upon returning to the shore he was talking "gibberish," not making sense at all, according to his daughter. He had no noticeable weakness and was walking and moving fine. After 911 was called, medics evaluated the patient at the beach, and then transported the patient. Upon arrival, he had a generalized tonic-clonic seizure. The patient was given 2 mg of lorazepam intravenous push to abort his convulsions that lasted 5 min after which he had a post-ictal phase. The glucose blood check was 102.

What would you do next?

1. Cancel the code stroke as the patient had a seizure upon arrival to the ED and is accordingly not eligible for thrombolysis.
2. Cancel the code stroke because the patient is on coumadin and therefore is ineligible for thrombolysis.
3. Cancel the code stroke because the patient's history is too complicated to sort out in time to return to the office where patients are waiting.
4. Continue to evaluate the patient, do the computed tomography (CT), and order some lab tests.

You order a STAT lab work-up including a prothrombin time (PT), and a dilantin level. You examine the patient. His pulse is regular at a rate of 80 beats per minute. His blood pressure is 120/70. He has no carotid bruits; heart exam shows regular heart rhythm and no murmurs. Peripheral pulses are symmetric.

On mental status exam, he is awake, but aphasic. He speaks in neologisms when you ask him questions, uttering words that are not part of the vocabulary. He does not follow orders, although he appears to attend to you when you address him. He keeps attempting to swallow repeatedly. There is no hemi-spatial neglect. Cranial nerve (CN) exam shows intact eye movements and eye closure to visual threats is less from the right visual field. There is no facial paresis and the remainder of the CN examination is intact. On motor exam there is intact strength, tone, and bulk and no pronator drift. Sensory exam is not reliable owing to the aphasia, but he appears to withdraw symmetrically from noxious stimulation. Reflexes are brisk; Babinski responses are equivocal. The patient does not comply with the cerebellar exam because of his aphasia.

A CT of the brain is done and shows no acute ischemic changes and no evidence of hemorrhage. There is an old lacunar stroke in the left putamen (Fig. 1A, *arrow*), and focal encephalomalacia in the posterior area of the left parietal lobe (Fig. 1B,C, *arrows*). No acute changes. The CT is shown in Fig. 1.

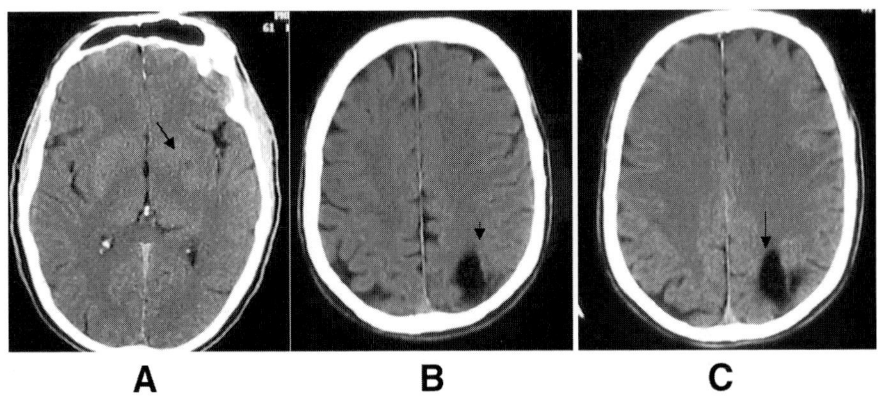

Fig. 1. Noncontrast brain CT done about 2.5 h after stroke symptom onset.

The dilantin level retruns at 8.5, which is subtherapeutic. The PT/international normalized ratio (INR) is 1.3. Upon re-questioning the daughter, you learn that the patient had reduced the dose of dilantin from 300 mg to 200 mg daily over the last few weeks aiming to taper the medication; you give the patient a boosting dose of 500 mg intravenous dilantin drip over 10 min. The time is now 12:10 PM. What will you do next?

1. Just wait and observe whether the patient will improve after giving the dilantin dose.
2. Prepare to administer recombinant tissue plasminogen activator (rt-PA) because aphasia cannot be caused by seizures.
3. Arrange for a immediated magnetic resonance imaging (MRI) brain image, to include a diffusion-weighted sequence because you are not sure yet if the patient has a new stroke.
4. Administer t-PA intravenously, as you are running out of the 3-h time window, which will end at 12:30 PM (in 20 min), as the patient might have a stroke.

You decide to treat the patient with intravenous t-PA. You do not want to delay the patient by going to MRI, which may be done later. You order the t-PA from pharmacy and you mix it as follows: the patient is 70 kg so you calculate the total dose (0.9mg/kg) to be 63 mg. You administer 10% of the total dose, which is 6.3 mg intravenously, as a bolus over 1 min and then hang the remaining 56.7 mg (90%) to be given as an intravenous drip over 1 h.

The patient starts to improve and he is able to express few words that make sense, but still has neologisms and frequent paraphasic errors. The MRI of the brain is done and shows no evidence of acute stroke (*see* the diffusion sequences in Fig. 2, which are negative for any acute restricted diffusion), however you can see the old stroke with chronic bleeds (*see* the gradient echo sequence in Fig. 3: the black arrow on the right and the left point to hypointensities, which signify chronic blood).

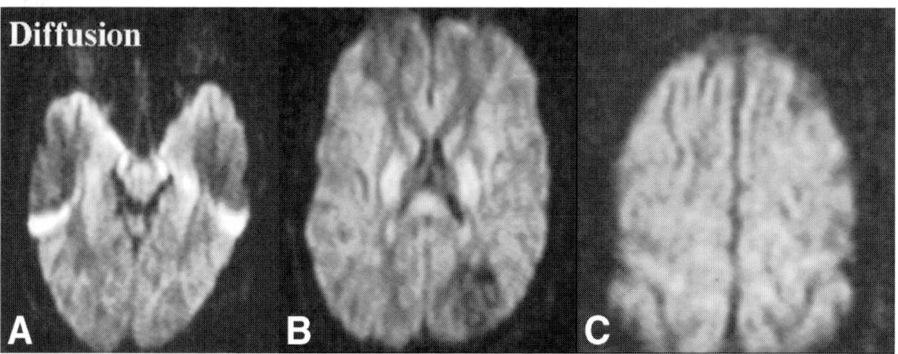

Fig. 2. Diffusion-weighted MRI done about 3.5 h after stroke symptom onset.

An magnetic resonance angiography (MRA) and magnetic resonance venography (MRV) are done and are shown Fig. 4. The MRA looks normal. The MRV shows chronically partially thrombosed superior saggital sinus with multiple venous collaterals (arrows point to a decreased caliber and an absent anterior portion of the superior saggittal sinus).

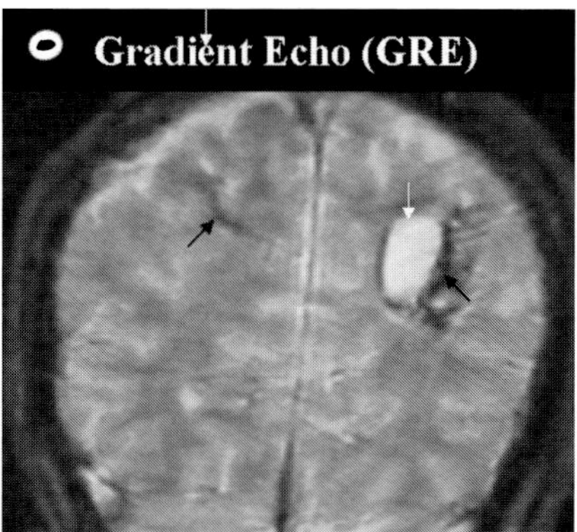

Fig. 3. Gradient echo coronal MRI showing evidence of prior hemorrhage.

An MR of the neck with special fat saturation sequences is negative with no evidence of dissection. Extracranial carotid ultrasound is normal.

The patient completely resolves back to normal and his neurological exam is normal with fluent and appropriate speech. You think that the diagnosis is probably seizure and not stroke as the diffusion was totally normal, though you cannot completely rule out the possibility of having re-perfused the ischemic brain tissue post t-PA. Note that the MRI machine used did not have a perfusion sequence capability, which if present might have helped in showing decreased perfusion in stroke or increased perfusion in seizure.

The patient does well and has no complications. His coumadin dose is adjusted to reach therapeutic PT/INR levels. His dilantin dose is increased back to 300 mg orally daily, with a discharge blood dilantin level of 14 (therapeutic). His neurological exam is normal on discharge.

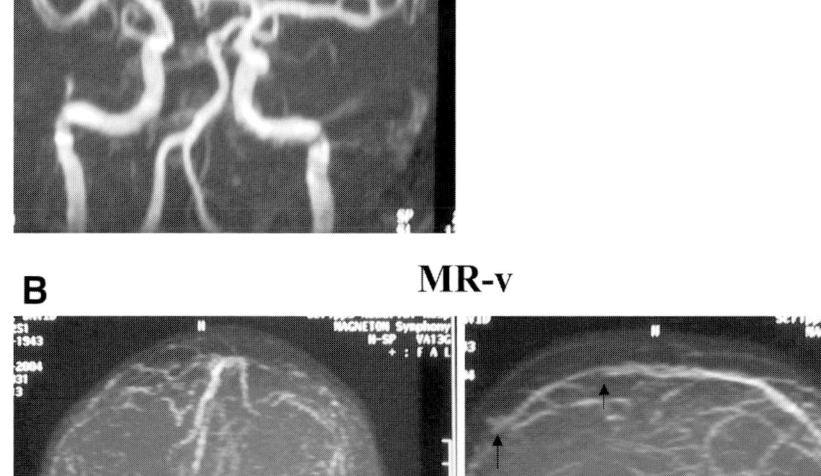

Fig. 4. (A) MRA and **(B)** MR-v taken 5 h after stroke onset. Note normal arterial flow and chronic narrowing of the superior sagittal sinus.

COMMENT

Most neurology offices are not organized to accommodate lengthy physician absences for emergencies, as obstetrical and cardiology offices are; patients are generally scheduled for weeks in advance, and may resent missing their neurologist, even if the absence is for an emergency. On the other hand, this case illustrates the typically complicated scenario that only a skilled neurologist can decipher. The patient was at risk for a carotid dissection because the symptoms began while surfing. Pure aphasia is unusual as a seizure manifestation, so initially the suspicion was for ischemic event.

Seizure at onset is listed as a contraindication for stroke thrombolysis (*see* Chapter 18). In this case, however, the patient manifested focal neurological findings first, and only suffered a generalized convulsion later, during medic transport. Hence, in this case the generalized seizure did not occur at onset, but well after the onset of the event. In any event, there appears to be no risk of thrombolytic therapy when given to post-ictal patients. Hemorrhage generally occurs in the area of ischemia, and because the post-ictal patient would have not ischemia, there would be little to no risk. On the other hand, elderly patients may harbor predisposing lesions, such as silent microbleeds, that could pose a hemorrhage risk. Therefore, one should not hesitate to administer thrombolytic therapy to an appropriate young (< 70-yr-old) patient with seizure after onset, or in situations where it is not clear that the focal deficit is ischemia-related vs post-ictal, but one should proceed with caution in the older patient.

Case 13

You are called on the code stroke pager to the cardiac care unit (CCU), for a code stroke involving a 60-yr-old right-handed African-American man with a past medical history of hypertension, chronic atrial fibrillation on coumadin, coronary artery disease, status post-pacemaker and, 6 d ago, coronary artery bypass surgery. The patient began to exhibit acute expressive aphasia and right-sided weakness that was noticed by his CCU nurse when she saw him today at 5:00 pm; patient was last seen to be at his normal baseline at 4:30 PM that day.

What will you do next?

1. Cancel the code stroke as the patient has had surgery 6 d ago and is not eligible for thrombolytic therapy.
2. Cancel the code stroke as the patient is on coumadin therapy and he is accordingly ineligible to thrombolytic therapy.
3. Evaluate the patient further.

The patient is stable with a pulse of 140, blood pressure 185/101. He has no carotid bruits and on auscultation he has irregularly irregular heart sounds and no murmurs. His pulses were palpable and symmetric. His neurological exam reveals a frustrated middle-aged looking man with inability to express any words, although he phonates sounds. He follows simple but not complex commands appropriately. Cranial nerve exam shows intact eye movements, no visual field deficits, right central facial paresis, and otherwise unrevealing. Motor exam shows intact strength except in right-hand finger extensors in which the strength was slightly reduced. Tone and bulk were intact. The patient had mild pronator drift of the right hand. Sensory exam was not very reliable but the patient had evidence of right sensory hemineglect on double sensory stimulation. His reflexes were slightly brisker on the right side with a right Babinski sign. Cerebellar exam shows intact finger to nose and heal to shin but slower rapid alternating movements on the right hand. Gait was not tested because of complete bed rest.

The computed tomography (CT) of the brain is done and is shown in Fig. 1. There are two hyperdense dot signs in the left sylvian fissure to which the white arrowheads point to in Fig. 1A, and the magnified image Fig. 1B. This sign possibly signifies small clots in the branches of the sylvian segment of the left middle cerebral artery (MCA).

The result of the prothrombin time (PT)/international normalized ratio (INR) come back and the INR is 1.3. You exclude the patient from intravenous tissue plasminogen activator (t-PA) because of the recent major surgery, but wonder if any interventional therapy may be feasible. You call interventional radiology. They advise against intra-arterial (IA) thrombolysis with t-PA because they also fear the complications of bleeding from the cardiac surgery, but they suggest the

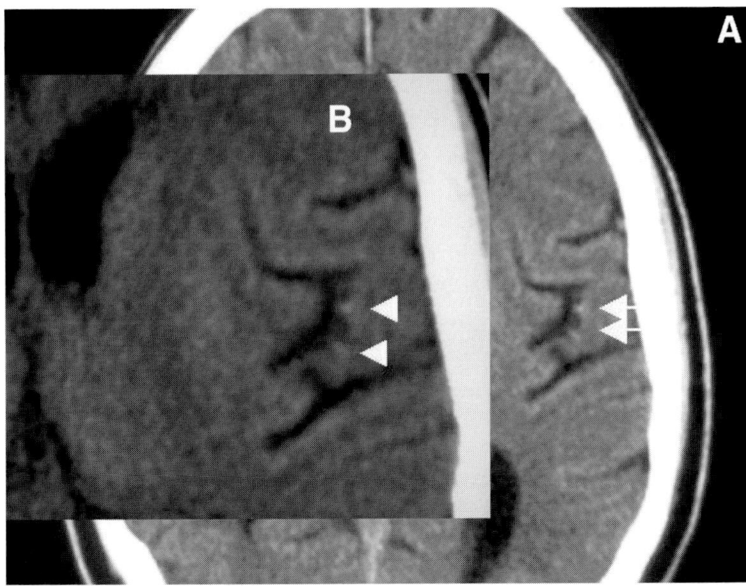

Fig. 1. Noncontrast head CT within 3 h of stroke symptom onset shows two hyperdense MCA "dot" signs in the sylvian fissure.

option of mechanical thrombolysis and you decide to go for that. After calling in the interventional team and preparing the procedure room, the procedure starts 6 h from onset of the stroke symptoms.

The cerebral angiogram is shown in Fig. 2. There is an occlusion of the M2 segment (Fig. 2A) of the left MCA as shown by the arrow. Snaring with a microcather and local IA injection of abciximab (Reopro) results in minimal recanalization (Fig. 2B, *arrow*).

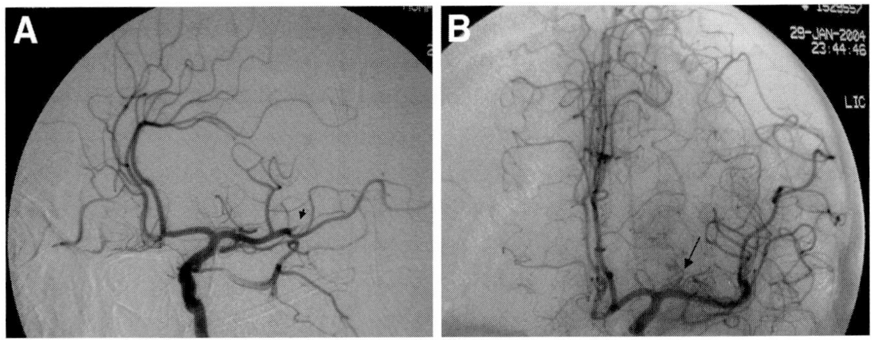

Fig. 2. Intracerebral angiogram of the left middle and anterior cerbral artery about 7 h after stroke symptom onset. **(A)** before and **(B)** after mechanical removal of the MCA embolus.

The procedure is associated with complicating injury to the vascular wall of the M2 branch with some extravasation of contrast into the subarachnoid space. This is shown on the CT done post-angiogram, which is shown in Fig. 3 as pointed by the arrows in Fig. 3A,B.

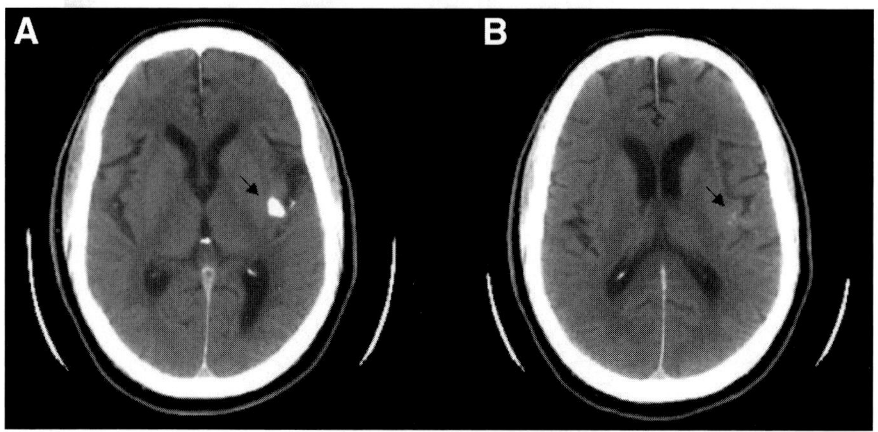

Fig. 3. Noncontrast brain CT following the angiogram reveals a leakage of angiographic dye into the left insular cortex.

Clinically, the patient is slightly worse after the angiogram; he still can phonate without uttering words but has an additional receptive component to his aphasia, has slight increase in the right-sided weakness and right hemispatial visual neglect.

Over the following days the patient improves: his strength normalizes and he starts to express some words and phrases appropriately; the neglect resolves. Speech, physical, and occupational therapy are consulted.

Evaluation of the stroke etiology includes carotid duplex ultrasound imaging, which show no stenosis and an echocardiogram that shows moderate dilatation of the left ventricle (LV) with severely depressed systolic function, septal dyskinesis, and mildly enlarged left atrium. No thrombi are visualized.

The patient is discharged on coumadin for his atrial fibrillation after control of his PT.

A repeat CT is done before discharge and is shown below with evidence of resolution of the contrast which had extravasated, and evolution of the stroke with a hypodensity in the left lentiform nucleus (Fig. 4A), in the left frontal operculum and more superiorly in the left frontal lobe (Fig. 4B,C).

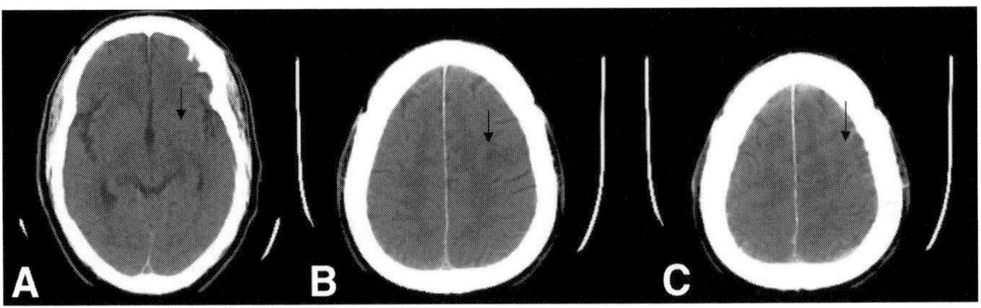

Fig. 4. Computed tomography following mechanical thrombolysis.

COMMENT

IA therapy for acute stroke remains experimental (*see* Chapters 10 and 11). Even in the best centers with the most dedicated teams, there is generally some delay in mobilizing the angiography team and suite. Since the brain deteriorates with every passing minute, in generally interventional therapy has a lower chance of benefiting the patient. For this reason, intravenous thrombolytic therapy should be used preferentially in all patients who qualify. Unfortunately, this patient was excluded from intravenous therapy because of the recent thoracotomy. The use of mechanical embolectomy in place of IA thrombolysis may or may not become an accepted modality; this patient suffered a complication, and studies are currently underway (2004) to determine the safety and efficacy of mechanical embolectomy for acute stroke. The use of small quantities of IA thrombolytic should be safe in patients with recent major surgery, as very little material would escape the cerebral circulation. On the other hand, if mechanical techniques are proven safe and as effective, it would make sense to avoid the infusion of any lytic agents.

Index

P

R

S